Courage to Change-Captain's Log Accountability Journal

by

Brian Wellbrock

authorHOUSE®

AuthorHouse™
1663 Liberty Drive, Suite 200
Bloomington, IN 47403
www.authorhouse.com
Phone: 1-800-839-8640

First published by AuthorHouse   1/27/2010

ISBN: 978-1-4343-6096-0 (sc)

Library of Congress Control Number: 2008902817

Printed in the United States of America
Bloomington, Indiana

This book is printed on acid-free paper.

Table of Contents

Introduction

You have just been promoted!

How many of you have felt like stowaways on your own ship (your life)? It's time to take the helm of your ship and be the Captain God designed you to be. Your health, your life, is far too valuable to be beaten and battered by the storms. The Captain's Log is a reference guide and daily record of how well you are running your ship.

Your life is your ship, this program is the sails, and YOU are the Captain. A Captain is responsible for his or her ship and its crew. A good Captain must always log why and what he or she does out of accountability. God is your Superior and as the two of you set sail on this healthy journey of self discovery and life change, He will show you how to navigate through the storms, push through the doldrums and fight off the pirates that try to steel, kill and destroy what is rightfully yours. He will give you the Courage to Change physically and spiritually!

Following the guidelines in the Captain's Log will give you the tools to lose 30 pounds in 12 weeks. Some of you don't need to lose that much but still need accountability in your exercise and eating habits. Many of you may have 40, 50, 100, or even 500 pounds to lose as you regain your health and become the Captain in your life. You see, your ship (your life) contains valuable cargo. It is the resting place for the God of the universe. Yes, of all the places in the universe for God to call home, He chose your body and your heart!

A bruised and battered ship with no one at the helm is blown wherever the wind takes it. Ah, but a ship led by the power of a living God and a strong and healthy courageous Captain (YOU) will travel to far away places and will discover treasures beyond your comprehension.

As you make healthy choices remember, the Captain's Log is not meant to create perfection. That is impossible for any Captain. But without a strategy or plan and a system of accountability a Captain is lost.

So, enjoy learning the basics of good health and putting them into action. Enjoy getting lean and boosting your energy the right way. Enjoy getting stronger both physically and spiritually. Enjoy becoming the Captain of your life! Wahoo! But most of all enjoy being loved by a God that loves you no matter what you do. And let His unconditional love fuel you to action!

The Train S.A.A.F.E. Method

A Captain must always think of safety. The Train S.A.A.F.E. Method was developed so you can safely train and maximize your potential. When all five categories are followed your life will change drastically and you will be an amazing Captain of your life. Many of the topics are covered in great detail in my book, "Courage to Change, to Believe, to Hope, to Act, to Live! Losing 30 pounds in 12 weeks."

SUPPORT

All of you were designed to be in healthy relationships with people. You weren't designed to go through changes in life alone. Support and encouragement is imperative with any goals whether physical, mental, Spiritual or any combination by like minded friends, family and/or colleagues. Your Faith in Action Team meetings as you cover the material in Courage to Change will help give you the support you need. They will also help uncover the negative support usually present on some level in your life trying to sabotage you.

ACCOUNTABILITY

Accountability must be present in your life while on this journey of healthy living. We encourage all individual clients, corporations, schools and churches to choose accountability partners and/or groups, individuals to whom you are accountable FOR and TO while making healthy choices. This is a must while persevering through the Courage to Change and living in the highest standard of excellence. The Captain's Log and your Courage to Change Life Application Journal will facilitate this. It is through support and accountability to yourself and others you will put into action what you are learning. Support and accountability is covered in detail in the A.S.K. Principle of Courage to Change.

APPLICATION

Application is the action following a learned principle or lesson. All programs, methodologies, high energy motivational seminars and physical training are taught with application as the ultimate goal. Without application, education of any kind is useless. You might get pumped up for a while but without application you have no idea what to do with your excitement.

Remember, Courage to Change is not solely a Bible study. Never was Courage to Change designed to be a "shelf-help" book, something you read then put on the shelf! It is an intensive program designed to help you put your 'Faith in Action!" Every weekly lesson plan must always be accompanied with action. It is in the weekly lesson plans and daily actions of good choices you take care of you and defeat the unhealthy lifestyle that has gotten you here! While you meet with others in fellowship and grow and heal with Courage to Change, you must be diligent with your nutrition, cardiovascular training, resistance training and flexibility. It is action God requires all of you to display as you take back control of you health and become the Captain of your life.

FUN

Join us as we take you on the fun-nest health trip you have ever been on! If you aren't having fun or at least learning how to have fun at healthy living you won't want to change. So let's get excited and have fun with life. Let out a huge smile and laugh as much as possible. Enjoy the amazingly incredible life God gave you and make every day a day of victory no matter what the day throws at you! Smile, smile, smile, smile, laugh, laugh, laugh, laugh, laugh!

EDUCATION

Many of you have grown up hearing the words God, family, and then career. But where do **"you"** fit into this picture. Is **"self"** important? Are **"you"** important? The answer is **YES**. Ultimately your life is about God, not you, but how can you truly serve and love others if you don't first love yourself? The second greatest commandment says to, "Love your neighbor **as yourself**." You are to have relationship with and love God as the greatest commandment but are commanded also to love yourself in Matthew 22:37, which then enables you to have relationship with and love others. How to love yourself through God's eyes is what Courage to Change is teaching you.

Education begins with pulling out of you that which is holding you back, then putting back in that which moves you forward. Your journey toward healthy living Begins with your relationship with God. But remember, everything you learn in Courage to Change must be accompanied with action! This formula describes how you can achieve successful healthy living!

Leadership training / Character building / Becoming the Captain of your life

+

Nutrition training

+

Cardiovascular training

+

Resistance training

+

Flexibility training

=

Successful healthy living

Program Basics

The following guidelines work as an initial **"cheat sheet"** as you get started with your nutrition and exercise.

Exercise basics:

Frequency:
Weight or resistance training 2-3 days per week
Cardiovascular training – 5-6 days per week for weight loss – 2-3 days per week for maintenance

Intensity: Heart rate during cardio
4 days per week – lower end of target heart rate zone
2 days per week – upper end of target heart rate zone
See heart rate chart toward back of Courage to Change for details

Time: How long do you do cardio?
Weight training days – cardio 30-45 minutes
Non-weight training days – cardio 45 minutes to 1 hour

Time: How long do you do resistance training?
45 minutes – 1 hour each time

Type: What kind of exercises?
Cross training is the best way to train. For beginners the stationary bike is recommended. Treadmill, Elliptical, and outdoor activities all work as long as the heart rate is achieved for the full duration of time. See cardio section of Courage to Change for more details.

Nutrition basics:
Eat 5-6 small meals per day
Eat a nutrient dense protein source in each meal
Stay away from sugar and bananas
Don't eat complex carbohydrates after 5 unless you have a late intense weight training session. Then you can have a little after your session.
No fried foods
Refer to the nutrition section and 7 day meal plan in Courage to Change for a more detailed look at your nutrition.

Putting nutrition, weight training and cardio together:
Weight training before cardio when doing it back to back.
When separate - cardio is best first thing in the morning and weights in afternoon/early evening – but schedule will sometimes dictate what actually happens. Everyone's life is different.

Always eat before weight training – 30-45 minutes before.
Never eat before cardio – wait 2 hours after you have eaten to do cardio.

When doing weight training and cardio together, again do weights first, then cardio but DO eat before you go.

These are the basics to get you started. You will learn about these in more detail as you study and review the sections on nutrition and exercise. Now it is time to begin your journey toward healthy living by having the Courage to Change. Each week you will be challenged physically, emotionally, and spiritually to grow and mature into the healthy image of God. Your Courage to Change journal will help guide you through the study material found in each week's reading assignments. It is all laid out for you with no guess work. I am excited for you.

Now go and get healthy!

Time to feast

Feast Food

"He prepares a table before me in the presence of my enemies..."
Psalms 23:5

Though you may think your favorite donuts, pizza, ice cream or cheese burgers are your enemies, they aren't! Maybe you think many of the fast food chain restaurants are your enemy. Nope, not them either. After my wife Silesia and I were married I thought the cream cheese and butter cream, raspberry filled wedding cake was my enemy. It wasn't either. The enemy IS the enemy along with his friends, fear, insecurity, timidity, hopelessness, unworthiness, doubt, guilt, shame, etc; all of which we all experience at one time or another regarding our health and body image. Here is the good news. As you heal spiritually, God is preparing a table for you to feast. But as you literally feast the enemies must watch from afar because they are no longer welcome at your table. How does that sound? Are you getting excited?

Throughout "Courage to Change", you have had many opportunities to change your belief system. I would encourage you as we journey into the food and nutrition portion of the Captain's Log to keep the beautiful attitude and open heart that is vital to your success. As you may know, what you eat can affect your results physically by as much as seventy percent. There are many differing views on diets and it is easy to feel overwhelmed. I desire to keep this simple, healthy, and result oriented.

Proper eating is actually a feast, a daily celebration of God's gift of life and health.

Basically, when we see our food as fuel and not as comfort then we can begin to learn some simple rules. God is there at all times to comfort you and to fuel your spirit. He is also there to help you with the courage to fuel your body with a healthy balanced approach to food.

God gave us everything we need to eat right and take care of ourselves. Eating foods in their natural state, the way He made them is best for optimal results. (Funny how God must have known that.) It is important to understand not all starches and other carbohydrates were created equal. Though man-made breads, bagels, pastas, crackers, and tortillas are low fat foods, they are typically processed, usually bleached and have a much higher glycemic index, meaning it takes your body out of its fat burning zone. Much of their nutritional values, like important vitamins and minerals have been depleted during these processes which actually makes them empty calories. Though there are healthy man-made foods, for the most part when at the grocery store ask yourself, "is it **man-made or God-made**."

As I previously stated there are some man-made carbohydrates that are healthy but **naturally occurring**, complex carbohydrates are best for leaning down and being healthy. They include: brown rice, wild and long grain rice, kidney beans, black beans, pinto beans, yams, small potatoes, couscous, all natural whole oats (oatmeal), and grits. There are many whole or natural grains as

3

well. A basic list to get you started is in the grocery list portion of this book. Examples of healthy man-made meal replacements are shown later in this section.

What Is Nutrition?
The Education You Have Been Starving For!

Nutrition means the processes by which an animal or a plant uses food to repair wasted tissues and promote growth and development. When we implement a proper nutrition plan and regular exercise program into our lives, our bodies will grow stronger, have more energy, last longer, fully develop, and give us mind power through a change in our chemical makeup. In other words, WE ARE WHAT WE EAT! Proper nutrition is a balance of the right kind and amounts of calories and the nutrients within those calories. *Our physical body is energy!* So how or where do we get our physical energy? From *Nutrition!* And what is nutrition? ***The foods we eat!*** Plain and simple! We have either poor nutrition or good nutrition. This education process will show you what good nutrition is, how simple the process actually is, and how to apply it to your life!

Metabolism

Metabolism is the sum of all the chemical reactions that take place in a living organism, or, more simply put, **the process by which our bodies burn and utilize the foods we ingest.** (Foods are chemicals.) Our goal is to raise our metabolisms enough to enhance the efficiency of our bodies' ability to burn, excrete, absorb, and store the foods we consume. OK, blah, blah, blah!

Your metabolism is like a constantly burning fire. When was the last time you built a fire out in the wilderness or even in your back yard? What did it take to start the fire, and what did it take to keep it going? First you had to start the fire with kindling and a match. Once the fire was slowly burning, what happened if you did not put any more wood or waited too long to put more wood on the fire? It went out, right! That is why you *frequently* add wood to the fire in order to keep it going. What would happen if you threw all of the wood on the fire all at once? It would smother it, right!

Your body works exactly the same way. The foods that we consume act the same way that the wood does in the burning fire. If we do not continue to nourish our bodies every few hours, our own fires will go out. Our metabolism will slow to a lethargic pace. If we consume too much food at one time, that too will smother our fire. Say, for example, a person consumes 5 pieces of food. Those pieces of food then make their way to the stomach and intestines for digestion. Starting in the mouth, the food is met and attacked by substances called enzymes. Let's pretend that 5 enzymes meet these 5 pieces of food and do their job perfectly! What happens if those 5 pieces change to 35 pieces of food and are met by those same 5 enzymes? In that case, the enzymes must work over time to break down all the extra food, thus slowing down the digestion process. The food stays in the stomach and intestines for a much longer period, we feel sluggish and lethargic, and our fire goes out once again! We need to build our fire hot enough to keep us warm indefinitely!

Nutrients

Nutrients are the chemical substances present in food that are used by the body for survival. Do not confuse nutrients with calories! Vitamins and minerals are nutrients but do not supply the body with energy! We get our calories from the food and the nutrients from the calories. Some foods are both nutrients and calories, as will be discussed shortly. If a food is **nutrient dense,** it contains large amounts of good-quality nutrients. If a food is not nutrient dense, then it contains poor or sparse amounts of nutrients. Foods that are not nutrient dense may be thought of as fillers. They fill us up but do not do much else for us!

Supplementation

Supplements are those nutrients that cannot be provided naturally in optimal daily amounts. Because of the constant abuse of our land by cultivation, our food supply does not always contain optimal amounts of some much-needed nutrients. So even if we eat healthy, our diet may still lack many nutrients. Nutrient supplementation is required to give us the amounts we need to be truly healthy human beings. Say on one of your imperfect days (we all have them) you are unable to get one of your meals in. In order to keep your fire going, you need to consume something with the right kind of calories and nutrients. Though it is best to get our calories from the food we eat, we sometimes must have an alternative.

However, supplementation rarely means extra calories; it generally means extra nutrients such as quality vitamins and minerals. For example, if corn is constantly grown in the same field year after year, each year the corn will require the same amount of nutrients to grow and survive. Each season the corn absorbs nutrients from the soil in order to flourish, and each year the soil is depleted more and more because of this constant demand. We are like the corn. We grow and may even look healthy, but many of us are empty and starving for nourishment on the inside—just like the child who grows up without any love! The child will grow on the outside but is like an empty shell longing to be filled on the inside.

Supplements go hand in hand with a quality nutritional meal plan.

Optional weight loss, muscle recovery and digestive supplements

There are many books that get into the specifics of vitamin and mineral supplementation. The following list will get you started and will help your muscles recover faster and be healthier as you train. I recommend studying up on supplementation by reading other books and possibly seeing a nutritionist or registered dietician (one who is also healthy and who is a big advocate of exercise and a balanced program; not just a "pill-popper! They are out there")

Vitamin C

Vitamin C is a must. It is needed for a strong immune system as you tax your body with exercise.

Fish Oil

Fish oil is a good supplement for when you are on a low fat diet. A low fat diet sometimes makes it hard to get all of your essential fatty acids in like your omega-3's.

L-Carnitine

L-Carnitine is an all-natural amino acid and is a metabolism booster or stimulator. It helps enhance your fat metabolism and reduces fat levels in your blood. It is the suggested natural alternative to all the harmful stimulants and fat burning products on the market these days. Contains no caffeine, ephedrine or other harmful stimulants. Weight loss products with stimulants should be avoided. Not only do they make your heart race like crazy and give you the shakes through a synthetic form of stimulation, they also over-stimulate your adrenal system which causes a physiological addiction. Your body becomes dependent on the artificial stimulation instead of your own body's ability to provide energy through your adrenal system.

L-Glutamine

L-Glutamine is all-natural and is the most prevalent amino acid in your muscle cell and is a great supplement for anyone who exercises regularly, especially resistance or weight training. L-Glutamine helps in muscle recovery and repair and promotes muscle development by causing an increase in your body's growth hormone. Remember: the more lean muscle you have the hotter your metabolism is; which means body fat is coming off – even when you are sleeping at night.

Chromium Picolinate

Chromium Picolinate is a popular all-natural mineral supplement due to its positive effects on blood sugar regulation. Since sugar is the most important thing to regulate in your diet when leaning down, this supplement is proven effective by helping regulate blood sugar and insulin levels; thus helping keep the body in its optimal fat burning zone and it also helps squelch those sugar cravings.

Glucosamine Chondroitin

Glucosamine Chondroitin is an all-natural aid to joint pain by acting as an anti-inflammatory and aids in cellular repair of connective tissue, specifically cartilage. It is great for those with arthritis and you fitness enthusiasts with sore joints, nooks and crannies.

Pro-Biotic / Acidophilus

If you eat good healthy food but don't have an efficient digestive system your body will not get the nutrients it needs. A Pro-Biotic is a natural supplement with live, healthy bacteria that helps aid the digestive system in breaking down food so your body can better utilize the food's nutrition.

Creatine Monohydrate

If your goal is to simply lose weight and to have a strong lean healthy body, this is a good supplement. Creatine Monohydrate is an all-natural supplement. It is a cell-volumizing compound made naturally in the body that supplies energy to your muscles. Make sure you drink plenty of water when taking this supplement because of how your muscle cells absorb optimal water supplies (cell-volumizing). Don't worry about bloating. Bloating is extra-cellular or outside the cell, like with a woman during her menstrual cycle. Cell-volumizing is intra-cellular or inside the cell. Since the richest source of Creatine is found in animal meat such as beef, chicken, fish and turkey, it is an important supplement for vegetarians that want a strong healthy body. It is a good supplement for anyone, men and women wanting good strong and healthy muscles. It isn't just for bodybuilders.

Calories

A calorie is a unit used in the study of metabolism and defined as the amount of heat required to raise the temperature of 1 kilogram of water 1 degree Celsius. *BLAH! BLAH! BLAH!* Now, what does this mean you ask? Just about everyone has heard some talk about working out to burn fat. What is fat? Fat is a calorie and nutrient and is used for long-term energy (discussed in more detail later). When you exercise, you notice that your temperature increases and causes perspiration (i.e., you get soaked); therefore, you are burning calories. GREAT! Calories are needed for a combination of energy, body structure, and regulation of the body's many functions. Calories are made up of three components: **(1) carbohydrates, (2) protein,** and **(3) fat.** These calories contain our needed nutrients and supply the fuel to keep our fires going!

Carbohydrates

A carbohydrate is a calorie and nutrient that provides the body with 4 calories per gram and short-term energy, not body structure or regulation. Carbohydrates need to be broken into three distinct groups: (1) complex carbohydrates, (2) simple carbohydrates, and (3) fiber.

The body stores **complex carbohydrates** in the form of **glycogen**. The areas that store glycogen are our muscle cells and liver. The glycogen in our muscles is there for a short-term energy reserve. Anytime your body is stressed with resistance, your body taps into the glycogen stores to supply the body with energy. Glycogen is to the body as "low gear" is to your car. That is why when you lift weights you are able to work out at a more intense level but for only a short time. Because of your body's inability to continue using oxygen at the higher intensity levels, you experience fatigue. When your body has burned up your oxygen, it is like taking the spark out of your spark plug (and you run out of gas!).

Only when your oxygen is used continuously at a lower intensity can you tap into the fat stores. Unfortunately, our glycogen stores *do* have a cap on them! This means anything over the cap is stored as fat! **Read that last sentence again**! The requirements suggested within your meal plan will help you learn the amounts you need to consume.

We get **simple sugars** from the fruits we eat and a number of different sweeteners. The reason simple carbohydrates are not a good substitute for complex carbohydrates is that most do not get stored in the body. Rather than being converted into glycogen and stored in the muscle cells and liver like the complex carbohydrate, the simple sugar is converted into blood sugar called **glucose,** which burns very quickly. It is like putting nitrous oxide in your fuel tank—it burns like crazy for a short time, and then fizzles out.

Those of you who consume too much fruit throughout the day probably experience a temporary fruit buzz, then get tired a short time later. Now you know why! The simple sugar found in fruit is called **fructose** and should be the main source of simple sugars consumed each day. If consumed in moderation, table sugar **(sucrose)** may be used in tea, on breakfast cereals, and for some cooking. Try to think of the term *simple* as just that! SIMPLE! Because it does not get stored in the body! We need approximately 2–4 servings of fruit each day. This is only a guideline! If you weigh 400 pounds, you need to consume more. Your meal plan requirements provide you with the correct amount.

The third form of carbohydrate is **fiber**. Fiber is to the body as Liquid Drano is to your pipes! Those of you who consume large salads throughout the day in an attempt to be healthy have good intentions but are starving your bodies of calories. Fiber is considered dead calories because we cannot digest it. The only place a person's body can digest fiber is in the large intestine, where bacteria called intestinal micro flora live. Unlike livestock, humans do not have enzymes that can break down fibrous vegetables.

If you have ever noticed corn in your stool at one time or another, this is because of the fiber surrounding the kernel and because of inadequate chewing. Make sure you chew your food thoroughly so that even though the calories are lost, the nutrients within the calories are utilized. Eat as many different colors of vegetables as possible. The different colors are created by the many different kinds of vitamins and minerals that our bodies will use! So please do not think that eating a huge salad is sufficient for your carbohydrate intake each day. Though you will be absorbing most of the wonderful vitamins and minerals, you will not get any energy and will simply see most of those meals come out the other end a while later!

Protein

A protein is a calorie and nutrient that provides the body with 4 kilo-calories per gram as well as all three of the body's functions; it is paramount to our survival! Protein supplies the body with energy, structure, and regulation! The solid human body is 75% protein! Americans consume way too much non-nutrient-dense protein. Eating a lot of red meat does give a person quality protein but also supplies the body with tremendous amounts of saturated fat. Nutrient-dense protein comes from egg whites, chicken and turkey breasts, tuna, ostrich, and most fish. *Very lean* cuts of pork loin, pot roast, and other red meat are also good sources of nutrient-dense protein, but pay close attention to the fat content when purchasing these products. Try to limit the amount of red meat you consume. A person trying to lose weight (body fat) should not consume any red meat until her or his fitness goals are reached.

Even a person who consumes 100% of his or her daily intake of protein may still be **protein deficient**. That may seem puzzling, but let me explain! The building blocks of protein are substances called **amino acids.** An **essential amino acid** is one that *cannot* be produced by the human body in sufficient amounts and therefore needs to be included in the diet. There are approximately 9 essential amino acids. The **nonessential amino acid** is one that *can* be produced in the body in sufficient amounts. There are approximately 11 nonessential amino acids. Without a balance of all the different kinds of amino acids we will be protein deficient.

Your meal plan gives you a balance of foods that will enable you to consume the right amounts of amino acids. All of the previously mentioned proteins have different kinds and amounts of these amino acids. *Why do we need the different kinds of foods containing proteins? Why not just eat a lot of chicken?* In answering these questions, we must understand what **protein synthesis** is and how it works.

Protein synthesis occurs after our body has broken down the consumed protein into its amino acids. Protein synthesis is the body's ability to take the amino acids from the previously consumed protein and rebuild them into a protein that is then used by the body (a factory, so to speak). The body simply breaks the protein down, then builds it back up by reconnecting the different amino acids to again form a protein. **But ingesting only a couple of main sources of protein limits the amount of amino acids our body has to make its own protein.** It is like baking bread without adding enough yeast. The loaf will bake but will not grow and develop into a beautiful peace of work.

Since protein is a part of everything—muscle and other cells, hair, skin, teeth, enzymes, hormones, etc.—we need to make sure we consume the right amounts. Proper protein intake increases structural growth through cell regeneration, improves regulation by the different, more efficient hormones and other functions at work, and increases some energy from the amino acids present in the blood stream! *Remember, we are what we eat!*

Lipids (Fats/Oils)

Fats are calories and nutrients that provide our body with structure and long-term energy. Fat can also be thought of as the body's shock absorber, insulator, or protection device. Fat is stored in our body in the form of **adipose tissue.** Unlike the complex carbohydrate, which has a cap on the amount the body can store as glycogen, our fat stores are limitless. Anything in excess will again be stored as fat. Remember, that which is not burned is stored in some way.

How many of us have a junk drawer at home or in the office? We have to clean it out periodically to save what we need, dispose of the junk, and leave room for future stuff. Imagine if your junk drawer had no limit to the amount of things it could hold. You would soon get disorganized, wouldn't be able to find anything, would become slow and fall behind in your tasks, and would become frustrated. With the right amount of body fat and fat taken into the body, a person's body can find and organize the nutrients it needs to function properly, can carry out important tasks with ease and efficiency, and can help improve cognitive abilities and increase confidence levels. The analogy means that your junk drawer would be organized and used for important things!

We must understand what junk is and what is necessary for proper functioning. Body fat exceeding 15% for males and 20% for females is excess junk in our junk drawer. We must discard these impurities through proper nutrition and regular exercise.

So how do we monitor the amount and kinds of fat we ingest? Your meal plan has you at either a maintenance phase, a fat-loss phase, or a building phase. Those of you who are in a fat-loss phase specifically want to keep your fat intake lower (around 10 grams per day) until you reach your desired goals. At that time you can have more variety and higher amounts of fat. You may go as high as 20–30 grams per day on a maintenance and building phase; they require different amounts of calories in general. Keep the amount of **saturated fat** you consume to a minimum. Saturated fat is a lipid that remains solid at room temperature. Most saturated fat is found in animal products. Always cut off the excess saturated fat *before* cooking! Even if you cut it off after cooking, much of the fat will have soaked into the meat while it was being cooked. Remember, much of the saturated fat will turn liquid when cooked, so it is hard to see, and will soak into the food very easily.

Most of the fat we consume should be **unsaturated**. Unsaturated fat comes in two forms: monounsaturated or polyunsaturated. These unsaturated fats are considered oils. An **oil** is a lipid that remains liquid at room temperature. **Monounsaturated fat** is found in olive and canola oils. **Polyunsaturated fat** is found in corn, safflower, and soybean oils. Use these kinds of oils to cook with rather than lard or butter. The calories add up quickly! Get in the habit of using as little oil as possible. Use it only to coat your cooking pan.

Though we need to limit the amount of fat in our diet, we do need some fatty acids to be healthy. **Essential fatty acids** are found in the two types of unsaturated fats. Omega 3 is a polyunsaturated fat found in fish and is the most important fatty acid. Omega 6 (poly) and Omega 9 (mono) are also essential fatty acids we need to consume. These are found in the different oils we use in cooking. Remember, though these fats are essential, not much is needed to satisfy your body's needs. If you notice that you have dry, scaly skin, poor wound healing, or liver abnormalities, see your physician and add more fish or hemp-seed oil into the diet. Your body might just be lacking some of the essential fatty acids. Too little fat may also cause growth failure in infants.

Cholesterol and **cortisol** (sterols) are types of fat (lipids) needed in the body as precursors to the regulation of different hormones in the body. Cholesterol is the most abundant steroid in the body. Cholesterol is found in animals but not in plants. That is why vegetarians must be careful to supply their bodies with the right nutrients. Egg yolks provide cholesterol. Though researchers have found that eating the yolk in eggs is not as harmful as once thought, try to keep the whole egg–to–egg white ratio at 2:5.

Fighting the Fat

So now that we know all there is to know about fat, (not really) how do we get rid of the darn stuff in our bodies? Since fat is a long-term energy source and is the most concentrated source of energy (9 kilo-calories per gram), it also takes the longest to burn off. But do not let this discourage you! Body-fat burning is the easiest form of exercise there is; it just takes longer! Fat burning is easier because it requires much less resistance than other types of exercise.

Remember the complex carbohydrate. It was like putting your car in "low gear"—you get great strength and power but run out of gas much more quickly. Fat burning is like putting your car in "overdrive" and going on a nice long trip. Your trip may take longer, but your gas mileage is much more efficient because you have used less energy. Think about it! When do you use more gas: in the city going from stop to 50 or 60 to stop again consistently, or on an interstate with the cruise control on 70? Your body is exactly the same way! Your meal plan basically takes you on a trip. Your destination is 30-60 minutes away. You are in overdrive on the interstate (90–100 rpm on the bike) and are driving on a flat surface and not up hills (manual level 1, 2, or 3). Periodically you glance down to see how much gas you have left, just as you monitor your heart rate to keep it in the targeted range your meal plan has provided. Enjoy the ride!

Remember, though tiring, fat burning should not be exhausting. There is a big difference! If you get out of breath and cannot talk comfortably, you are doing too much! If your heart rate goes above its highest recommended level, you may as well forget about burning fat! What does it mean to be above your maximum target heart rate zone? Why are you not burning fat? Just because you are working hard does not mean you are burning sufficient amounts of fat! During high-intensity workouts your body begins burning carbohydrates instead of fat! This means you are tapping back into your glycogen stores when your heart rate is too high! Your intentions are good, but you burn a lot of calories (glycogen), not fat specifically. If a person eats a healthy diet and always does high-intensity workouts where the heart rate goes up and down sporadically, he or she will still burn fat, just not as efficiently. I want you to have **optimal circumstances** for whatever goal or goals you are trying to reach!

So, how far do you take it? How much body fat are you supposed to have? We know that a healthy male's body fat should be between 10-15% and a woman's between 15-20% (a 12 pound margin for both). Of course, every person's results vary, but when you follow this plan *closely*, approximately 1% of body fat per week will come off. If you are a man who begins with 45% body fat and wants to reach 12%, then it will take approximately 33 weeks to get where you want to be. If you are a woman who begins at 34% body fat and wants to get down to 15%, then it will take you a minimum of 19 weeks to get there. Since life makes it difficult to create optimal conditions, it may take longer. Who cares? Remember that your confidence comes from God, *not* the end result of your goals. So do the best you can. If you do it right your body has *no alternative* but to respond.

You can take your body to whatever level you desire as long as you remember that you are enhancing the outer expression of your inner beauty and Godliness. The funny thing is that as you move forward, lose weight, learn about yourself, and increase your physical confidence, your inner beauty will be affected simultaneously. It is impossible to strengthen yourself physically and not strengthen yourself emotionally and spiritually in the process if you do it right. All parts of you are interlaced, coexisting to give you life. Your inner beauty is a direct result of how you take care of yourself physically; they must work together.

Vitamins & Minerals

Vitamins are nutrients (not calories) that provide the body with regulation. Vitamins do not provide the body with any energy or structure, only regulation. Do not think that by taking vitamins and minerals your energy will increase right away. However, the vitamins will aid your energy levels indirectly by helping to regulate the body's many systems, thus increasing the utilization of calories and nutrients taken in.

Fat-soluble vitamins include:

A	**Retinol**
D	**Cholecalciferol**
E	**Tocopherol**
K	**Phylloquinone**
	Menaquinone

Water-soluble vitamins include:

C	**Ascorbic acid**
B1	**Thiamine**
B2	**Riboflavin**
B3	**Niacin**
B5	**Pantothenic acid**
B6	**Pyridoxine**
B12	**Cobalamine**
Folate	
Biotin	

Minerals are nutrients (not calories) that provide the body with structure and regulation but not energy. Like the vitamin, minerals will indirectly aid energy levels by helping to regulate the many systems of the body.

The minerals needed in larger amounts (expressed in grams) are:

Sodium chloride	**Potassium**	**Magnesium**
Calcium	**Phosphorus**	**Sulfur**

The trace minerals (expressed in milligrams) are:

Iron	**Zinc**	**Iodine**
Selenium	**Copper**	**Manganese**
Fluoride	**Chromium**	**Molybdenum**

Vitamins

Vitamins	*Food Source*	*Function*
Vitamin A (fat soluble) *Retinol*	Fish, liver, eggs, fortified milk, carrots, tomatoes, apricots, cantaloupe	Promotes good vision, helps in the maintenance and formation of new and healthy skin.
Vitamin C (water soluble) **Ascorbic acid**	Citrus fruits, strawberries, tomatoes	Helps build a strong immune system; aids in healing wounds; promotes healthy gums, teeth, and capillaries; aids in iron absorption and maintains normal connective tissue.
Vitamin D (fat soluble) *Cholecalciferol*	Fortified milk, fish; produced by the human body when exposed to sunlight	Promotes strong bones and teeth; also is necessary for absorption of calcium. Moderate sun is good for you! Enjoy it!
Vitamin E (fat soluble) **Tocopherol**	Nuts, vegetable oils, whole grains, olives, asparagus, spinach	Helps protect tissue against oxidation; helps in the formation of red blood cells; also aids the body in absorbing vitamin K.
Vitamin K (fat soluble) *Phylloquinone/Menaquinone*	Cauliflower, broccoli, cabbage, spinach, cereals, soybeans, beef liver	The human body produces approximately 50% of its needs; aids in blood clotting; absorption of vitamin K is greatly enhanced by the consumption of vitamin E.
Vitamin B1 (water soluble) *Thiamine*	Whole grains , dried beans, lean meats (especially pork), fish	Helps initiate the release of energy from carbohydrates; also very important for a healthy brain, nerve cells, and proper functioning of the heart.
Vitamin B2 (water soluble) *Riboflavin*	Nuts, dairy products, liver	Helps initiate the release of energy from various foods; interacts with other B vitamins and benefits protein synthesis.
Vitamin B3 (water soluble) *Niacin*	Nuts, dairy products, liver	Helps initiate the release of energy from various foods; involved in synthesis of DNA; aids in normal functioning of skin, nerves, and digestive system; acts as a diuretic by flushing out liquids; may leave reddish tint on skin.
Vitamin B5 (water soluble) *Pantothenic acid*	Whole grains, dried beans, eggs, nuts	Helps initiate the release of energy from various foods; helps produce various materials throughout the body.
Vitamin B6 (water soluble) *Pyridoxine*	Whole grains, dried beans, eggs, nuts	Aids in protein synthesis through an increase in the chemical reactions of proteins and amino acids; aids in proper functioning of the brain and formation of red blood cells.
Vitamin B12 (water soluble) *Cobalamine*	Liver, beef, eggs, milk, shellfish	Aids in protein synthesis through an increase in the formation of red blood cells; helps the body's nervous system function normally.
Folate (water soluble)	Leafy green vegetables, liver, beans, grains, wheat bran	An active agent with B12 in the production of hemoglobin (the oxygen-carrying protein of the blood found in red blood cells); is also important in the production of DNA.
Biotin (water soluble)	Yeast, eggs, liver, milk	Aids in metabolizing proteins and carbohydrates; important in the formation of essential fatty acids.

Minerals

Mineral	*Food Source*	*Function*
Calcium *Ca*	Milk and milk products, sardines and salmon eaten with bones, dark leafy vegetables, shellfish, hard water	In conjunction with exercise calcium increases bone density, size, and strength; aids in the prevention of osteoporosis; helps maintain and regulate heartbeat, blood clotting, muscle contraction, and nerve conduction. Absorption is limited without resistance training!
Potassium *K*	Potatoes, oranges, bananas, dried fruits, peanut butter, coffee, tea, cocoa, dried beans and peas, yogurt, molasses, meat	Important in the process of muscle contraction and promoter of regular heartbeat; regulates transfer of nutrients to cells throughout the body; also helps regulate blood pressure and controls water balance in the tissues and cells of the body.
Sodium *Na*	Table salt, salt as an additive in prepared foods, baking soda	Aids in regulation of blood pressure (major contributor to high blood pressure if consumed in high amounts); plays an integral role in the regulation of water balance throughout the body.
Magnesium *Mg*	Raw leafy green vegetables, wheat bran, whole grains, nuts, soybeans, bananas, apricots, spices	Helps calcium in the promotion of bone growth, muscle contraction, and nerve conduction; also promotes regular heart rhythm.
Phosphorus *P*	Meats, poultry, fish, cheese, egg yolks, dried peas and beans, milk and milk products, soft drinks, nuts	Phosphorus is present in almost all foods; aids in bone growth and strengthening of teeth; also important in energy metabolism (the burning of calories for fuel).
Chloride *Cl*	Fish, table salt	Most commonly seen in the form of table salt (NaCl); aids in the water balances of the body; forms hydrochloric acid in the stomach to aid in digestion.
Chromium *Cr*	Meat, cheese, whole grains, dried beans and peas, peanuts	Important for glucose (blood sugar) metabolism; has been said to be a cofactor for insulin; a person who craves sugar or sweets is likely to have a chromium deficiency. Chromium supplements such as chromium picolinate help lean the body down when taken in conjunction with regular exercise.
Copper *Cu*	Beef and pork liver, dried beans, raisins, nuts, shellfish, chocolate, corn oil margarine	Crucial in the formation of red blood cells; cofactor in absorbing iron into blood cells; also aids in the production of several respiratory enzymes.
Fluoride *Fl*	Fluoridated water and the foods cooked in it, fish, tea, gelatin, toothpaste (though not a food)	Helps prevent the onset of osteoporosis by contributing to solid bone and tooth formation. Absorbed best when taken in conjunction with resistance training.
Iodine *I*	Primary source is iodized salt; others are seafood, products made from seaweed, vegetables grown in iodine-rich soil, vegetable oil	Aids in the normal functioning of the thyroid gland; necessary for normal cell function; promotes healthier skin, hair, and nails; prevents goiter (an enlargement or swelling of the thyroid gland found especially in Switzerland and the Savoy Alps).
Selenium *Se*	Egg yolks, fish, chicken, red meat, tomatoes, shellfish, tuna, garlic	Works in conjunction with vitamin E to fight cell damage by oxygen-derived compounds; the more oxygen one's body can utilize, the faster tissues heal, thus promoting a stronger, healthier body.
Manganese *Mn*	Whole grains, vegetables, fruits, instant coffee, tea, egg yolks, beets, cocoa powder	Helps prevent the onset of osteoporosis by promoting normal bone growth and development; also important for normal reproduction and cell function.

Zinc *Zn*	Eggs, poultry, crab meat, liver, beef, whole-wheat bread, oysters	Helps maintain an acute sense of smell and taste; aids in normal body growth and sexual development; crucial for fetal growth and wound healing.
Iron *Fe*	Red meat, egg yolks, liver, kidneys, green leafy vegetables, dried fruits, beans, peas, nuts, enriched grain products	Since iron is a part of many proteins and enzymes throughout the body, it aids the body in metabolizing (building) proteins; also an essential part of the formation of hemoglobin (the oxygen-carrying factor in the blood). Women especially need to monitor their iron intake owing to loss of blood during menstruation and possible pregnancy.
Molybdenum *Mo*	Dark green vegetables, cereal grains, beans, peas, organ meats	Helps maintain normal cell function.
Sulfur *S*	Cabbage, onions, soybean oil	Though sulfur by itself is not used as a nutrient by the human body, when combined with vitamin B1 it helps stabilize protein molecules in the body. Examples: hair, nails, skin. Also may be used in treating rheumatism, gout, and bronchitis.

Remember, many vitamins and minerals are not properly used by the body without regular exercise. **That is why there is no miracle pill or magic potion to make us healthy. <u>Proper nutrition will not work efficiently without regular exercise.</u>** One such example is calcium. Calcium is a positively charged ion that we need for strong bones. But is simply taking calcium supplements enough to supply what the body needs? No. People who take calcium supplements but do not exercise have good intentions but are wasting a lot of money and may still be afflicted with osteoporosis! Basically you have expensive urine.

Why is this? At rest and without exercise your bones have more of a neutral charge. **Only with exercise, specifically resistance training, does your bone produce a negative charge that will attract the positively charged calcium you ingest.** A great example of this is with the astronauts who are nutritionally well provided for while in space. Even though they have great nutrition they still see significant and immediate losses of bone strength and bone density upon leaving the Earth's atmosphere. This is because they are weightless and have no resistance acting on their bodies and the calcium is not being absorbed into the bone properly. NASA now supplies the astronauts with resistance training equipment on each shuttle to help prevent the onset of osteoporosis.

So you see, you must have a balance of everything! There is no quick fix! But if we integrate a total health "Courage to Change" program through nutrition, supplementation, cardiovascular and resistance exercise, flexibility, relaxation, stress management, love, and companionship, we have no choice but to achieve greatness within ourselves!

Water

Water is perhaps the most important thing we consume. **Water makes up approximately 60% of our body.** It is needed for body structure and regulation but not energy. Water and other nutrients work in conjunction with one another, and water is number one in helping transport nutrients throughout the body. If we do not drink enough water, it is like driving a car without any oil in the engine or liquid in the radiator. Water acts as a solvent, keeps our temperature down, lubricates our joints, flushes impurities out through our feces more efficiently, and transports our nutrients from one cell to the next. ***Dehydration** is one result of not drinking enough water. A burning sensation during urination may be the result of dehydration. When we urinate, the fluid actually contains very small solid materials. Water dilutes those solid particles in the urine.*

How much water should a person drink? Experts have developed many formulas to answer this question. I have come up with a formula of my own: <u>**You are not drinking enough water if you do not have the constant urge to go to the bathroom or notice any coloration in your urine!**</u> This extremely scientific formula took years to develop but is finally available to you. **Urine should always be crystal clear!** Seriously though, each person should drink at least half of their body weight in ounces of water per day. Keep water in a 1-quart sipper with you all the time to ensure that you drink enough water every day. Without water our nutrients will not arrive at their destination.

Alcohol

Even though some forms of alcohol have been shown to lower a person's blood pressure, it remains one of the most useless nutrients we can ingest. Alcohol does supply the body with energy but gives us ***zero nutrient value.*** We suggest limiting alcohol consumption to 2 beverages per week. Not only does alcohol lack any nutrient value, it also causes dehydration. To give you an idea how harmful alcohol is, I will compare it to pure fat! Pure fat contains 9 kilo-calories per gram and has the highest concentration of energy. Alcohol contains 7 kilo-calories per gram—only two kilo-calories less than pure fat—and has no nutrient value. You may as well sit down with a spoon and a tub of lard. Since it has no nutrient value, where do the calories go? **The belly and the butt!** Most of the calories consumed from alcohol get stored as fat! Aside from the dreaded hangover, alcohol frequently causes liver failure and in pregnant women may cause birth defects and Fetal Alcohol Syndrome.

Food Label Reading

Now, don't panic! Food label reading is very easy. You simply need to know what to look for! Many educators who teach nutritional food label reading take a lot of time to show you how to calculate the percentages of calories, but this approach just complicates matters and confuses the consumer. I want you to focus on number of grams and number of calories. <u>Do not worry about the percentage</u>. A person wanting to be healthy should buy foods with no more than 3–5 grams per serving of fat. All foods are labeled with information for one serving. So how do you figure out how many calories come from each nutrient? Simple! Just multiply the number of grams per serving by the nutrient's concentration of energy. *What?* What is the concentration of energy for the four different kinds of calories?

Carbohydrates	**4 kilo-calories per gram**
Protein	**4 kilo-calories per gram**
Alcohol	**7 kilo-calories per gram**
Fat	**9 kilo-calories per gram**

So if the food label reads *10 grams (g) of fat, 16 g of protein, and 27 g of carbohydrates,* how many calories come from each of these? The number of grams of fat (10) is multiplied by 9, which equals 90 calories of fat per serving. You multiply 16 grams of protein by 4 to give you 64 calories of protein per serving. The 27 grams of carbohydrates are multiplied by 4 to give you 108 calories of carbohydrates per serving. If you add the three together, the total number of calories comes to 262 for one serving of that product. For some reason, many products are a little off from the figure you will reach. But it should always be very close! Since this particular product has 10 grams of fat per serving, you know not to buy it.

Another item to look for is the sugar content. Say the previously mentioned food had 0 grams of fat but the other contents remained the same. However, below the total carbohydrates the label says 25 grams of sugar. **The low fat content makes this item look attractive, but if you look closely, all but 2 grams of the carbohydrates comes from pure sugar! That particular product has poor nutrient density.** Remember, sugar is not a complex carbohydrate and does not get stored in the body unless it is as fat! It mainly promotes tooth decay.

Many products try to trick you into thinking they are healthy because they have little to no fat and high carbohydrate content. Simply check that the sugar content is below 5–10 grams. If a label says 25 g of carbohydrates, 5 g of sugar, 3 g of fat, and 16 g of protein, then that food is something you may purchase. Right now Courage to Change suggests certain food criteria, but once you reach your desired goals and have the control you have longed for, you can apply all these guidelines to your life and do it on your own! This is why you need to learn to read a food label.

When to eat in relation to exercise? The million dollar question!

1. A.M. Just Cardio

When doing **ONLY** cardio in the morning right after waking up, **DO NOT** eat before your workout! If you do, the food you just ate will immediately be converted into energy. The food will be burned for fuel rather than your body fat! We don't want that!

2. A.M. Just Strength Training

When doing only strength training, **ALWAYS** eat something 30–45 minutes before the workout. Your body burns sugar during strength training and needs the extra blood sugar for a good workout. Not eating before you workout can have serious consequences including nausea and vertigo.

3. A.M. Strength Training and Cardio

ALWAYS do strength training first, and **DO eat** before you go. Eating before your workout will give you the energy you need for strength training but will be burned off before it is time to do your cardio for fat burning. This is a win-win situation! This doesn't mean a huge meal. Something small 30-45 minutes before will do it.

4. P.M. Just Cardio (anytime during the day after your first meal)

Do not eat anything for 2 hours prior to your cardio workout. Again, if you do you will be burning what you ate instead of your body fat.

5. P.M. Just Strength Training (anytime during the day after your first meal)

Follow guidelines as specified in number 2.

6. P.M. Strength Training and Cardio (anytime during the day after your first meal)

Follow guidelines as specified in number 3.

Though starchy complex carbohydrates are not recommended in the afternoon and evening hours, when you cut them out depends on when you do your weight training session. Those of you who do your weight training in the evening hours need to consume *one* serving of complex carbohydrates, along with protein and vegetables within 1 hour following a weight training workout. Your muscles need the energy following the workout.

For weight loss purposes no more than 3-4 servings of complex starches should be consumed per day and they should all be consumed before 4p.m.

The exception = If you do your intense weight training sessions late in the evening before bedtime it is a good idea to consume *one* serving of a good complex carbohydrate, along with protein and vegetables. Remember: a little goes a long way!

Sample Grocery List

This grocery list will give you basic guidelines as you take care of your nutritional needs. Anything beyond the basics for most of you as you begin the exercise and nutrition portion of Courage to Change can be overwhelming. So stick to the basics, at least for the first 12 weeks or so.

Complex Carbohydrates and Substitutions

Malt-O-Meal   **Total**
Cream of Wheat   **Special K**
Oatmeal

Or other high-grain, high-fiber, low-fat, low- or no-sugar cereal with less than 2 grams of fat.

Skim Milk or Rice Dream   A vanilla-flavored nondairy drink made from rice.

Rice   Large box (brown, long-grain, or wild)
Potatoes (small)   Red, brown, or sweet potatoes **(yams are best)**
Whole Wheat Pasta Shell or rotini—durum semolina, spinach, tomato, or rainbow

Beans   Kidney   (canned is easiest, natural is healthiest)
                   Black
                   Pinto
                   Lima

Low-fat cottage cheese (Cottage Cheese has a lot of protein but still has some carbs)

Corn

Nutrient-Dense Protein and Substitutions

Chicken Breasts   Boneless and skinless
Turkey Breasts   Boneless and skinless
Extra-Lean Pork Loin
Extra-Lean Red Meat (keep to a minimum)

Fish   Tuna steak   Shrimp   Swordfish
                   Any white fish   Scallops   Mahi-Mahi
                   Halibut   Crab   Walleye
                   Cod   Orange Roughy   Crappie
                   Haddock   Pollack   Whiting Filet
                   Salmon (keep to a minimum)

Eggs   Large (Egg Beaters work well too, but real eggs are better!)

Tofu

Simple Sugars and Substitutions

Oranges	**Pears**	**Grapes (keep to a minimum, loaded with sugar)**
Apples	**Peaches**	**Cantaloupe (1 cup per serving)**
Tangerines	**Berries** ½ cup or choice of other fruits	

½ Grapefruit
No bananas or juice (too much sugar)

Fibrous Foods and Substitutions

Fibrous Vegetables   Lots of dark green, red, yellow, and purple. Veggies are your friend! Frozen are easier to prepare in a hurry. Corn is starchy and should be treated as a complex carbohydrate. Eating vegetables raw is healthiest because the enzymes in the vegetables are killed during the cooking process. Enzymes help break down food for better digestion and nutrient absorption in the body.

Instead of using high sodium seasonings, flavor your food with other foods: green peppers, yellow peppers, red peppers, onions, fresh basil, parsley, pepper, garlic, rosemary, ginger, and thyme. Use the spices God gave you to lose weight, entice your taste buds, and be healthy!

Veggie Burgers or soy meat: Morning Star Farm patties. These do not have hydrogenated or partially hydrogenated oils in them. Good for an alternative midmorning snack.

Optional Items

Non-fat dressings—your favorites
Smart Temptations Cilantro, Spicy Brown Mustard
A-1 Steak Sauce, Lime and Sun-Dried Tomatoes
Chunky Picante Sauce
Heinz 57 Sauce
Honey Dijon, Ranch

All-natural dressings and foods found in stores like Whole Foods are best. They aren't loaded with all the preservatives most store bought brands have. The battle against harmful pesticides, preservatives, hormones and other chemicals in our foods and the treatment of animals is for another time. If you are a vegetarian – go for it. Bottom line: I believe **100%** that certain animals are here for us to nourish our bodies with wonderful, much needed protein, but we must respect these animals and all of God's creation with kindness and responsibility.

Food Storage

If you travel or are on the road with your job, remember to set yourself up for success, not failure. It is difficult to get your food when you are on the road, but having your food prepared in advance and with you in a cooler will help. To heat up your food, simply stop at a 7-11 or other convenience store and use the microwave.

Purchase a Playmate cooler, medium size—make sure that the cooler is large enough to hold all of your meal containers for one full day. If possible, get one with a replaceable water/ice bottle so you do not have to mess with the ice.

1-qt. water bottle or sipper
3–4 serving-size microwavable containers
1–2 small containers for dressings, etc.

Quick and easy Preparation Suggestions

The following ideas for preparation are ideas for quick and easy on the go people. There are so many healthy recipe books out there these days. As long as you stick to the guidelines of portion control in this book have fun finding recipes you like. Also, be looking for my Courage to Change recipe book, "Feast Food" in the near future.

You are learning time management. The less time you spend cooking, the more time you can spend with your family doing other things. One idea is to get the entire family involved in the cooking. The kids may even have good preparation ideas. This will bring the family together and teach the kids good habits. Once you get the hang of it, you will only need a few hours once a week to prepare for the entire week. **Taking 3–4 hours on a Sunday to prepare your week's food will actually save endless hours of cooking throughout the week.** Think about it! Most time in the kitchen is spent cleaning, throwing away trash, and doing the dishes. Doing these chores before and after each meal gets old fast. When food is prepared in advance, all you need to do is reheat the food and then throw the containers in the dishwasher. Those of you who do not have dishwashers can take two minutes to clean your container immediately after finishing. In a large family, each member can be responsible for his or her own dishes. **This is all part of learning self control and learning to manage your time efficiently.**

Pre-preparing your food and making things like casseroles is important because when do you make bad choices? When you are hungry! Sometimes the last thing you want to do when you get home is cook. You are tired, hungry, have to take care of home and family responsibilities and want nourishment right away. This is why many of you go to cereal or tons of pre-made carbs and breads, because they are easy and available. Prepare in advance for those nights when you know you will be tired and hungry.

Here is a list of ideas to help get you started. These are very simple and are certainly NOT gourmet.

Vegetables

In a large mixing bowl, combine green beans, okra, and/or broccoli. You may use as much of any of these vegetables that you desire. The frozen vegetable medley package is a quick and easy alternative. You may use PictSweet as a wonderful seasoning blend and add onions, celery, parsley, or green or red peppers to add even more flavor. Cover the bowl with a paper towel and microwave for about 5 minutes on high. Split into two servings and place in serving-size containers. Most of the time I toss the vegetables I have chosen right in with the pasta or rice and cook it all together. Whether in the microwave or on the stove, it all cooks at the same rate. It saves time and uses fewer containers while cooking.

Rice

Prepare according to instructions on label. You can make up to ½ box and keep in the refrigerator for up to one week. You can also add rice to the vegetables as described above. Experiment with different kinds of rice. I have found brown rice to be the "cleanest" through the body. Once in a while I will purchase Uncle Ben's long-grain and wild rice, mix with brown rice and vegetables, and cook everything together. The reason I dilute the long-grain and wild rice with the brown rice is because of the incredibly high sodium content in Uncle Ben's and similar products. The difference is significant:

White rice: 5 milligrams of sodium per serving
Uncle Ben's long-grain and wild rice: 620 milligrams of sodium per serving—**WOW!**

Canned Tuna Fish in Water

Tuna can be mixed with rice, salsa, and veggies. It makes a nice light snack that actually fills you up for a while. Out of the three main complex carbohydrates, beans, rice, and potatoes, I prefer rice to be eaten with tuna. Experiment a little and try different ways of fixing tuna! **Eating Tuna will send your metabolism through the roof!!! (You want that.)**

Chicken and Fish

Place on plate and cover with a paper towel. Defrost separately in microwave. Cook separately for about 2 minutes. After meat has cooled down, cut into bite-size pieces and place in the veggie-rice mix. Baked or grilled is also tasty. If you have a lot to cook, I suggest purchasing a large, inexpensive aluminum-foil roaster to cook all of the chicken or fish at once. You can cook the fish and chicken at the same time, but in different containers. I usually bake at approximately 350 degrees. The time will vary depending on the amount of food in the oven. If the taste of fish gets old, crush up Cornflakes or Total or a similar cereal. Use that for breading, bake, and ENJOY! When you do this, decrease the amount of complex carbohydrates (rice, pasta, potatoes) eaten with the meat.

Potatoes, yams and Pasta

Potato: Stick the potato several times with a paring knife. Bake in microwave for about 2½ minutes. Turn on other side and microwave for another 2½ minutes. Eat it separately with a little seasoning or cut into bite-size pieces and place in serving container with veggies of choice. Cover and store in refrigerator.

Pasta: Place desired amount of pasta in a saucepan and cover with water. Bring to boil, reduce heat, and simmer until pasta is limp. Remove, drain excess water, and add to the veggie/fish container. Add everything together or keep separate. Cover and refrigerate.

Miscellaneous Foods: Pour fat-free dressing or picante sauce into small container. In the morning, place all containers in your cooler and have a healthy day.

Snacks & Meal Replacements

Snacks should ONLY be eaten if you are ravenous and feel you NEED more!

SNACKS MAY BE EATEN AS A TREAT IN THE EARLY EVENING HOURS, BETWEEN 7:30 and 10:30 P.M. If possible, just go to bed. You are probably eating at this time out of habit!

The following snack and meal replacement ideas are for those days you feel you need more and for those imperfect days when it is impossible for you to get all of your meals in! Additional information is provided in the fast-food section.

Snacks

During the first two weeks, you will probably feel full a lot of the time. This is normal! Your metabolism needs some time to adjust to the different foods and amounts of foods you are taking in. The key to jump-starting your metabolism is to eat, not starve yourself. I guarantee that after two weeks of following this meal plan "religiously", you will begin to be hungry and crave a snack once in a while. This just means that your metabolism is rising and body fat is coming off.

1. 4 or 5 low- or no-salt pretzels—dip in nonfat Smart Temptations dressings, nonfat ranch dressing, or your favorites. Remember that these items usually contain a lot of sodium. Use sparingly!

2. Soft-shell taco—wet one side of a 6-inch nonfat flour or corn tortilla. Add the following ingredients: pieces of chicken breast meat, nonfat mozzarella cheese, broccoli, coleslaw, cilantro lime dressing or nonfat Honey Dijon (my favorite!). Roll and hold together with a toothpick, then heat in the microwave for 1 minute.

3. One serving Malt-O-Meal (3 tsp.)

4. One cup of your favorite nonfat frozen yogurt. Enjoy!

5. "Mock rice pudding":   ½ cup rice
                                  2 egg whites
                                  3 tbsp. brown sugar
Put ingredients in cereal bowl, mix, cover with a paper towel, and microwave for 3 minutes.

6. One serving of a hearty low-sodium, nonfat vegetable soup

Remember: if you are carbohydrate sensitive or have problems with your insulin, snacks should consist of protein.

Meal Replacements

We all have imperfect days, sometimes frequently! But remember, when practicing a balanced lifestyle, when one aspect of your life is off, the rest will carry you through! Taking control of your self means not running from problems but being able to work with and around them more efficiently! Though I suggest that you get your calories from regular food, those imperfect days may require you to get nourishment by supplementation. So in addition to nutrient supplementation such as vitamins and minerals, you may take something with quality calories as well. You want a meal replacement to be quick and easy but also to contain many nutrients and calories you need for energy. The following list includes some examples of meal replacements!

Remember that we want you to eat! So it is imperative that you get all your meals in every day. Being hungry is a healthy sign! It means your metabolism is rising and your calories are being used instead of being stored as fat!

On days that seem like conspiracies against you, do not panic! Carry an apple or a low-fat health bar (Pure Protein Bar or UltraMet) that is as low as possible in sugar. If it is high in sugar you will be regenerated for a short time but will crash and crash hard, a short time later! *Keeping a health bar in your purse or brief case does not give you permission to eat it! It is there only for emergencies!* Remember, it is more important for you to consume *some* food at your designated time rather than to go without any.

There are many meal replacement products on the market that are good for supplementing your nutritional requirements. Below are simply a few popular brands that have proven effective. Remember: you must always consult your physician before starting any meal plan or exercise program. There are many meal replacement products on the market that are good for supplementing your nutritional requirements.

Protein meal replacements / shakes for men and women

Men

Lean Body
Calories: 230
Fat: 1.5g
Carbohydrates: 12g
Sugars: 1g
Protein: 42g

Myoplex Original
Calories: 270
Fat: 3 grams
Carbohydrates: 23 grams
Sugar: 3 grams
Protein: 42 grams

Met-Rx
Calories: 260
Fat: 3 grams
Carbohydrates : 18 grams
Sugar: 6 grams
Protein: 40 grams

Women

Lean Body for Her
Calories: 200
Fat: 1g
Carbohydrates: 19g
Sugars: 1g
Protein: 30g

Myoplex Light
Calories: 180
Fat: 2 grams
Carbohydrates: 17 grams
Sugar: 3 grams
Protein : 24 grams

Mealplex
Calories: 180
Fat: 2 grams
Carbohydrates: 17 grams
Sugar: 2 grams
Protein : 24 grams

There are many other popular brands. Just take notice of the different caloric needs for men and women and you'll be fine. Scout your area for the best buys and cheapest prices. Ordering on line is sometimes cheaper. Just Google the names of the products and you will find them.

The following pre-made protein meal replacement is great for on the go people who spend a lot of time in their vehicle, as well as teachers, court reporters and others who may not be able to take breaks throughout the day.

Myoplex Light / pre-made drink
Calories: 190
Fat: 2.5 grams
Carbohydrates : 20 grams
Sugar: 1 grams
Protein: 24 grams

There are numerous brands now. Find the ones you like. You may need to experiment a little. Not everyone has the same tastes.

Protein Bar meal replacements - For emergencies on those days that are difficult to get a meal in when you need to. Keep these bars in your desk, brief case or purse so you can stay nourished when time gets away from you. Choose one closest to your particular nutritional needs. Be careful on how many bars you eat in a day. Some of the protein bars taste just like a candy bar. They have come a long way. Even though they may be high in protein, many of them have a lot of saturated fat. Again, protein bars should be eaten in emergencies. The protein drinks are better because they are closer to what you need to accomplish your goals. Too many bars and you will hinder your weight loss and will starve your body of much needed fiber and other nutrients. With that being said, protein bars also seem to save my life sometimes. When I am busy and have back to back training classes for 4-5 hours plus some drive time they are perfect if I don't have other food available. Just be responsible with them.

Strive
Calories: 200
Fat: 9 grams
Carbohydrates: 25 grams
Sugar: 0 grams
Protein: 20 grams

Carb Solutions
Calories: 240
Fat: 11 grams
Carbohydrates: 15 grams
Sugar: 1 grams
Protein: 23 grams

Trio-plex
Calories: 327
Fat: 7 grams
Carbohydrates: 36 grams
Sugar: 9 grams
Protein: 30 grams

Pure Protein
Calories: 310
Fat: 9 grams
Carbohydrates: 26 grams
Sugar: 10 grams
Protein: 31 grams

U-Turn
Calories: 300
Fat: 8 grams
Carbohydrates: 26 grams
Sugar: 12 grams
Protein: 30 grams

Fast Food

The following is a list of healthy nutritional options from the most popular fast food restaurants. When on the go during those days that seem like conspiracies against you, eating at a fast food restaurant can still be a healthy alternative to your meal plan guidelines. Vacations and business travel also make it hard to eat healthy while driving or flying to your destination. The following fast food restaurants are everywhere, including major airports and do have healthy choices if you know what to look for.

Water, Water, Water! Always order water with your meals. Stay away from all regular OR diet soft drinks. Your body is only properly hydrated and replenished from drinking water. This will also save you a ton of money over the long haul.

McDonalds
Grilled Caesar Salad with low fat balsamic Vinaigrette
Grilled California Cobb (without bacon) with low fat balsamic Vinaigrette
Grilled Chicken Sandwich or McGrill without bun or mayo

Combine a side salad with one of the chicken sandwich options without bun or mayo for a whole meal.

Wendy's
A good meal would be the following:

Hot stuffed Baked Potato with broccoli –
NO cheese, use fat free ranch or other low calorie dressing sparingly for flavor
Eat only half of the potato, ask for extra broccoli if you want to
Ultimate chicken grill with NO bun or mayo

Spinach Chicken Salad or Mandarin Chicken Salad with Balsamic Vinaigrette or honey mustard – use dressing sparingly, avoid the bacon as much as possible.

Burger King
Chicken Caesar salad, don't eat cheese, sweet onion vinaigrette dressing
Side salad, sweet onion vinaigrette dressing

Grilled Chicken Whopper without bun or mayo
Grilled Sante-Fe Chicken without bun or mayo
Grilled Savory Mustard Chicken without bun or mayo
Grilled Smokey Barbecue Chicken

Combine a side salad with one of the chicken sandwich options without bun or mayo for a whole meal.

Chick-Fil-A
Chargrilled chicken garden salad
Southwest chargrilled salad
Dressings: Fat free Dijon honey mustard, light Italian

Chargrilled chicken cool wrap with fat free Dijon honey mustard or light Italian.
Ask without cheese! The flour tortilla isn't the best because it is processed and a high glycemic carbohydrate with low nutritional value but it is still better than eating fried chicken and waffle fries! ☺

Boston Market
Hand carved rotisserie turkey
Sides: new potatoes, broccoli

Southwest grilled chicken salad with light Italian or balsamic vinaigrette, no cheese

Jack in the Box
Asian Chicken Salad with Low fat balsamic Vinaigrette, without Wonton strips or Roasted slivered almonds

Side Salad with grilled chicken breast

Subway, Quizno's and other sandwich shops
If you want to go in these places and just order the meat and vegetables that go in the sandwich feel free but stay away from all bread, mayo and secret sauces, even the whole wheat buns. The bread has way too many carb-calories and will turn your body off of its efficient fat metabolism. These shops usually have side garden salads available. Order the salad with extra chicken or turkey breast from the main menu.

Why is it more important for you to consume some food than to go without any? If you are forced to eat at a fast-food restaurant, the food may not be quite as healthy as the food you were intending to eat, but it is good enough to keep your metabolism going. Your metabolism may slow down a little but will not go out completely, as it would if you did not eat anything. Your body has a hard time starting your metabolism without healthy, nourishing food. But remember: eat at a fast-food restaurant only in an emergency situation, and just do the best you can! **Perfection is not a human quality! Striving for perfection can be!** When you understand this, you won't feel the pressure to succeed—you will just do it!

How to Order when Dining Out

It is possible to stay on your program while eating at a restaurant.

When ordering in any restaurant, ask the chef to prepare your meal using little or no oil or butter. They can do it with steam or on the grill, and as an added bonus, it is delicious! You must get in the habit of asking for exactly what you want. If you ask only for no oil or butter, the chef may oblige you, but many dishes will still come to you covered in cheese, so be specific when ordering. And remember: Your taste buds are going to learn what is good and what is not. Eating out is about atmosphere, socializing, creating a mood, and romance. Who came up with the idea that eating fat-soaked food is an essential part of the dining process? Enjoying the moment and taking care of yourself simultaneously is the right way to go!

Let me give you an example of how to eat in a restaurant if leaning down is one of your current fitness goals. Let's use the Macaroni Grille as the restaurant of choice. There are hundreds of restaurants like the Macaroni Grille. They may specialize in many different tastes from many different cultures, but the concept is the same. First, smile at the server and ask how he or she is. Then simply tell the server you are on a special health plan and your food has to be prepared a certain way. This approach is better than just blurting out some recipe and demanding that the server do what you ask. Be nice and you will be treated with respect and will usually get what you want. Remember, in order to be served by anyone in any situation, you must first be willing to "serve" *them* with love, respect, and kindness. On those occasions when you get a less than willing wait person, you still need to serve them the same way. Your gift of kindness could lift them spiritually and turn their day around.

Next, ask that the bread and olive oil not be brought to the table. Tell them you don't need it. You can do it! Ask your companions to help out and respect your wishes. When you become the one not needing to lose weight and are with someone else who is making the effort, support what they are trying to accomplish and pass up the bread also!

Once that issue is out of the way, order a nice bowl of angel hair pasta or rice with *no* sauce. Ask that one tablespoon of olive oil be mixed in with the pasta for some flavor and consistency. For additional flavor, ask for basil to be lightly sprinkled over the pasta along with two juicy diced tomatoes. Finally, ask for a grilled chicken breast, topped with additional basil, to be cut up and placed over the tomatoes atop the pasta, along with 4 or 5 jumbo shrimp, lightly sautéed with almost no butter or oil. Some fresh lemon squeezed on top tastes great as well.

If eating a salad, ask for a garden salad with a variety of greens, no cheese or croutons, and nonfat dressing. If they do not have nonfat dressing, then ask for something like honey-mustard or low-calorie vinaigrette. If you are hungry for other vegetables, ask for them raw or steamed as a side dish. If you have vegetables mixed with your pasta, you will end up eating way too much of the pasta to get to the vegetables. Restaurants such as Macaroni Grille want to give you tons of food to maximize the value of your meal. Don't forget that ½ cup of most complex carbohydrates is one serving. Most bowls of pasta you would get at a restaurant have up to 4 or 5 servings—way too many calories in one sit-down meal. Take the rest home with you and enjoy it in another meal. But you do want to eat all the chicken, shrimp, and vegetables.

By taking care of yourself in public and not just at home, you have the opportunity to influence the people around you in a positive way. I have had people come to my table from other parts of the restaurant just to ask me what I ordered and if it was on the menu. I order what I want and the restaurant usually makes it perfectly. I have had chefs come out in person to ask me if it was prepared to my satisfaction. Yes, it is often a struggle. But whoever said we weren't supposed to struggle, even with the things we know will benefit us? It seems to me that the things that benefit us most are also the things we struggle with most. Knowing Christ is a struggle in itself because the world doesn't understand it and persecutes us for it. Just do the best you can, and if you fall, hold yourself accountable, dust yourself off, and by the grace of God begin again.

Oh, and don't forget! A bare minimum 20% gratuity should be given to your server for serving what you requested. They deserve it! And even if they don't, plant the seed!

Steps to take when traveling:

1. Make a commitment to stay on your program.
2. Take your courage to change book and journal and Bible with you.
3. Carry protein bars with you at all times.
4. Call ahead of time if you are flying and ask for the carb sensitive meal or the one for diabetics. Even if you aren't diabetic this meal will help you stay in your fat burning zone.
5. When entering other time zones <u>do your best</u> to keep on the same time schedule of eating and sleeping.
6. Drink tons of water. The air in an airplane is dryer than the desert (true fact)!
7. Be confident in your ability to locate and order healthy food from a restaurant.
8. If staying with friends or family make your intentions known of your commitment to stay healthy. Offer to buy groceries if you need to or if it applies.
9. When driving make periodic stops to stretch for a few minutes. If you are on a time crunch then do it when you stop for a restroom break.
10. When flying make frequent trips to the rest room and stretch for a few minutes at a time.
11. Get your workout in before you leave so your body will be more relaxed as you travel.
12. Choose hotels that have a fitness facility of some kind.
13. When staying with friends or family for extended periods locate a local fitness facility or be prepared to train where you are staying without equipment. Either way be prepared.
14. Have fun and feast!

The following pages contain a sample 7 day Meal Plan for both men & women

The following meal plans are only a guideline and are in no way intended to diagnose, treat or prevent any sickness, disease or affliction. The number of daily calories is designed for a person on an aggressive exercise program like the one in this book. Cardiovascular exercise should be done 45 minutes- 1 hour 5-6 days per week with 3 days per week weight training alone or with your Courage to Change training team. A bear minimum of 350 calories should be burned every day you do cardio. If you can't do it all at one time at first then break it into 2-3 different sessions throughout each day so you burn 350 calories per day. Eventually you will be able to do it in one session. The equipment you use should give you an estimate of how many calories you burned in your session.

Remember: These are only guidelines. As always consult your physician before starting any exercise or nutrition plan. You don't have to follow each day exactly. Mix up the days as they pertain to your likes and dislikes. Be creative and find different ways of preparing your meals so you don't get bored eating the same foods the same ways every day.

Female 100-130 pounds

	Day 1	Day 2	Day 3	Day 4	Day 5	Day 6	Day 7
Breakfast	1 Cup Cream of Wheat 1 Cup skim milk 3 egg whites 1 small apple	1 Cup Oatmeal 1 Cup skim milk 3 egg whites 1 small peach	1 Cup skim milk 1 small apple Rice omelet: 3 egg whites scrambled with ½ cup brown rice and chunky salsa	1 serving Special K 1 Cup skim milk 3 egg whites 1 cup strawberries	1 Cup Malt-o-meal 1 Cup skim milk 3 egg whites ½ grapefruit	1 Cup Grits or Grape nuts 1 Cup skim milk 3 egg whites 1 cup cantaloupe	1 Cup Total no raisins 1 Cup skim milk 3 egg whites 1 small apple
Mid-morning Snack	Protein Shake, Blended with 16 oz water	Protein Shake, Blended with 16 oz water	Protein Shake, Blended with 16 oz water	Protein Shake, Blended with 16 oz water	Protein Shake, Blended with 16 oz water	Protein Shake, Blended with 16 oz water	Protein Shake, Blended with 16 oz water
Lunch	3 ½ ounces chicken breast 1 small yam Broccoli 1 small apple	3 ½ ounces turkey breast 2 very small new potatoes Broccoli 1 small apple	3 ½ ounces chicken breast 1 small yam Broccoli 1 small apple	3 ½ ounces lean steak ½ cup brown rice Spinach salad 1 small apple	3 ½ ounces lean pork loin 1 small yam Broccoli ½ grapefruit	3 ½ ounces chicken breast ½ cup black beans Broccoli 1 small apple	3 ½ ounces chicken breast 1 small yam Broccoli 1 small apple
1st Mid Afternoon Snack	4 ounces tuna Broccoli or large salad ½ cup brown rice	4 ounces crab Broccoli or large salad 1 cup brown rice	4 ounces tuna Broccoli or large salad 1 cup brown rice	4 ounces Albacore in water Broccoli or large salad 1 cup brown rice	4 ounces tuna Broccoli or large salad 1 cup brown rice	4 ounces tuna Broccoli or large salad 1 cup brown rice	4 ounces tuna Broccoli or large salad 1 cup brown rice
2nd Mid Afternoon Snack	1 orange	1 orange	1 peach	1 orange	1 orange	1 Pear	1 orange
Dinner	3 ½ ounces Tilapia Broccoli or large salad	3 ½ ounces Swordfish Broccoli or large salad	3 ½ ounces Shrimp Broccoli or large salad	3 ½ ounces Halibut Broccoli or large salad	3 ½ ounces Atlantic Cod Broccoli or large salad	3 ½ ounces Mahi-Mahi or Scallops Asparagus Bell peppers	Splurge meal: Have fun and make your splurge meal memorable with friends and family once per week! Enjoy!
Late Evening Snack	None	None	None	None	None	None	None
Approximate Daily Caloric breakdown	Calories: 1454 Protein: 137 Carbohydrates: 212 Fat: 9	Calories: 1454 Protein: 137 Carbohydrates: 212 Fat: 9	Calories: 1454 Protein: 137 Carbohydrates: 212 Fat: 9	Calories: 1454 Protein: 137 Carbohydrates: 212 Fat: 9	Calories: 1454 Protein: 137 Carbohydrates: 212 Fat: 9	Calories: 1454 Protein: 137 Carbohydrates: 212 Fat: 9	No guilt No shame I am in control of my eating!

Female 130-150 pounds

	Day 1	Day 2	Day 3	Day 4	Day 5	Day 6	Day 7
Breakfast	1 Cup Cream of Wheat 1 Cup skim milk 3 egg whites 1 small apple	1 Cup Oatmeal 1 Cup skim milk 3 egg whites 1 small peach	1 Cup skim milk 1 small apple Rice omelet: 3 egg whites scrambled with ½ cup brown rice and chunky salsa	1 serving Special K 1 Cup skim milk 3 egg whites 1 cup strawberries	1 Cup Malt-o-meal 1 Cup skim milk 3 egg whites ½ grapefruit	1 Cup Grits or Grape nuts 1 Cup skim milk 3 egg whites 1 cup cantaloupe	1 Cup Total no raisins 1 Cup skim milk 3 egg whites 1 small apple
Mid-morning Snack	Protein Shake, Blended with 16 oz water	Protein Shake, Blended with 16 oz water	Protein Shake, Blended with 16 oz water	Protein Shake, Blended with 16 oz water	Protein Shake, Blended with 16 oz water	Protein Shake, Blended with 16 oz water	Protein Shake, Blended with 16 oz water
Lunch	5 ounces chicken breast 1 small yam Broccoli	5 ounces turkey breast 2 very small new potatoes Broccoli	5 ounces chicken breast 1 small yam Broccoli	5 ounces lean steak ½ cup brown rice Spinach salad	5 ounces lean pork loin 1 small yam Broccoli	5 ounces chicken breast ½ cup black beans Broccoli	5 ounces chicken breast 1 small yam Broccoli
1st Mid Afternoon Snack	1-6 ounce can tuna in water Broccoli or large salad ¼ cup brown rice	1-6 ounce can crab in water Broccoli or large salad ¼ cup brown rice	1-6 ounce can tuna in water Broccoli or large salad ¼ cup brown rice	1-6 ounce can Albacore in water Broccoli or large salad ¼ cup brown rice	1-6 ounce can tuna in water Broccoli or large salad ¼ cup brown rice	1-6 ounce can tuna in water Broccoli or large salad ¼ cup brown rice	1-6 ounce can tuna in water Broccoli or large salad ¼ cup brown rice
2nd Mid Afternoon Snack	½ small apple	½ small apple	½ small apple	½ small apple	½ small apple	½ small apple	½ small apple
Dinner	7 ounces Tilapia Mixed veggies or large salad	7 ounces Swordfish Mixed veggies or large salad	7 ounces Shrimp Mixed veggies or large salad	7 ounces Halibut Mixed veggies or large salad	7 ounces Atlantic Cod Mixed veggies or large salad	7 ounces Mahi-Mahi or Scallops Asparagus Bell peppers	Splurge meal: Have fun and make your splurge meal memorable with friends and family once per week! Enjoy!
Late Evening Snack	None	None	None	None	None	None	None
Approximate Daily Caloric breakdown	Calories: 1483 Protein: 173 Carbohydrates: 174 Fat: 11	Calories: 1483 Protein: 173 Carbohydrates: 174 Fat: 11	Calories: 1483 Protein: 173 Carbohydrates: 174 Fat: 11	Calories: 1483 Protein: 173 Carbohydrates: 174 Fat: 11	Calories: 1483 Protein: 173 Carbohydrates: 174 Fat: 11	Calories: 1483 Protein: 173 Carbohydrates: 174 Fat: 11	No guilt No shame I am in control of my eating!

Female 150-170 pounds

	Day 1	Day 2	Day 3	Day 4	Day 5	Day 6	Day 7
Breakfast	1 Cup Cream of Wheat 1 Cup skim milk 5 egg whites 1 small apple	1 Cup Oatmeal 1 Cup skim milk 5 egg whites 1 small peach	1 Cup skim milk 1 small apple Rice omelet: 5 egg whites scrambled with ½ cup brown rice and chunky salsa	1 serving Special K 1 Cup skim milk 5 egg whites 1 cup strawberries	1 Cup Malt-o-meal 1 Cup skim milk 5 egg whites ½ grapefruit	1 Cup Grits or Grape nuts 1 Cup skim milk 5 egg whites 1 cup cantaloupe	1 Cup Total no raisins 1 Cup skim milk 5 egg whites 1 small apple
Mid-morning Snack	Protein Shake, Blended with 16 oz water	Protein Shake, Blended with 16 oz water	Protein Shake, Blended with 16 oz water	Protein Shake, Blended with 16 oz water	Protein Shake, Blended with 16 oz water	Protein Shake, Blended with 16 oz water	Protein Shake, Blended with 16 oz water
Lunch	7 ounces chicken breast Broccoli	7 ounces turkey breast Broccoli	7 ounces chicken breast Broccoli	7 ounces lean steak Spinach salad	7 ounces lean pork loin Broccoli	7 ounces chicken breast Broccoli	7 ounces chicken breast Broccoli
1st Mid Afternoon Snack	1-6 ounce can tuna in water Broccoli or large salad	1-6 ounce can crab in water Broccoli or large salad	1-6 ounce can tuna in water Broccoli or large salad	1-6 ounce can Albacore in water Broccoli or large salad	1-6 ounce can tuna in water Broccoli or large salad	1-6 ounce can tuna in water Broccoli or large salad	1-6 ounce can tuna in water Broccoli or large salad
2nd Mid Afternoon Snack	Protein Shake, Blended with 16 oz water	Protein Shake, Blended with 16 oz water	Protein Shake, Blended with 16 oz water	Protein Shake, Blended with 16 oz water	Protein Shake, Blended with 16 oz water	Protein Shake, Blended with 16 oz water	Protein Shake, Blended with 16 oz water
Dinner	7 ounces Tilapia Mixed veggies or large salad Small handful Strawberries	7 ounces Swordfish Mixed veggies or large salad Small handful Blueberries	7 ounces Shrimp Mixed veggies or large salad Small handful Strawberries	7 ounces Halibut Mixed veggies or large salad Small handful Strawberries	7 ounces Atlantic Cod Mixed veggies or large salad Small handful Strawberries	7 ounces Mahi-Mahi or Scallops Asparagus Bell peppers Small handful Raspberries	Splurge meal: Have fun and make your splurge meal memorable with friends and family once per week! Enjoy!
Late Evening Snack	None	None	None	None	None	None	None
Approximate Daily Caloric breakdown	Calories: 1513 Protein: 205 Carbohydrates: 140 Fat: 14	Calories: 1513 Protein: 205 Carbohydrates: 140 Fat: 14	Calories: 1513 Protein: 205 Carbohydrates: 140 Fat: 14	Calories: 1513 Protein: 205 Carbohydrates: 140 Fat: 14	Calories: 1513 Protein: 205 Carbohydrates: 140 Fat: 14	Calories: 1513 Protein: 205 Carbohydrates: 140 Fat: 14	No guilt No shame I am in control of my eating!

Female 170-200 pounds

	Day 1	Day 2	Day 3	Day 4	Day 5	Day 6	Day 7
Breakfast	1 Cup Cream of Wheat 1 Cup skim milk 4 egg whites 1 small apple	1 Cup Oatmeal 1 Cup skim milk 4 egg whites 1 small peach	1 Cup skim milk 1 small apple Rice omelet: 4 egg whites scrambled with ½ cup brown rice and chunky salsa	1 serving Special K 1 Cup skim milk 4 egg whites 1 cup strawberries	1 Cup Malt-o-meal 1 Cup skim milk 4 egg whites ½ grapefruit	1 Cup Grits or Grape nuts 1 Cup skim milk 4 egg whites 1 cup cantaloupe	1 Cup Total no raisins 1 Cup skim milk 4 egg whites 1 small apple
Mid-morning Snack	Protein Shake, Blended with 16 oz water	Protein Shake, Blended with 16 oz water	Protein Shake, Blended with 16 oz water	Protein Shake, Blended with 16 oz water	Protein Shake, Blended with 16 oz water	Protein Shake, Blended with 16 oz water	Protein Shake, Blended with 16 oz water
Lunch	5 ounces chicken breast ½ cup brown rice Broccoli	5 ounces turkey breast ½ cup Kidney Beans Broccoli	5 ounces chicken breast ½ cup brown rice Broccoli	5 ounces lean steak 1 small yam Spinach salad	5 ounces lean pork loin ½ cup wild rice Broccoli	5 ounces chicken breast ½ cup black beans Broccoli	5 ounces chicken breast ½ cup brown rice Broccoli
1st Mid Afternoon Snack	1-6 ounce can tuna in water Broccoli or large salad ½ small apple	1-6 ounce can crab in water Broccoli or large salad ½ small apple	1-6 ounce can tuna in water Broccoli or large salad ½ orange	1-6 ounce can Albacore in water Broccoli or large salad ½ small apple	1-6 ounce can tuna in water Broccoli or large salad ½ small apple	1-6 ounce can tuna in water Broccoli or large salad ½ small apple	1-6 ounce can tuna in water Broccoli or large salad ½ small apple
2nd Mid Afternoon Snack	Protein Shake, Blended with 16 oz water	Protein Shake, Blended with 16 oz water	Protein Shake, Blended with 16 oz water	Protein Shake, Blended with 16 oz water	Protein Shake, Blended with 16 oz water	Protein Shake, Blended with 16 oz water	Protein Shake, Blended with 16 oz water
Dinner	7 ounces Tilapia Mixed veggies or large salad	7 ounces Swordfish Mixed veggies or large salad	7 ounces Shrimp Mixed veggies or large salad	7 ounces Halibut Mixed veggies or large salad	7 ounces Atlantic Cod Mixed veggies or large salad	7 ounces Mahi-Mahi or Scallops Asparagus Bell peppers	Splurge meal: Have fun and make your splurge meal memorable with friends and family once per week! Enjoy!
Late Evening Snack	None	None	None	None	None	None	None
Approximate Daily Caloric breakdown	Calories: 1525 Protein: 194 Carbohydrates: 153 Fat: 13	Calories: 1525 Protein: 194 Carbohydrates: 153 Fat: 13	Calories: 1525 Protein: 194 Carbohydrates: 153 Fat: 13	Calories: 1525 Protein: 194 Carbohydrates: 153 Fat: 13	Calories: 1525 Protein: 194 Carbohydrates: 153 Fat: 13	Calories: 1525 Protein: 194 Carbohydrates: 153 Fat: 13	No guilt No shame I am in control of my eating!

Female 200-250 pounds

	Day 1	Day 2	Day 3	Day 4	Day 5	Day 6	Day 7
Breakfast	1 Cup Cream of Wheat 1 Cup skim milk 4 egg whites 1 small apple	1 Cup Oatmeal 1 Cup skim milk 4 egg whites 1 small peach	1 Cup skim milk 1 small apple Rice omelet: 4 egg whites scrambled with ½ cup brown rice and chunky salsa	1 serving Special K 1 Cup skim milk 4 egg whites 1 cup strawberries	1 Cup Malt-o-meal 1 Cup skim milk 4 egg whites ½ grapefruit	1 Cup Grits or Grape nuts 1 Cup skim milk 4 egg whites 1 cup cantaloupe	1 Cup Total no raisins 1 Cup skim milk 4 egg whites 1 small apple
Mid-morning Snack	Protein Shake, Blended with 16 oz water	Protein Shake, Blended with 16 oz water	Protein Shake, Blended with 16 oz water	Protein Shake, Blended with 16 oz water	Protein Shake, Blended with 16 oz water	Protein Shake, Blended with 16 oz water	Protein Shake, Blended with 16 oz water
Lunch	3 ½ ounces chicken breast ½ cup brown rice Broccoli 1 small apple	3 ½ ounces turkey breast ½ cup Kidney Beans Broccoli 1 small apple	3 ½ ounces chicken breast ½ cup brown rice Broccoli 1 small apple	3 ½ ounces lean steak 1 small yam Spinach salad 1 small apple	3 ½ ounces lean pork loin ½ cup wild rice Broccoli ½ grapefruit	3 ½ ounces chicken breast ½ cup black beans Broccoli 1 small apple	3 ½ ounces chicken breast ½ cup brown rice Broccoli 1 small apple
1st Mid Afternoon Snack	1-6 ounce can tuna in water Broccoli or large salad	1-6 ounce can crab in water Broccoli or large salad	1-6 ounce can tuna in water Broccoli or large salad	1-6 ounce can Albacore in water Broccoli or large salad	1-6 ounce can tuna in water Broccoli or large salad	1-6 ounce can tuna in water Broccoli or large salad	1-6 ounce can tuna in water Broccoli or large salad
2nd Mid Afternoon Snack	Protein Shake, Blended with 16 oz water	Protein Shake, Blended with 16 oz water	Protein Shake, Blended with 16 oz water	Protein Shake, Blended with 16 oz water	Protein Shake, Blended with 16 oz water	Protein Shake, Blended with 16 oz water	Protein Shake, Blended with 16 oz water
Dinner	7 ounces Tilapia Mixed veggies or large salad Small handful Strawberries	7 ounces Swordfish Mixed veggies or large salad Small handful Blueberries	7 ounces Shrimp Mixed veggies or large salad Small handful Strawberries	7 ounces Halibut Mixed veggies or large salad Small handful Strawberries	7 ounces Atlantic Cod Mixed veggies or large salad Small handful Strawberries	7 ounces Mahi-Mahi or Scallops Asparagus Bell peppers Small handful Raspberries	Splurge meal: Have fun and make your splurge meal memorable with friends and family once per week! Enjoy!
Late Evening Snack	None	None	None	None	None	None	None
Approximate Daily Caloric breakdown	Calories: 1557 Protein: 185 Carbohydrates: 178 Fat: 13	Calories: 1557 Protein: 185 Carbohydrates: 178 Fat: 13	Calories: 1557 Protein: 185 Carbohydrates: 178 Fat: 13	Calories: 1557 Protein: 185 Carbohydrates: 178 Fat: 13	Calories: 1557 Protein: 185 Carbohydrates: 178 Fat: 13	Calories: 1557 Protein: 185 Carbohydrates: 178 Fat: 13	No guilt No shame I am in control of my eating!

Female 250-300 pounds

	Day 1	Day 2	Day 3	Day 4	Day 5	Day 6	Day 7
Breakfast	1 Cup Cream of Wheat 1 Cup skim milk 3 egg whites	1 Cup Oatmeal 1 Cup skim milk 3 egg whites	1 Cup skim milk Rice omelet: 3 egg whites scrambled with ½ cup brown rice and chunky salsa	1 serving Special K 1 Cup skim milk 3 egg whites 1 cup	1 Cup Malt-o-meal 1 Cup skim milk 3 egg whites	1 Cup Grits or Grape nuts 1 Cup skim milk 3 egg whites	1 Cup Total no raisins 1 Cup skim milk 3 egg whites
Mid-morning Snack	Protein Shake, Blended with 16 oz water	Protein Shake, Blended with 16 oz water	Protein Shake, Blended with 16 oz water	Protein Shake, Blended with 16 oz water	Protein Shake, Blended with 16 oz water	Protein Shake, Blended with 16 oz water	Protein Shake, Blended with 16 oz water
Lunch	7 ounces chicken breast ½ cup brown rice Broccoli ½ small apple	7 ounces turkey breast ½ cup Kidney Beans Broccoli ½ small apple	7 ounces chicken breast ½ cup brown rice Broccoli ½ small apple	7 ounces lean steak 1 small yam Spinach salad ½ small apple	7 ounces lean pork loin ½ cup wild rice Broccoli ¼ grapefruit	7 ounces chicken breast ½ cup black beans Broccoli ½ small apple	7 ounces chicken breast ½ cup brown rice Broccoli ½ small apple
1st Mid Afternoon Snack	1-6 ounce can tuna in water Broccoli or large salad	1-6 ounce can crab in water Broccoli or large salad	1-6 ounce can tuna in water Broccoli or large salad	1-6 ounce can Albacore in water Broccoli or large salad	1-6 ounce can tuna in water Broccoli or large salad	1-6 ounce can tuna in water Broccoli or large salad	1-6 ounce can tuna in water Broccoli or large salad
2nd Mid Afternoon Snack	Protein Shake, Blended with 16 oz water	Protein Shake, Blended with 16 oz water	Protein Shake, Blended with 16 oz water	Protein Shake, Blended with 16 oz water	Protein Shake, Blended with 16 oz water	Protein Shake, Blended with 16 oz water	Protein Shake, Blended with 16 oz water
Dinner	7 ounces Tilapia Mixed veggies or large salad	7 ounces Swordfish Mixed veggies or large salad	7 ounces Shrimp Mixed veggies or large salad	7 ounces Halibut Mixed veggies or large salad	7 ounces Atlantic Cod Mixed veggies or large salad	7 ounces Mahi-Mahi or Scallops Asparagus Bell peppers	Splurge meal: Have fun and make your splurge meal memorable with friends and family once per week! Enjoy!
Late Evening Snack	3 ½ ounces Chicken	3 ½ ounces Chicken	3 ½ ounces Turkey	3 ½ ounces Chicken	3 ½ ounces Chicken	3 ½ ounces Turkey	None
Approximate Daily Caloric breakdown	Calories 1613 Protein 228 Carbohydrates 137 Fat 15	Calories 1613 Protein 228 Carbohydrates 137 Fat 15	Calories 1613 Protein 228 Carbohydrates 137 Fat 15	Calories 1613 Protein 228 Carbohydrates 137 Fat 15	Calories 1613 Protein 228 Carbohydrates 137 Fat 15	Calories 1613 Protein 228 Carbohydrates 137 Fat 15	No guilt No shame I am in control of my eating!

Female 300-400 pounds

	Day 1	Day 2	Day 3	Day 4	Day 5	Day 6	Day 7
Breakfast	1 Cup Cream of Wheat 1 Cup skim milk 3 egg whites 1 small apple	1 Cup Oatmeal 1 Cup skim milk 3 egg whites 1 small peach	1 Cup skim milk 1 small apple Rice omelet: 3 egg whites scrambled with ½ cup brown rice and chunky salsa	1 serving Special K 1 Cup skim milk 3 egg whites 1 cup strawberries	1 Cup Malt-o-meal 1 Cup skim milk 3 egg whites ½ grapefruit	1 Cup Grits or Grape nuts 1 Cup skim milk 3 egg whites 1 cup cantaloupe	1 Cup Total no raisins 1 Cup skim milk 3 egg whites 1 small apple
Mid-morning Snack	Protein Shake, Blended with 16 oz water	Protein Shake, Blended with 16 oz water	Protein Shake, Blended with 16 oz water	Protein Shake, Blended with 16 oz water	Protein Shake, Blended with 16 oz water	Protein Shake, Blended with 16 oz water	Protein Shake, Blended with 16 oz water
Lunch	3 ½ ounces chicken breast ½ cup brown rice Broccoli	3 ½ ounces turkey breast ½ cup Kidney Beans Broccoli	3 ½ ounces chicken breast ½ cup brown rice Broccoli	3 ½ ounces lean steak 1 small yam Spinach salad	3 ½ ounces lean pork loin ½ cup wild rice Broccoli	3 ½ ounces chicken breast ½ cup black beans Broccoli	3 ½ ounces chicken breast ½ cup brown rice Broccoli
1st Mid Afternoon Snack	1-6 ounce can tuna in water Broccoli or large salad 1 small apple	1-6 ounce can crab in water Broccoli or large salad 1 small apple	1-6 ounce can tuna in water Broccoli or large salad 1 orange	1-6 ounce can Albacore in water Broccoli or large salad 1 small apple	1-6 ounce can tuna in water Broccoli or large salad 1 small apple	1-6 ounce can tuna in water Broccoli or large salad 1 small apple	1-6 ounce can tuna in water Broccoli or large salad 1 small apple
2nd Mid Afternoon Snack	Protein Shake, Blended with 16 oz water	Protein Shake, Blended with 16 oz water	Protein Shake, Blended with 16 oz water	Protein Shake, Blended with 16 oz water	Protein Shake, Blended with 16 oz water	Protein Shake, Blended with 16 oz water	Protein Shake, Blended with 16 oz water
Dinner	7 ounces Tilapia Mixed veggies or large salad Small handful Strawberries	7 ounces Swordfish Mixed veggies or large salad Small handful Blueberries	7 ounces Shrimp Mixed veggies or large salad Small handful Strawberries	7 ounces Halibut Mixed veggies or large salad Small handful Strawberries	7 ounces Atlantic Cod Mixed veggies or large salad Small handful Strawberries	7 ounces Mahi-Mahi or Scallops Asparagus Bell peppers Small handful Raspberries	Splurge meal: Have fun and make your splurge meal memorable with friends and family once per week! Enjoy!
Late Evening Snack	3 ½ ounces Chicken	3 ½ ounces Chicken	3 ½ ounces Turkey	3 ½ ounces Chicken	3 ½ ounces Chicken	3 ½ ounces Turkey	None
Approximate Daily Caloric breakdown	Calories: 1711 Protein: 208 Carbohydrates: 189 Fat: 15	Calories: 1711 Protein: 208 Carbohydrates: 189 Fat: 15	Calories: 1711 Protein: 208 Carbohydrates: 189 Fat: 15	Calories: 1711 Protein: 208 Carbohydrates: 189 Fat: 15	Calories: 1711 Protein: 208 Carbohydrates: 189 Fat: 15	Calories: 1711 Protein: 208 Carbohydrates: 189 Fat: 15	No guilt No shame I am in control of my eating!

Male 100-130 pounds

	Day 1	Day 2	Day 3	Day 4	Day 5	Day 6	Day 7
Breakfast	1 Cup Cream of Wheat 1 Cup skim milk 5 egg whites 1 small apple	1 Cup Oatmeal 1 Cup skim milk 5 egg whites 1 small peach	1 Cup skim milk 1 small apple Rice omelet: 5 egg whites scrambled with ½ cup brown rice and chunky salsa	1 serving Special K 1 Cup skim milk 5 egg whites 1 cup strawberries	1 Cup Malt-o-meal 1 Cup skim milk 5 egg whites ½ grapefruit	1 Cup Grits or Grape nuts 1 Cup skim milk 5 egg whites 1 cup cantaloupe	1 Cup Total no raisins 1 Cup skim milk 5 egg whites 1 small apple
Mid-morning Snack	Protein Shake, Blended with 16 oz water	Protein Shake, Blended with 16 oz water	Protein Shake, Blended with 16 oz water	Protein Shake, Blended with 16 oz water	Protein Shake, Blended with 16 oz water	Protein Shake, Blended with 16 oz water	Protein Shake, Blended with 16 oz water
Lunch	½ chicken breast 1 small yam Broccoli 1 small apple	2 ounces Turkey breast 2 very small new potatoes Broccoli 1 small apple	½ chicken breast 1 small yam Broccoli 1 small apple	2 ounces lean steak ½ cup brown rice Spinach salad 1 small apple	2 ounces lean pork loin 1 small yam Broccoli ½ grapefruit	½ chicken breast 1 cup black beans Broccoli 1 small apple	½ chicken breast 1 small yam Broccoli 1 small apple
1ˢᵗ Mid Afternoon Snack	3 1/2 ounces tuna Broccoli or large salad ½ cup brown rice	3 1/2 ounces crab Broccoli or large salad ½ cup brown rice	3 1/2 ounces tuna Broccoli or large salad ½ cup brown rice	3 1/2 ounces Albacore in water Broccoli or large salad ½ cup brown rice	3 1/2 ounces tuna Broccoli or large salad ½ cup brown rice	3 1/2 ounces tuna Broccoli or large salad ½ cup brown rice	3 1/2 ounces tuna Broccoli or large salad ½ cup brown rice
2nd Mid Afternoon Snack	1 orange	1 Tangerine	1 Peach	1 orange	1 orange	1 Pear	1 orange
Dinner	3 ½ ounces Tilapia Broccoli or large salad 1 small apple	3 ½ ounces Swordfish Broccoli or large salad 1 small apple	3 ½ ounces Shrimp Broccoli or large salad 1 small apple	3 ½ ounces Halibut Broccoli or large salad 1 small apple	3 ½ ounces Atlantic Cod Broccoli or large salad 1 small apple	3 ½ ounces Mahi-Mahi or Scallops Asparagus Bell peppers Small handful raspberries	Splurge meal: Have fun and make your splurge meal memorable with friends and family once per week! Enjoy!
Late Evening Snack	None	None	None	None	None	None	None
Approximate Daily Caloric breakdown	Calories: 1544 Protein: 137 Carbohydrates: 239 Fat: 8	Calories: 1544 Protein: 137 Carbohydrates: 239 Fat: 8	Calories: 1544 Protein: 137 Carbohydrates: 239 Fat: 8	Calories: 1544 Protein: 137 Carbohydrates: 239 Fat: 8	Calories: 1544 Protein: 137 Carbohydrates: 239 Fat: 8	Calories: 1544 Protein: 137 Carbohydrates: 239 Fat: 8	No guilt No shame I am in control of my eating!

Male 130-150 pounds

	Day 1	Day 2	Day 3	Day 4	Day 5	Day 6	Day 7
Breakfast	1 Cup Cream of Wheat 1 Cup skim milk 5 egg whites 1 small apple	1 Cup Oatmeal 1 Cup skim milk 5 egg whites 1 small peach	1 Cup skim milk 1 small apple Rice omelet: 5 egg whites scrambled with ½ cup brown rice and chunky salsa	1 serving Special K 1 Cup skim milk 5 egg whites 1 cup strawberries	1 Cup Malt-o-meal 1 Cup skim milk 5 egg whites ½ grapefruit	1 Cup Grits or Grape nuts 1 Cup skim milk 5 egg whites 1 cup cantaloupe	1 Cup Total no raisins 1 Cup skim milk 5 egg whites 1 small apple
Mid-morning Snack	Protein Shake, Blended with 16 oz water	Protein Shake, Blended with 16 oz water	Protein Shake, Blended with 16 oz water	Protein Shake, Blended with 16 oz water	Protein Shake, Blended with 16 oz water	Protein Shake, Blended with 16 oz water	Protein Shake, Blended with 16 oz water
Lunch	5 ounces chicken breast 1 small yam Broccoli 1 small apple	5 ounces Turkey breast 2 very small new potatoes Broccoli 1 small apple	5 ounces chicken breast 1 small yam Broccoli 1 small apple	5 ounces lean steak ½ cup brown rice Spinach salad 1 small apple	5 ounces lean pork loin 1 small yam Broccoli ½ grapefruit	5 ounces chicken breast 1 small yam Broccoli 1 small apple	5 ounces chicken breast 1 small yam Broccoli 1 small apple
1st Mid Afternoon Snack	1-6 ounce can tuna in water Broccoli or large salad ½ cup brown rice	1-6 ounce can crab in water Broccoli or large salad ½ cup brown rice	1-6 ounce can tuna in water Broccoli or large salad ½ cup brown rice	1-6 ounce can Albacore in water Broccoli or large salad ½ cup brown rice	1-6 ounce can tuna in water Broccoli or large salad ½ cup brown rice	1-6 ounce can tuna in water Broccoli or large salad ½ cup brown rice	1-6 ounce can tuna in water Broccoli or large salad ½ cup brown rice
2nd Mid Afternoon Snack	1 orange	1 Tangerine	1 Peach	1 orange	1 orange	1 Pear	1 orange
Dinner	3 ½ ounces Tilapia Broccoli or large salad	3 ½ ounces Swordfish Broccoli or large salad	3 ½ ounces Shrimp Broccoli or large salad	3 ½ ounces Halibut Broccoli or large salad	3 ½ ounces Atlantic Cod Broccoli or large salad	3 ½ ounces Mahi-Mahi or Scallops Asparagus Bell peppers	Splurge meal: Have fun and make your splurge meal memorable with friends and family once per week! Enjoy!
Late Evening Snack	None	None	None	None	None	None	None
Approximate Daily Caloric breakdown	Calories: 1618 Protein: 179 Carbohydrates: 204 Fat: 10	Calories: 1618 Protein: 179 Carbohydrates: 204 Fat: 10	Calories: 1618 Protein: 179 Carbohydrates: 204 Fat: 10	Calories: 1618 Protein: 179 Carbohydrates: 204 Fat: 10	Calories: 1618 Protein: 179 Carbohydrates: 204 Fat: 10	Calories: 1618 Protein: 179 Carbohydrates: 204 Fat: 10	No guilt No shame I am in control of my eating!

Male 150-170 pounds

	Day 1	Day 2	Day 3	Day 4	Day 5	Day 6	Day 7
Breakfast	1 Cup Cream of Wheat 1 Cup skim milk 4 egg whites 1 small apple	1 Cup Oatmeal 1 Cup skim milk 4 egg whites 1 small peach	1 Cup skim milk 1 small apple Rice omelet: 4 egg whites scrambled with ½ cup brown rice and chunky salsa	1 serving Special K 1 Cup skim milk 4 egg whites 1 cup strawberries	1 Cup Malt-o-meal 1 Cup skim milk 4 egg whites ½ grapefruit	1 Cup Grits or Grape nuts 1 Cup skim milk 5 egg whites 1 cup cantaloupe	1 Cup Total no raisins 1 Cup skim milk 4 egg whites 1 small apple
Mid-morning Snack	Protein Shake, Blended with 16 oz water	Protein Shake, Blended with 16 oz water	Protein Shake, Blended with 16 oz water	Protein Shake, Blended with 16 oz water	Protein Shake, Blended with 16 oz water	Protein Shake, Blended with 16 oz water	Protein Shake, Blended with 16 oz water
Lunch	7 ounces chicken breast 1 small yam Broccoli 1 small apple	7 ounces Turkey breast 2 very small new potatoes Broccoli 1 small apple	7 ounces chicken breast 1 small yam Broccoli 1 small apple	7 ounces lean steak ½ cup brown rice Spinach salad 1 small apple	7 ounces lean pork loin 1 small yam Broccoli ½ grapefruit	7 ounces chicken breast 1 small yam Broccoli 1 small apple	7 ounces chicken breast 1 small yam Broccoli 1 small apple
1st Mid Afternoon Snack	1-6 ounce can tuna in water Broccoli or large salad	1-6 ounce can crab in water Broccoli or large salad	1-6 ounce can tuna in water Broccoli or large salad	1-6 ounce can Albacore in water Broccoli or large salad	1-6 ounce can tuna in water Broccoli or large salad	1-6 ounce can tuna in water Broccoli or large salad	1-6 ounce can tuna in water Broccoli or large salad
2nd Mid Afternoon Snack	1 orange	1 Tangerine	1 Peach	1 orange	1 orange	1 Pear	1 orange
Dinner	7 ounces Tilapia Broccoli or large salad	7 ounces Swordfish Broccoli or large salad	7 ounces Shrimp Broccoli or large salad	7 ounces Halibut Broccoli or large salad	7 ounces Atlantic Cod Broccoli or large salad	7 ounces Mahi-Mahi or Scallops Asparagus Bell peppers	Splurge meal: Have fun and make your splurge meal memorable with friends and family once per week! Enjoy!
Late Evening Snack	None	None	None	None	None	None	None
Approximate Daily Caloric breakdown	Calories: 1656 Protein: 206 Carbohydrates: 181 Fat: 12	Calories: 1656 Protein: 206 Carbohydrates: 181 Fat: 12	Calories: 1656 Protein: 206 Carbohydrates: 181 Fat: 12	Calories: 1656 Protein: 206 Carbohydrates: 181 Fat: 12	Calories: 1656 Protein: 206 Carbohydrates: 181 Fat: 12	Calories: 1656 Protein: 206 Carbohydrates: 181 Fat: 12	No guilt No shame I am in control of my eating!

Male 170-200 pounds

	Day 1	Day 2	Day 3	Day 4	Day 5	Day 6	Day 7
Breakfast	1 Cup Cream of Wheat 1 Cup skim milk 3 egg whites ½ small apple	1 Cup Oatmeal 1 Cup skim milk 3 egg whites ½ small peach	1 Cup skim milk ½ small apple Rice omelet: 3 egg whites scrambled with ½ cup brown rice and chunky salsa	1 serving Special K 1 Cup skim milk 3 egg whites ½ cup strawberries	1 Cup Malt-o-meal 1 Cup skim milk 3 egg whites ¼ grapefruit	1 Cup Grits or Grape nuts 1 Cup skim milk 3 egg whites ½ cup cantaloupe	1 Cup Total no raisins 1 Cup skim milk 3 egg whites ½ small apple
Mid-morning Snack	Protein Shake, Blended with 16 oz water	Protein Shake, Blended with 16 oz water	Protein Shake, Blended with 16 oz water	Protein Shake, Blended with 16 oz water	Protein Shake, Blended with 16 oz water	Protein Shake, Blended with 16 oz water	Protein Shake, Blended with 16 oz water
Lunch	5 ounces chicken breast 1 small yam Broccoli	5 ounces Turkey breast 2 very small new potatoes Broccoli	5 ounces chicken breast 1 small yam Broccoli	5 ounces lean steak ½ cup brown rice Spinach salad	5 ounces lean pork loin 1 small yam Broccoli	5 ounces chicken breast 1 small yam Broccoli	5 ounces chicken breast 1 small yam Broccoli
1ˢᵗ Mid Afternoon Snack	1-6 ounce can tuna in water Broccoli or large salad	1-6 ounce can crab in water Broccoli or large salad	1-6 ounce can tuna in water Broccoli or large salad	1-6 ounce can Albacore in water Broccoli or large salad	1-6 ounce can tuna in water Broccoli or large salad	1-6 ounce can tuna in water Broccoli or large salad	1-6 ounce can tuna in water Broccoli or large salad
2nd Mid Afternoon Snack	Protein Shake, Blended with 16 oz water	Protein Shake, Blended with 16 oz water	Protein Shake, Blended with 16 oz water	Protein Shake, Blended with 16 oz water	Protein Shake, Blended with 16 oz water	Protein Shake, Blended with 16 oz water	Protein Shake, Blended with 16 oz water
Dinner	7 ounces Tilapia Mixed veggies or large salad	7 ounces Swordfish Mixed veggies or large salad	7 ounces Shrimp Mixed veggies or large salad	7 ounces Halibut Mixed veggies or large salad	7 ounces Atlantic Cod Mixed veggies or large salad	7 ounces Mahi-Mahi or Scallops Asparagus Bell peppers	Splurge meal: Have fun and make your splurge meal memorable with friends and family once per week! Enjoy!
Late Evening Snack	None	None	None	None	None	None	None
Approximate Daily Caloric breakdown	Calories: 1695 Protein: 231 Carbohydrates: 162 Fat: 13	Calories: 1695 Protein: 231 Carbohydrates: 162 Fat: 13	Calories: 1695 Protein: 231 Carbohydrates: 162 Fat: 13	Calories: 1695 Protein: 231 Carbohydrates: 162 Fat: 13	Calories: 1695 Protein: 231 Carbohydrates: 162 Fat: 13	Calories: 1695 Protein: 231 Carbohydrates: 162 Fat: 13	No guilt No shame I am in control of my eating!

Male 200-250 pounds

	Day 1	Day 2	Day 3	Day 4	Day 5	Day 6	Day 7
Breakfast	1 Cup Cream of Wheat 1 Cup skim milk 5 egg whites 1 small apple	1 Cup Oatmeal 1 Cup skim milk 5 egg whites 1 small peach	1 Cup skim milk 1 small apple Rice omelet: 5 egg whites scrambled with ½ cup brown rice and chunky salsa	1 serving Special K 1 Cup skim milk 5 egg whites 1 cup strawberries	1 Cup Malt-o-meal 1 Cup skim milk 5 egg whites ½ grapefruit	1 Cup Grits or Grape nuts 1 Cup skim milk 5 egg whites 1 cup cantaloupe	1 Cup Total no raisins 1 Cup skim milk 5 egg whites 1 small apple
Mid-morning Snack	Protein Shake, Blended with 16 oz water	Protein Shake, Blended with 16 oz water	Protein Shake, Blended with 16 oz water	Protein Shake, Blended with 16 oz water	Protein Shake, Blended with 16 oz water	Protein Shake, Blended with 16 oz water	Protein Shake, Blended with 16 oz water
Lunch	3 ½ ounces chicken breast 1 small yam Broccoli ½ small apple	3 ½ ounces Turkey breast 2 very small new potatoes Broccoli ½ small apple	3 ½ ounces chicken breast 1 small yam Broccoli ½ small apple	3 ½ ounces lean steak ½ cup brown rice Spinach salad ½ small apple	3 ½ ounces lean pork loin 1 small yam Broccoli ¼ grapefruit	3 ½ ounces chicken breast 1 small yam Broccoli ½ small apple	3 ½ ounces chicken breast 1 small yam Broccoli ½ small apple
1st Mid Afternoon Snack	1-6 ounce can tuna in water Broccoli or large salad	1-6 ounce can crab in water Broccoli or large salad	1-6 ounce can tuna in water Broccoli or large salad	1-6 ounce can Albacore in water Broccoli or large salad	1-6 ounce can tuna in water Broccoli or large salad	1-6 ounce can tuna in water Broccoli or large salad	1-6 ounce can tuna in water Broccoli or large salad
2nd Mid Afternoon Snack	Protein Shake, Blended with 16 oz water	Protein Shake, Blended with 16 oz water	Protein Shake, Blended with 16 oz water	Protein Shake, Blended with 16 oz water	Protein Shake, Blended with 16 oz water	Protein Shake, Blended with 16 oz water	Protein Shake, Blended with 16 oz water
Dinner	7 ounces Tilapia Mixed veggies or large salad	7 ounces Swordfish Mixed veggies or large salad	7 ounces Shrimp Mixed veggies or large salad	7 ounces Halibut Mixed veggies or large salad	7 ounces Atlantic Cod Mixed veggies or large salad	7 ounces Mahi-Mahi or Scallops Asparagus Bell peppers	Splurge meal: Have fun and make your splurge meal memorable with friends and family once per week! Enjoy!
Late Evening Snack	None	None	None	None	None	None	None
Approximate Daily Caloric breakdown	Calories: 1755 Protein: 225 Carbohydrates: 185 Fat: 12	Calories: 1755 Protein: 225 Carbohydrates: 185 Fat: 12	Calories: 1755 Protein: 225 Carbohydrates: 185 Fat: 12	Calories: 1755 Protein: 225 Carbohydrates: 185 Fat: 12	Calories: 1755 Protein: 225 Carbohydrates: 185 Fat: 12	Calories: 1755 Protein: 225 Carbohydrates: 185 Fat: 12	No guilt No shame I am in control of my eating!

Male 250-300 pounds

	Day 1	Day 2	Day 3	Day 4	Day 5	Day 6	Day 7
Breakfast	1 Cup Cream of Wheat 1 Cup skim milk 7 egg whites ½ small apple	1 Cup Oatmeal 1 Cup skim milk 7 egg whites ½ small peach	1 Cup skim milk ½ small apple Rice omelet: 7 egg whites scrambled with ½ cup brown rice and chunky salsa	1 serving Special K 1 Cup skim milk 7 egg whites ½ cup strawberries	1 Cup Malt-o-meal 1 Cup skim milk 7 egg whites ¼ grapefruit	1 Cup Grits or Grape nuts 1 Cup skim milk 7 egg whites ½ cup cantaloupe	1 Cup Total no raisins 1 Cup skim milk 7 egg whites ½ small apple
Mid-morning Snack	Protein Shake, Blended with 16 oz water	Protein Shake, Blended with 16 oz water	Protein Shake, Blended with 16 oz water	Protein Shake, Blended with 16 oz water	Protein Shake, Blended with 16 oz water	Protein Shake, Blended with 16 oz water	Protein Shake, Blended with 16 oz water
Lunch	7 ounces chicken breast ½ cup brown rice Broccoli	7 ounces Turkey breast ½ cup Kidney Beans Broccoli	7 ounces chicken breast ½ cup brown rice Broccoli	7 ounces lean steak ½ small yam Spinach salad	7 ounces lean pork loin ½ cup wild rice Broccoli	7 ounces chicken breast ½ cup brown rice Broccoli	7 ounces chicken breast ½ cup brown rice Broccoli
1st Mid Afternoon Snack	1-6 ounce can tuna in water Broccoli or large salad	1-6 ounce can crab in water Broccoli or large salad	1-6 ounce can tuna in water Broccoli or large salad	1-6 ounce can Albacore in water Broccoli or large salad	1-6 ounce can tuna in water Broccoli or large salad	1-6 ounce can tuna in water Broccoli or large salad	1-6 ounce can tuna in water Broccoli or large salad
2nd Mid Afternoon Snack	Protein Shake, Blended with 16 oz water	Protein Shake, Blended with 16 oz water	Protein Shake, Blended with 16 oz water	Protein Shake, Blended with 16 oz water	Protein Shake, Blended with 16 oz water	Protein Shake, Blended with 16 oz water	Protein Shake, Blended with 16 oz water
Dinner	7 ounces Tilapia Mixed veggies or large salad	7 ounces Swordfish Mixed veggies or large salad	7 ounces Shrimp Mixed veggies or large salad	7 ounces Halibut Mixed veggies or large salad	7 ounces Atlantic Cod Mixed veggies or large salad	7 ounces Mahi-Mahi or Scallops Asparagus Bell peppers	Splurge meal: Have fun and make your splurge meal memorable with friends and family once per week! Enjoy!
Late Evening Snack	5 ounces Chicken	5 ounces Chicken	5 ounces Turkey	5 ounces Chicken	5 ounces Chicken	5 ounces Turkey	None
Approximate Daily Caloric breakdown	Calories 1901 Protein 283 Carbohydrates 145 Fat 16	Calories 1901 Protein 283 Carbohydrates 145 Fat 16	Calories 1901 Protein 283 Carbohydrates 145 Fat 16	Calories 1901 Protein 283 Carbohydrates 145 Fat 16	Calories 1901 Protein 283 Carbohydrates 145 Fat 16	Calories 1901 Protein 283 Carbohydrates 145 Fat 16	No guilt No shame I am in control of my eating!

Male 300-400 pounds

	Day 1	Day 2	Day 3	Day 4	Day 5	Day 6	Day 7
Breakfast	1 Cup Cream of Wheat 1 Cup skim milk 10 egg whites ½ small apple	1 Cup Oatmeal 1 Cup skim milk 10 egg whites ½ small peach	1 Cup skim milk ½ small apple Rice omelet: 10 egg whites scrambled with ½ cup brown rice and chunky salsa	1 serving Special K 1 Cup skim milk 10 egg whites ½ cup strawberries	1 Cup Malt-o-meal 1 Cup skim milk 10 egg whites ¼ grapefruit	1 Cup Grits or Grape nuts 1 Cup skim milk 10 egg whites ½ cup cantaloupe	1 Cup Total no raisins 1 Cup skim milk 10 egg whites ½ small apple
Mid-morning Snack	Protein Shake, Blended with 16 oz water	Protein Shake, Blended with 16 oz water	Protein Shake, Blended with 16 oz water	Protein Shake, Blended with 16 oz water	Protein Shake, Blended with 16 oz water	Protein Shake, Blended with 16 oz water	Protein Shake, Blended with 16 oz water
Lunch	7 ounces chicken breast ½ cup brown rice Broccoli	7 ounces Turkey breast ½ cup Kidney Beans Broccoli	7 ounces chicken breast ½ cup brown rice Broccoli	7 ounces lean steak ½ small yam Spinach salad	7 ounces lean pork loin ½ cup wild rice Broccoli	7 ounces chicken breast ½ cup brown rice Broccoli	7 ounces chicken breast ½ cup brown rice Broccoli
1st Mid Afternoon Snack	1-6 ounce can tuna in water Broccoli or large salad	1-6 ounce can crab in water Broccoli or large salad	1-6 ounce can tuna in water Broccoli or large salad	1-6 ounce can Albacore in water Broccoli or large salad	1-6 ounce can tuna in water Broccoli or large salad	1-6 ounce can tuna in water Broccoli or large salad	1-6 ounce can tuna in water Broccoli or large salad
2nd Mid Afternoon Snack	Protein Shake, Blended with 16 oz water	Protein Shake, Blended with 16 oz water	Protein Shake, Blended with 16 oz water	Protein Shake, Blended with 16 oz water	Protein Shake, Blended with 16 oz water	Protein Shake, Blended with 16 oz water	Protein Shake, Blended with 16 oz water
Dinner	7 ounces Tilapia Mixed veggies or large salad	7 ounces Swordfish Mixed veggies or large salad	7 ounces Shrimp Mixed veggies or large salad	7 ounces Halibut Mixed veggies or large salad	7 ounces Atlantic Cod Mixed veggies or large salad	7 ounces Mahi-Mahi or Scallops Asparagus Bell peppers	Splurge meal: Have fun and make your splurge meal memorable with friends and family once per week! Enjoy!
Late Evening Snack	7 ounces Chicken	7 ounces Chicken	7 ounces Turkey	7 ounces Chicken	7 ounces Chicken	7 ounces Turkey	None
Approximate Daily Caloric breakdown	Calories: 2011 Protein: 306 Carbohydrates: 147 Fat: 17	Calories: 2011 Protein: 306 Carbohydrates: 147 Fat: 17	Calories: 2011 Protein: 306 Carbohydrates: 147 Fat: 17	Calories: 2011 Protein: 306 Carbohydrates: 147 Fat: 17	Calories: 2011 Protein: 306 Carbohydrates: 147 Fat: 17	Calories: 2011 Protein: 306 Carbohydrates: 147 Fat: 17	No guilt No shame I am in control of my eating!

Time to Exercise

You are a winner!

"Take a deep breath," I suggested
as sweat dripped from her brow.
"You've got to breathe deeply and fill the lungs
as if to sing aloud!"

One more set, I knew she could do it,
if she just believed
she'd know she'd get through it!

So she dug a little deeper
and she continued to perspire,
and she tuned everything out,
even the people she inspired!

She could feel her muscles working,
her lungs burning with desire.
She knew she could do it;
it was hers to aspire!

She could feel her form slipping,
but her determination kept her straight.
Her muscles were fatiguing
by the force of her own body weight!

"Thirty more seconds," I said with true vision,
"and treat yourself right, it is your decision!
Make yourself strong both inside and out
And let's tear down those walls of guilt and doubt!"

And so people were watching,
but she didn't care.
She was working her tail off—
her fat, "Beware!"

As the countdown came closer
and the end was near,
she knew that God's greatness
had taken the place of fear!

The buzzer went off
as she finished with strife
She let her heart slow
as she pondered her life!

"It all makes sense now,"
she said with a grin.
"You don't train half way—
you train to WIN!"

Exercise
Two Kinds: Cardiovascular & Strength Training

Cardiovascular Training

Time to get lean!

1. **For weight loss**, cardiovascular exercise should be done 45 minutes to 1 hour, 5–6 days per week, along with strength training.
2. **For maintenance**, cardiovascular exercise should be done 45 minutes to 1 hour, 2–3 days per week, along with strength training.
3. **Cross-training**, or incorporating different types of cardiovascular exercise into your program, will help your body respond more effectively and will battle the boredom that so many people face.

Example for weight loss: 45 minutes -1 hour - Monday, Wednesday, Friday = stationary bike or spinning class, elliptical. Tuesday, Thursday, Saturday = treadmill, cross trainer, Stairmaster, or group exercise class designed for fat loss.

How it's broken down

Stationary Bike: (my suggestion for fat burn for beginners)

Frequency: 3 times per week. Individuals with knee problems should consider doing most of their cardio throughout the week on the stationary bike or other non-impact exercise machine. I will discuss why I prefer the stationary bike in a few minutes.

Duration or amount of time spent each session: 45 minutes to 1 hour. If you are just starting an exercise program and cannot finish the entire session, don't worry about it—just do the best you can. Within 3 weeks you should be able to finish with no problem.

Intensity or level of resistance: manual setting of levels or whatever your fitness level can handle to keep desired heart rate in its target zone. You will need to monitor your progress because your body is going to get stronger. This means that it will eventually take more resistance, or faster RPMs, to get your heart rate where it should be.

Heart rate: find your <u>target heart rate zone</u> on the following page. To find your heart rate during exercise, find your pulse at the neck, count for 6 seconds, and then add a 0. The resulting number is what your heart rate is at that particular moment. Many stationary bikes and other cardio equipment have heart-rate monitors built into their computers. Although I would like you to learn how to find and figure out your heart rate on your own, feel free to use the heart-rate monitors.

Note: Spinning classes are great too! Many athletic clubs or recreation centers offer spinning classes in which an instructor will take you through an entire hour of a bike workout while stimulating your mind and emotions at the same time. Find the instructors you like best. They are not all the same! Remember: Without emotional and spiritual stimulation, your fitness routine becomes boring, mundane, and repetitious, and you will quit! I have seen it a thousand times!

Treadmill: (best for getting rid of cellulite), Cross-Trainer, Stairmaster, and Group Exercise Classes

Frequency: 2-3 times per week. Those of you with bad knees or joint problems should limit the amount of higher-impact exercise you perform.

Duration or amount of time spent each session: Find a speed that is difficult but easy enough for you to do 45 minutes to 1 hour. Work up to jogging 45 minutes to 1 full hour. As a beginner, 3.8 miles per hour is a good speed to try. This is a higher-impact exercise than the stationary bike and will tire you out faster. So you will have to pace yourself.

Intensity or level of resistance (grade of elevation): Begin with no elevation on the treadmill.

Your joints, muscles, tendons, ligaments, and other bodily tissues must get used to it. This is why I suggest the stationary bike so you can complete your entire cardio session. If you cannot continue to jog or walk at a faster rate, then slow down and walk until you recover a little.

Other types of aerobic exercise include Tae Bo and Cardio Kickboxing. They are both great forms of exercise, but should never take the place of resistance training. They are an aggressive form of cardiovascular exercise and should be used in moderation when trying to lose weight—no more than 2–3 times per week for cardio. The other days should be lower-intensity workouts such as the stationary bike. The following page will explain why.

In summary, the optimal type of cardio when your specific goal is fat loss is a lower-intensity workout. Again, I will explain why on the following page, which shows the calorie breakdown at different levels of exercise intensity.

RHR = resting heart rate
To find your resting heart rate, find your pulse at the neck first thing in the morning and count the number of beats for 1 minute. Find the number of beats you count on the vertical axis of the chart, then find your age on the horizontal axis and locate the point at which the two meet. For example, if you are 55 and have a resting heart rate of 65, your target heart-rate (THR) zone for optimal fat burn will be 127 to 151. The next page explains the importance of proper heart-rate training.

Target Heart Rate Zone
Age

	10yrs	15yrs	20yrs	25yrs	30yrs	35yrs	40yrs	45yrs	50yrs	55yrs	60yrs	65yrs	70yrs	75yrs	80yrs	85yrs	90yrs
45 RHR	147.3 to 186.9	144.2 to 182.6	141.1 to 178.3	138 to 174	134.9 to 169.7	131.8 to 165.4	128.7 to 161.1	125.6 to 156.8	122.5 to 152.5	119.4 to 148.2	116.3 to 143.9	113.2 to 139.6	110.1 to 135.3	107 to 131	103.9 to 126.7	100.8 to 122.4	97.7 to 118.1
50 RHR	149.2 to 187.6	146.1 to 183.3	143 to 179	139.9 to 174.7	136.8 to 170.4	133.7 to 166.1	130.6 to 161.8	127.5 to 157.5	124.4 to 153.2	121.3 to 148.9	118.2 to 144.6	115.1 to 140.3	112 to 136	108.9 to 131.7	105.8 to 127.4	102.7 to 123.1	99.6 to 118.8
55 RHR	151.1 to 188.3	148 to 184	144.9 to 179.7	141.8 to 175.4	138.7 to 171.1	135.6 to 166.8	132.5 to 162.5	129.4 to 158.2	126.3 to 153.9	123.2 to 149.6	120.1 to 145.3	117 to 141	113.9 to 136.7	110.8 to 132.4	107.7 to 128.1	104.6 to 123.8	101.5 to 119.5
60 RHR	153 to 189	149.9 to 184.7	146.8 to 180.4	143.7 to 176.1	140.6 to 171.8	137.5 to 167.5	134.4 to 163.2	131.3 to 158.9	128.2 to 154.6	125.1 to 150.3	122 to 146	118.9 to 141.7	115.8 to 137.4	112.7 to 133.1	109.6 to 128.8	106.5 to 124.5	103.4 to 120.2
65 RHR	154.9 to 189.7	151.8 to 185.4	148.7 to 181.1	145.6 to 176.8	142.5 to 172.5	139.4 to 168.2	136.3 to 163.9	133.2 to 159.6	130.1 to 155.3	127 to 151	123.9 to 146.7	120.8 to 142.4	117.7 to 138.1	114.6 to 133.8	111.5 to 129.5	108.4 to 125.2	105.3 to 120.9
70 RHR	156.8 to 190.4	153.7 to 186.1	150.6 to 181.8	147.5 to 177.5	144.4 to 173.2	141.3 to 168.9	138.2 to 164.6	135.1 to 160.3	132 to 156	128.9 to 151.7	125.8 to 147.4	122.7 to 143.1	119.5 to 138.8	116.5 to 134.5	113.4 to 130.2	110.3 to 125.9	107.2 to 121.6
75 RHR	158.7 to 191.1	155.6 to 186.8	152.5 to 182.5	149.4 to 178.2	146.3 to 173.9	143.2 to 169.6	140.1 to 165.3	137 to 161	133.9 to 156.7	130.8 to 152.4	127.7 to 148.1	124.6 to 143.8	121.5 to 139.5	118.4 to 135.2	115.3 to 130.9	112.2 to 126.6	109.1 to 122.3
80 RHR	160.6 to 191.8	157.5 to 187.5	154.4 to 183.2	151.3 to 178.9	148.2 to 174.6	145.1 to 170.3	142 to 166	138.9 to 161.7	135.8 to 157.4	132.7 to 153.1	129.6 to 148.8	126.5 to 144.5	123.4 to 140.2	120.3 to 135.9	117.2 to 131.6	114.1 to 127.3	111 to 123
85 RHR	162.5 to 192.5	159.4 to 188.2	156.3 to 183.9	153.2 to 179.6	150.1 to 175.3	147 to 171	143.9 to 166.7	140.8 to 162.4	137.7 to 158.1	134.6 to 153.8	131.5 to 149.5	128.4 to 145.2	125.3 to 140.9	122.2 to 136.6	119.1 to 132.3	116 to 128	112.9 to 123.7
90 RHR	164.4 to 193.2	161.3 to 188.9	158.2 to 184.6	155.1 to 180.3	152 to 176	148.9 to 171.7	145.8 to 167.4	142.7 to 163.1	139.6 to 158.8	136.5 to 154.5	133.4 to 150.2	130.3 to 145.9	127.2 to 141.6	124.1 to 137.3	121 to 133	117.9 to 128.7	114.8 to 124.4
95 RHR	166.3 to 193.9	163.2 to 189.6	160.1 to 185.3	157 to 181	153.9 to 176.7	150.8 to 172.4	147.7 to 168.1	144.6 to 163.8	141.5 to 159.5	138.4 to 155.2	135.3 to 150.9	132.2 to 146.6	129.1 to 142.3	126 to 138	122.9 to 133.7	119.8 to 129.4	116.7 to 125.1
100 RHR	168.2 to 194.6	165.1 to 190.3	162 to 186	158.9 to 181.7	155.8 to 177.4	152.7 to 173.1	149.6 to 168.8	146.5 to 164.5	143.4 to 160.2	140.3 to 155.9	137.2 to 151.6	134.1 to 147.3	131 to 143	127.9 to 138.7	124.8 to 134.4	121.7 to 130.1	118.6 to 125.8
105 RHR	170.1 to 195.3	167 to 191	163.9 to 186.7	160.8 to 182.4	157.7 to 178.1	154.6 to 173.8	151.5 to 169.5	148.4 to 165.2	145.3 to 160.9	142.2 to 156.6	139.1 to 152.3	136 to 148	132.9 to 143.7	129.8 to 139.4	126.7 to 135.1	123.6 to 130.8	120.5 to 126.5
110 RHR	172 to 196	168.9 to 191.7	165.8 to 187.4	162.7 to 183.1	159.6 to 178.8	156.5 to 174.5	153.4 to 170.2	150.3 to 165.9	147.2 to 161.6	144.1 to 157.3	141 to 153	137.9 to 148.7	134.8 to 144.4	131.7 to 140.1	128.6 to 135.8	125.5 to 131.5	122.4 to 127.2

Calorie breakdown during exercise

When doing cardiovascular exercise designed for fat loss, we want our calories from fat to be burned. A nice thing about the body is that it burns fat more efficiently toward the lower end of your THR zone. This is because of how much oxygen is being used by the body. The higher your heart goes, the faster your oxygen is used up, thus not allowing the free flow of oxygen to burn the body fat.

Think of a candle. If you place a glass over the candle, the flame uses up the oxygen and then dies. The same goes for your body fat. That is why I used 62 percent of your maximum heart rate on the lower end of your THR zone. Your THR zone is the optimal heart rate for what you want to accomplish, which in this case is fat loss. At 62 percent, you will maximize your fat-burning ability because oxygen will always be present. The following chart shows the breakdown of calories burned during exercise and how your level of intensity affects this.

Intensity	Carbohydrates	Protein	Fat
Healthy heart = 50-60% of max heart rate	10%	5%	85%
Temperate = 60–70% of max heart rate	10%	5%	85%
Aerobic = 70–80% of max heart rate	60%	5%	35%
Threshold = 80–90% of max heart rate	80%	5%	15%
Red line = 90–100% of max heart rate.	90%	5%	5%

Remember: There are two types of aerobic exercise—one is for fat loss, and the other is higher-intensity exercise that will help get you into great shape but doesn't burn as much fat while you are doing it. Our body has two main fuel tanks. We must learn how and why and when to tap into each one. As you can see in the chart, the higher your intensity or heart rate goes, the more sugar or carbohydrates are burned rather than body fat. Even at 70 percent of your maximum heart rate, the amount of sugar that is burned jumps to a whopping 60 percent. At 70 percent of your maximum heart rate, only 35 percent of what you are burning is body fat.

Allow your high-intensity workouts to come from resistance training, where sugar is greatly needed. Keep your cardio, on average, at a lower intensity to optimize fat loss. However, as I stated earlier, it is important to "up" the intensity two to three times per week. If you want to do something like Tae Bo, then do it. Billy Banks' workouts are incredible forms of fitness, and he is very inspiring. But his workouts, like any other type of workout, must be incorporated into a balanced program. How you put everything together is how you find results and achieve success for the rest of your life.

When doing cardiovascular exercise, you should monitor how your body is recovering after cardio and resistance training. If you want to maximize your workouts, then take your resting heart rate each morning. You will notice that it varies from day to day. If it is higher than usual, that means your body is tired, and you may want to consider doing a lower-intensity cardio workout such as the stationary bike that day. If your resting heart rate is good and low, it means your body is rested and can handle something a little more intense such as running, step class, Tae Bo, cardio kickboxing, or the Stairmaster. Remember that for optimal fat burn during cardio, your heart is best kept toward the lower end of the THR zone. But do "up" the intensity once in a while so your body doesn't get too used to the same thing all the time. I don't want you to just lose weight; I want you to be in great shape too!

Why the Bike?

When in a sitting position, and with little or no resistance, your body has optimal opportunity to utilize its fat stores due to its *sustained elevated heart rate.* Though you want to cross-train or do different types of cardio, the bicycle is the most effective fat burner when you first start a program. Why? Because it is probably the only exercise your body can handle for more than 20 minutes. Yes, researchers have found that the treadmill burns a lot more calories than the stationary bike. But what is more desirable? Jogging for 20 minutes and dying, never optimally tapping into your fat stores, or biking for 45 minutes to 1 full hour, burning fat specifically for 40 minutes, and still being able to walk out of the gym?

When you are in an upright position, on the treadmill or stair climber or in a step or aerobics class, your body is undergoing weight-bearing exercise. Therefore, the workout has a higher impact on your muscles and joints. The higher the impact, the shorter the amount of time you can safely do the workout. You tire more quickly. Resistance during fat-burning exercise should be increased only enough to elevate your heart rate to within its target range (review the preceding page for your THR).

Don't get me wrong: Your body needs resistance. Moderate impact is great for the battle against osteoporosis, and proper resistance training is absolutely the best exercise for strong bones. But when you first start a program, your joints won't be able to handle much. And even if you start a program while in shape, always doing a high-impact form of exercise for your cardio will eventually tear up your knees and back from the constant pounding. Look at getting lean and in shape as a long-term (lifelong) goal. (Remember your covenant) You must look to the future and see how the present will affect it. So 3 times per week on the treadmill, or jogging outdoors, is enough. The others should be low or non-impact.

When adjusting your stationary bike to fit your body, a few steps should be taken. First, whether it is a recumbent or an upright bike, adjust the seat so *your knees are slightly bent.* Never ride the bike with your legs fully extended and no bend in the knees. If your knees are straight as you push and extend, then your knees tend to slightly hyperextend, putting unnecessary pressure on the backs of your knees. This is not good! Second, **if the bike you have selected has**

foot straps on it, adjust them so the pedal is under the middle of your foot rather than the toes. This is very important! Everyone has different foot sizes. Most of the time the strap is tight enough that the only part of your foot on the pedal is your toes. What happens when you push with your toes over and over again? Any time your knee extends over your toe, as when you push off with your toe, the force being generated is going not directly into your thigh (quads) but into your knee joint and patellar (kneecap) tendon.

This may seem like a trivial worry, but discomfort is one of the biggest reasons that people quit exercising. You need to feel good all the time and not experience all of the stereotypical negatives associated with exercise.

Now the good news: When you have achieved your weight- and fat-loss goals, you will be able to reduce the number of times you must ride or do cardio to **only 2 to 3 times per week** (that is, if you are doing weight training as well). If you do not do weight training (heaven forbid!), you need to do cardio 5 days per week even during a maintenance phase.

Your resistance training is very important. The more lean muscle mass your body has, the higher your metabolism will be. More information on resistance training is provided later.

Periodization

Periodization is a term used to describe the body's ability to adapt to a certain routine or program. Basically, if your body, mind, or spirit isn't learning anything, it begins to regress or die. When your body gets bored because it is used to doing the same thing over and over, your body will rebel against your exercise and will stop burning fat, getting stronger and gaining endurance. This is a very real phenomenon. God knew what He was doing when He created you. He built within you a need to learn and to be stimulated so you will stay on top of your game.

Whether it is in your job, at home with your family or your body; stagnation, indifference and automatic pilot inhibits or squelches your enthusiasm and results. It is a violation of your spirit to do the same mindless things over and over. Change, learning and being stimulated with newness and variety are critical in achieving any results in your life.

While on an exercise program I have shown how "cross-training" is important as well as monitoring and changing up your heart rate during cardiovascular training. **Those of you who have extreme weight loss goals and are doing cardio 5-6 days per week for months and months need to be very careful not to get stagnant. Make sure you are changing your type of cardio and are changing up and monitoring your heart rate.** I also recommend you take an entire week off of cardio every 90 days to give your body rest. Continue with your weight training though. It will be good for you mentally and spiritually as well to make sure you haven't let this program control you or become obsessive regarding your health. I have had clients hit a plateau (periodization) at the 90 day mark even while doing everything perfectly. Upon them stopping the cardio for one week they lost 2 pounds because of the change and rest their body experienced.

Resistance Training

Though resistance training provides numerous benefits to your body, it is still only one part of health! Don't be fooled when you see those attractive television commercials on the AB Flex or some other ridiculous Mr. Quick Fix schemes. You won't get abdominals like the people on those commercials by buying their product. You may tone your abs but will never see them because they are covered by fat. Fighting the fat takes nutrition, cardiovascular and resistance exercise, flexibility, supplementation, and consistency. So how does resistance training play its role in helping you become healthy, and how does it tie in to nutrition, flexibility, relaxation, and supplementation?

Exercises that require resistance affect your muscles in a very positive way. The immediate benefit of resistance training is that your body becomes more attractive to you. Your body develops a long, slender, and firm musculature. The muscles throughout your body appear smooth and toned. Your abdominals and lower back become taut and hold your body erect and proud. The muscles in your middle back become strong and support your spine. Your body's ability to move is enhanced by the muscles' ability to contract and relax upon request. Your body begins to trust you again; it gets stronger, increases its stamina, and allows you to utilize oxygen more efficiently. Your head is held higher, your shoulders are squared, and your stance speaks of confidence and grace. These are some of the basic reasons resistance training is important.

Resistance training enables you to shape the outer part of your body so that it can be one with your inner self. Many of us believe that it doesn't matter what we look like on the outside, that all that matters is how we love, express ourselves, and interact with others. **This is not true. It is a lie, a stronghold.** Why do we have a physical body if we are supposed to ignore it? And aren't the chemicals that are partly responsible for our emotions made up of the same proteins that make up most of the muscle in our body? Therefore, how we tone and shape our muscles does have an impact on our ability to express love and all the other wonderful emotions.

As discussed earlier, protein synthesis is our body's way of utilizing the different proteins we ingest in a way that will make us healthier. When we perform resistance training exercises, our muscles (made up of proteins) are torn down. Our body then protects itself by using rest and the protein from our nutrition to build that torn muscle tissue up so that it is even stronger. Without resistance training, our body never truly understands what to do with the protein we consume. It just does the best it can, which is usually less than adequate. So resistance training is crucial in aiding our body's ability to utilize nutritious foods.

It would take perhaps another 200 pages to explain the different routines, muscles emphasized, and techniques involved with weight training so I will stick with the most important elements of resistance training to help get you started.

The **FITT** principle is a good way to monitor your exercise regimen. **Frequency** is how often you train certain muscles; **intensity** refers to the level of effort during a specific exercise (that is, the number of repetitions performed, 100% being the highest intensity possible for one repetition); **time** is the duration of any given exercise you perform (referring mostly to the interval, or rest between sets, of a specific exercise), and **type** refers to the purpose of the exercise, or region of the body to be worked, and the techniques required to accomplish it (for example, the type of exercise needed for maximum calcium recruitment, which is important for treating osteoporosis, is discussed below). The following table will give you an idea how these elements all work together but differ according to your goals.

Goals

	Tone	Lose Fat	Build Muscle	Power Lifting
Frequency	Each muscle twice per week	5 days per week	Each muscle no more than once every 5 days	Each muscle no more than once a week
Intensity	3–4 exercises per muscle; 10–20 repetitions at 60–75% intensity.	62–86% of target heart rate zone, low resistance; refer to your cardio page	3–4 exercises per muscle; 6–12 repetitions at 75–90%. intensity	1–2 exercises per muscle; 1–5 repetitions at 90-100% intensity
Time	45–90-second rest intervals	40 minutes to 1 hour	2½- to 3-minute rest intervals	3-minute or longer rest intervals
Type	Exercises targeting each muscle of the body; all kinds of exercises may be used	Stationary bike, treadmill, stair climber, aerobics class; refer to your cardio page	Exercises targeting each muscle of the body; all kinds of exercises may be used	Pressing exercises such as bench press, squat, power clean, clean and jerk, leg press, and shoulder press

The **Type** of exercise comprises hundreds of different techniques. The body is very dynamic with different angles and demands. **Since there are so many different types of exercises make sure you get help learning the various exercises and techniques necessary to accomplish your goals.** One very important thing to learn is the type of exercises needed to help build bone strength while gaining muscle strength at the same time. As discussed earlier, there are specific exercises that promote the body's ability to absorb calcium. When pressing, as in a bench press, your bones undergo compressive force. This force is called *axial loading* and recruits calcium into the bone more efficiently than a fly movement. Pressing exercises such as lunges, bench press, shoulder press, squats, and leg press promote calcium absorption. Other exercises are great for the muscles and their development but are less effective in battling the onset of osteoporosis.

Resistance Training as it Relates to Stress

Without resistance exercise, the muscles never truly contract and never truly relax. They operate at about 50% capacity, and that's it. When a muscle fully contracts through its full range of motion, it becomes fatigued. The fibers then require more oxygen, which increases circulation of oxygen-rich blood to the muscles being worked. The key to any relaxation technique is breathing, so the more oxygen our muscles receive, the better chance we have of relaxing throughout the day. Through resistance training our muscles learn the difference between complete relaxation and full contraction and receive better-oxygenated blood thus relaxing more efficiently. When our body is able to relax, our mind will follow close behind it. One always affects the other, significantly. As an added bonus, the more lean muscle your body has the more body fat you will lose during cardiovascular training. This again proves that everything affects everything else.

Resistance training and its effect on relaxation also has a lot to do with a person's flexibility. Your muscles have elastic properties. The more resistance training you do, the more elastic your muscles can become, thus increasing and enhancing your ability to stretch.

Specific guidelines and benefits of strength training

The best form of exercise for overall health, longevity, and injury prevention.

1. Strength training should be done a *minimum* of 45 minutes to 1 hour, 2–3 times per week.
2. Research shows that doing strength training before cardio burns more fat—*YEAH!*
3. Increases muscle strength and tone so you function better and have beautiful muscles.
4. Increases bone strength and battles the onset of osteoporosis. *(No broken hips if I can help it!)*

Note: Free weights should always be implemented into a strength training program—this type of training teaches better body function and also burns more calories.

Specific Guidelines for Stretching and flexibility

The best form of exercise for relaxation and just plain making you feel wonderful.

1. **Stretching should always be done in conjunction with strength training and cardiovascular exercise.**
2. Never stretch too hard when muscles are cold! Stretching should be done (a) after a proper warmup; (b) during and after strength training; (c) before and after cardiovascular training; and (d) anytime you feel tight, sore, or stressed out (*passive* stretching in this case)! *(It will make you feel better, I PROMISE!)*
3. Stretching reduces muscle stiffness and soreness associated with exercise and excessive traveling.

4. Stretching significantly reduces physical and emotional stress by loosening the muscles and surrounding tissues of the body. **(An absolute must in feeling your best.)**

If you want a personalized resistance training or flexibility regimen, Courage to Change can assess your needs and goals and formulate one for you. We can either train you in person with our amazing one on one and group personal training or send you a new program to follow every month through our web-site:

www.courage2change.org

If you are in the Houston area or want to schedule a seminar, call to set up an appointment if you haven't already done so at 936-827-7552.

Visualization

"Seeing with the eyes of faith"

While doing your cardiovascular exercise on the bike or on something at which you can maintain your balance, I want you to periodically close your eyes. I want you to picture yourself butt naked in front of a mirror and I want you to visualize what you want to look like. You must be realistic and it must be a true representation of your inner beauty and Godliness. I want you to (in your mind) turn to the side, to the back, the other side, look up and down and shape and mold yourself into a healthy, confident person in the Lord.

"Now faith is being sure of what we hope for and certain of what we do not see."
Hebrews 11:1

Part of exercising your Faith and being certain of what you do not see in the present is by going into the future and taking hold of a goal and bringing it into the present. Though you must always accept where you are at any given moment, every one of you with the power of Christ has the power to manifest almost anything you want in life as long as it is in God's will. And part of His will for you and everyone is to be healthy, confident and secure, free from oppression and self-afflicted sickness.

Picture yourself as a healthy individual and watch as God manifests it through your actions. Picture yourself as a good husband or wife and watch as God manifests it through your actions. Picture yourself crossing the finish line before you even run the race and watch as God manifests it through your actions. Go into the future and take hold of what is not currently seen, bring it into the present and watch as your Faith in the Lord increases by His Faithfulness to you.

If you believe in something strong enough and your actions support this belief, it already is and always will be. It has already happened. The goal of your faith, once it is tested and deemed genuine, is yours for the taking!

"For I know the plans I have for you," declares the Lord, "plans to prosper you and not
to harm you, plans to give you hope and a future." (Jeremiah 29:4)

While in college I competed in bodybuilding. Though not the healthiest sport because of many reasons, the discipline I learned was amazing. The hours I spent doing cardio became a powerful time of reflection and projecting confidence into me. I would sit on the bike and pedal every day with the hopes of transforming my body. I frequently kept my eyes closed and would picture myself on stage going through my routine and would in my mind sculpt my body. 12 weeks prior to the competition I did this and proceeded until competition day. I could at all times see the image in my mind of how I wanted to look. So the competition came and I won 1st place. My friend had gone to the competition and took some pictures. A few weeks later I received the pictures in the mail. As I looked them over I began to critique myself as I went from picture to picture. Then I came across one specific picture that boggled me. I realized later I had seen that picture somewhere before. It was the exact same picture I had seen in my mind 12 weeks prior to the competition. It was like it was manifested through my thoughts. It was so weird because I didn't know the Lord like I do now and didn't realize how powerful seeing through the eyes of faith actually was. I just did it. The below picture is the very one I saw in my mind, same pose, same smile, same everything.

All of you have the power of God in you, the power to manifest His abundance in your life before you actually do it. Visualize what you want and take it to the Lord. If it is in His will, see with the eyes of Faith, pay the price and take it! Your health is no different!

99.9% of you have no interest in taking fitness as far as I did. That's actually good because it isn't healthy. I have a more realistic and healthy approach to fitness as you have been reading about throughout this entire program. Body building in this context is vain, somewhat idolatrous and can lead to eating and other psychological disorders. That is a whole other book! The point is whatever your goal,

"You must first see it to achieve it!"

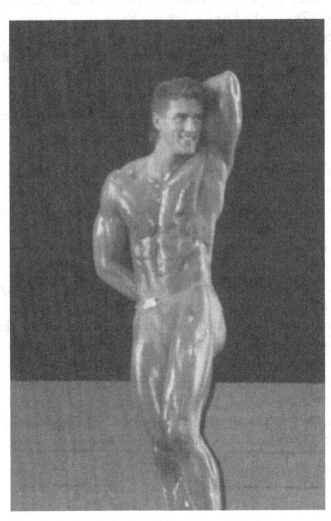

Advertising & Marketing

How much influence does the marketing industry have over you? To answer this question I did an experiment. I went to a grocery store to observe how they marketed different products. As I walked in, I was immediately greeted with a stand of fresh pastries, cookies, and cakes. I then proceeded to strategically position myself throughout the store. I went into every aisle, every corner, and every department.

To my amazement, from every spot I chose, in every direction I looked, I could see junk of some kind: chips, dip, soda, cookies, pastries, alcohol, crackers, candy bars. At the checkout counter I found more of the same, including *junk food for the mind*—magazines feeding us gossip, slander, turmoil, and indecency. These types of products cost the grocery store very little to make or buy, yet the cost is substantial for you and me. The grocery industry knows that Americans are impulse buyers. We go in need of a few items and leave with a bunch of junk that caught our eye when going down every aisle in the store.

Think of the aisles of frozen vegetables. Have you ever noticed what often hangs or is placed around them? JUNK! What is the first food people think of when they think of health food? Vegetables, right? This product placement encourages you the shopper to justify junk-food purchases by thinking, "I am treating myself well by buying healthy vegetables; therefore, I will reward myself with a treat." And why is the ice cream topping not by the ice cream? It is because the grocery store strategically places things on the other side of the store so that you will browse more to find what you are looking for. And as you look, you throw things you don't need in your cart out of impulse and visual stimulation.

Do not fall victim to the power of marketing and advertising. Learn to observe your surroundings, not just visually but with your brain taking control of what you allow to influence your decisions. Some experts say to stay around the edges of the grocery store, where you will find most of the fresh fruits and vegetables, meats and dairy products. I say, why let the grocery store dictate where you go? This approach is ludicrous. Besides, most grocery stores have just as much junk mixed in with the fresh produce as any other area in the store. Caramel toppings are stacked with the apples and fattening, high calorie dips are strategically placed with the vegetables. You need to believe in the strength of God in you enough to go anywhere and do anything without falling prey to manipulation and temptation which is exactly what is happening. You are being tempted to buy things that may taste good but are terrible for you. Break the ropes that hold you down and walk confidently through life. God is with you wherever you go. Next time you go to the grocery store, look around and observe how much temptation is around you. Acknowledge how things are marketed and how most people are easy targets. Then stand firm and make the decision to be strong enough to **"say no"** to the temptations around you. If you need to for a while, avoid those you struggle with. Over time you will be surprised by how far you've come.

6 Mandatory guidelines for optimal results

1. Carry a 1-quart sipper of water with you at all times—you must consume *at least half your body weight in ounces* of water per day. With exercise, you should consume 1 additional quart of water.

> You are not drinking enough water if:
>
> A. You do not have the constant urge to go to the bathroom
>
> B. You notice any coloration whatsoever in your urine

2. No juice/no bananas—these contain excessive amounts of fructose (natural sugars), which can easily be converted to fat when not utilized as energy. These are excess calories that tend to bloat you. How many of you have squeezed your own orange juice? How much juice did you get from one orange? One or two swallows, right? The average person needs 2–4 servings of fruit daily. By drinking a full glass of orange juice, you could consume up to twice your entire daily fruit requirement. That is way too many calories from sugar in one sitting.

3. No bread—even though low fat or nonfat, it seems to "hold" a bloat on the body! Many of you absolutely love bread. But it is important that you refrain from consuming it because bread is one of the worst things a person can eat when trying to lose body fat. Excess wheat (as in wheat bread) actually inhibits your body's ability to burn fat. So you would not only be bloated but would have a more difficult time burning fat during cardiovascular training. Once you reach your fitness goals, you can add a little bread back in the diet but not until then.

4. No butter, margarine, oil, or cream sauces, and no salad dressing—except nonfat, without "hydrogenated or partially hydrogenated" included in the ingredients (see grocery list).

5. When to do cardio and why?

Cardiovascular exercise is most effective first thing in the morning—200% more effective—because your body digests during the night and has more fat stores to draw on for energy in the morning. Since you do not eat during the night, your body burns calories to survive. The energy the body uses most in this process is glycogen (stored carbohydrate) in the muscle cells. Thus, the level of glycogen is lowest in the morning, and the fat stores can be tapped more quickly. Drink two glasses of cold water before the cardio. The type of cardio best for fat loss was discussed earlier. All you coffee drinkers don't panic— go for it! But no more than two cups in the morning before cardio. Caffeine actually increases your body's ability to burn fat by approximately 20%. This does not mean you should take a bunch of caffeine pills before your workouts! Anything that synthetically increases your heart rate can have harmful, or even fatal, side effects. We do not want that! Make sure your doctor gives you the OK before you drink anything with natural or artificial stimulants.

If morning cardio is not possible, then the cardio workout should follow weight training. Weight training is a higher-intensity form of exercise than cardiovascular training and should be done first because it requires carbohydrates for energy, whereas cardiovascular exercise requires both carbs and fat. During the first 15–20 minutes of cardiovascular exercise, the body burns carbohydrates for energy. It then taps into the fat stores. Since your body needs approximately 15–20 minutes of cardiovascular training before it begins to utilize fat stores, 45 minutes to 1 hour of cardio is necessary. The next *40* minutes are *PURE FAT BURN!* The only exception is the case of extreme weight lifting because the only time lactic acid is formed is when you use enough weight to be able to perform only 6 or fewer repetitions. Most soreness comes from pyruvic acid, not lactic acid. The presence of lactic acid inhibits the body's ability to burn fat efficiently. If this is you, then find a different time to get your cardio in for that day. If weight training is not your normal exercise routine, be sure to get your hour of cardiovascular training in for that day. An hour may seem like a lot, but fat burning is the easiest form of exercise there is! And don't forget that once you reach your desired body-fat goals you can decrease your amount of cardio to 2–3 days per week, provided you are maintaining a healthy diet.

6. Splurge Meals

Even while on a leaning down program you may have one splurge meal per week. This does not mean an entire day of splurging! It means you have *one meal* that includes a food you love. It will also begin to establish a pattern of control in your life. It is you who control when and how much you eat certain foods and will serve as a kind of reward or treat for doing so well. Of course the greatest reward comes when you don't even want the splurge meal. I have had clients ask me if they "had" to eat their splurge meal because of how good they felt eating healthy and clean. The answer is NO. You don't have to have a splurge meal but it is there to help you walk in the freedom and grace of God. Being too strict or going overboard with your health out of obligation is a form of legalism. Remember you are FREE from the bondage of good nutrition and exercise as you look to Jesus for your motivation. It is because of Him you offer your body as a living sacrifice, holy and pleasing to God.

But in this freedom, as your body becomes "cleaner," you will find that you do not crave the foods you once did. Those foods were a habit and a testament to the power of marketing and advertising. When you eat something that is loaded with preservatives, toxins, and fat, it slows your digestive process and you feel very lethargic. As you regain control of your life, you will begin to realize that your mind and commitment to yourself and God are far more powerful than any advertising!

Dynamic C2C Strength Training System™
Basic Theory, Terms, Q&A

You are about to begin the basics of the *Dynamic C2C Strength Training System*™. My next book will cover the material you are about to learn in detail, including 2 separate 12 week programs complete with pictures of every functional exercise, breathing techniques, stretching techniques, posture, and spinal alignment. Right now you are learning so much that going into detail would probably overwhelm you to the point of quitting and would add another 250 pages to this book. So we will keep to the basics in this book. Sound good?

In this section of Courage to Change you will cover common questions and answers (Q&A) that many people have regarding strength training. You will be given guidelines and a basic workable strength training program to follow.

Some basic theory behind a proper strength training program:

➤ Those of you who have exercised before; how many of you have been bored out of your mind at the gym you go to? How many plateaus have you hit; thus discouraging you from continuing on? It happens to most people who join a gym. I am not saying to not join a facility but you are about to learn the basics of how to train anywhere effectively by using the body God gave you.

➤ Proper training whether it is of a physical nature or spiritual nature requires individual attention to something while simultaneously understanding its affects on a corporate level! Let me explain.

➤ God did not design you in such a way as to make the rest of your body fall asleep while you work one muscle at a time. He designed you in such a way that as you may target one muscle or groups of muscles the rest of your body and nervous system is active and working to support you.

➤ Courage to Change is about freedom. When you train on an exercise machine you usually sit with your entire body supported with the exception of the one muscle you are targeting or isolating. Even those muscles you are targeting while working on machines have a fixed range of motion and don't have to provide any balance or stabilization because the machine does it all for you. You feel awkward and paralyzed. Where is the freedom here to move with balance, poise, grace and power? There is no freedom of movement at all. Plus it is horrible for your joints.

➤ Get ready as the *Dynamic C2C Strength Training System*™ takes you on a wonderful journey of rediscovering your body and how it moves. This section will cover the basics to get you started. You are an engineering marvel.

➤ The *Dynamic C2C Strength Training System*™ is designed for generally healthy people of all ages. Though your muscles WILL be beautiful, get firmer, stronger, and more flexible with *C2C*, this program is NOT a body building program! The vast majority of you simply want to be healthy, lose weight, get stronger, gain more energy, and learn how to use the amazing body God gave you.

➤ Even while targeting one muscle or group of muscles, in the *Dynamic C2C Strength Training System*™ your entire body will always be active at all times! Your nervous system will be stimulated, not just your individual muscles, thus gaining balance, coordination, core stabilization, and postural (spinal) alignment. You will accomplish this by using only free weights and occasionally a cable system.

➤ The exercises you will perform are designed for the following benefits:

- Posture
- Spinal alignment
- Core stabilization
- Balance
- Muscular strength and endurance
- Neuromuscular strength and endurance
- Cardiovascular strength and endurance
- Flexibility
- All of these are achieved as you use the *Dynamic C2C Strength Training System*™ principles and methodologies. Have fun learning to move. And as an added bonus you will look amazing!

➤ Choice of programs
- C2C 2-3 Program™
- 30/30 Program™

➤ Like with any exercise program, consult your physician before participating.

Terms & common questions & answers:

Q: What is a strength training exercise?
    A: A strength training exercise is a specific movement or movements with or without weight designed to work the muscles, joints, and other systems of the body in a way to enhance function, strength, tone, balance, flexibility, endurance, and bone density.

Q: What is a repetition?
    A: A repetition is performing an exercise one time.

Q: What is a set?
    A: A set is performing one exercise through a specified number of repetitions.

Q: What is a circuit?

    A: A circuit is performing 3 or more different exercises one right after the other with minimal rest between sets. The *Dynamic C2C Strength Training System*™ is a 5 exercise per circuit system.

Q: How long should everything take? (Repetitions, sets, circuits, rest between sets and circuits)

    A: Repetitions

        ❖ The speed (tempo) at which you perform each exercise varies slightly for each exercise and also varies based on a person's height. As a rule of thumb perform each exercise at a 2-1 or 3-1 ratio. For example, while performing a ball chest press you would count one thousand one, one thousand two (or to three if you want) on the down phase, and up quicker on the up phase (one thousand one). As a recap count to one thousand two or three on the down phase on all exercises and one thousand one on the up phase. All participants over 6'3" should add a one count to both numbers.

    A: Sets

        ❖ Each set should take no longer than 1 ½ minutes. Think about beginning each set at the 1 ½ minute mark. Also depends on exercise. Some take a little longer than others because some exercises require you to perform one side of your body at a time.

    A: Circuits

        ❖ Do your best to finish your entire circuit in 7 ½ minutes.

    A: Rest between sets

        ❖ If you finish your set before the 1 ½ minute mark then stretch and rest and begin your next set at 1 ½ minutes.

    A: Rest between circuits

        ❖ With the *Dynamic C2C Strength Training System*™ you will rest for 2 ½ minutes between circuits.

        ❖ This rest interval should be used wisely by stretching all the muscles you have worked in your circuit.

        ❖ Stretching should always be implemented into your *Dynamic C2C Strength Training System*™ regime.

    A: As a recap:

        ❖ Repetitions = down - one thousand two or three, up - one thousand one

        ❖ Sets = 1 ½ minutes

        ❖ Circuits = 7 ½ minutes

        ❖ Rest time = 2 ½ minutes (stretch time)

        ❖ Using this method of timing you will be able to finish an awesome functional workout in an hour or less, depending upon which program you choose to follow. Strength training should never go longer than 45 minutes to one hour in length. If you are a beginner and need more time between sets and/or circuits that is fine! <u>But stop at an hour even if you aren't finished.</u>

        ❖ With time you will be able to structure your sets and circuits according to these time guidelines.

Q: What is a fundamental exercise?

A: A fundamental exercise is an exercise that is fundamental to everyday living, everyday movement. You live in a three dimensional unstable environment and that is the environment in which you will train. That is why you will never use a machine with fixed movements. Though I list the muscles and exercises that target them, with the *Dynamic C2C Strength Training System*™ you will train movements' more than individual muscles. Like an individual link of a chain, a muscle by itself is useless if it doesn't contribute to overall body function. Your entire body must learn to function as a whole unit. The exercises I have chosen are fundamental to everyday functional living.

Q: What is a dynamic exercise?

A: A dynamic exercise is an exercise that involves using the upper and lower body simultaneously with multiple joints and muscles being worked during an exercise.

Q: How do I choose the right amount of weight for each exercise?

A: Each set of each exercise should be a <u>maximal effort</u>.

A: Choose a weight that by the time you get to your last 3 repetitions of each set you have difficulty finishing, without compromising technique. For example; if you are doing 15 repetitions while performing a ball chest press, the last 3 should be difficult to finish. If you could do 20-25 then you need to go heavier. If you could only get 8-10 then you need to go lighter.

A: It doesn't have to be exactly 15. 12-17 repetitions with maximal effort is best. Going under 10 repetitions with heavier weight is an intensity that few people enjoy.

Q: What if I can't finish the entire set with the weight I chose?

A: No problem! You will learn what weight works best for you over time. Your Captain's Log will remind you of the weights you use as you write them down.

A: The number of repetitions I have chosen for you in your *Dynamic C2C Strength Training System*™ workout is only a guideline. As a rule of thumb, as long as you choose a weight you can do 10 times with perfect form you are fine. If you can't do 10 repetitions or if your form is bad then you have gone too heavy and need to decrease the weight.

Q: What if I can't finish a whole circuit or workout?

A: No problem! You probably won't when you first begin. Just do the best you can and do what you can. This entire program is about freedom and grace as you learn how to use your beautiful body and build your endurance.

A: Be patient with yourself. You will eventually be able to finish. And don't forget to have fun! God is so proud of you for investing time, energy, and money into keeping His temple healthy!

Q: What if I can't do an exercise?

A: Most of the exercises I have chosen can be accomplished by all age groups and ability levels. There are always exceptions. If you can't do an exercise then choose a different exercise that works the same area - that you CAN do…and be patient with yourself!

Q: Who is a beginner?

    A: A beginner is someone who hasn't worked out at all for over 3 months. Just do the best you can when you begin your strength training regime. You probably won't be able to finish the entire workout. You will eventually!

Q: Who is an intermediate?

    A: An intermediate person is someone who has worked out a little here and there within the past 3 months whether cardio exercise or strength training.

Q: Who is advanced?

    A: An advanced person is someone who has done some kind of cardio exercise or weight training 2-3 times per week for at least 3 months.

Q: Do I need a 3rd day of strength training during each week on the C2C 2-3 Program™?

    A: Throughout my career the average client strength trains twice per week. My wife and I have seen tremendous results with twice per week. Those individuals who want to step it up a little and who want even more results do three times per week. Your *Dynamic C2C Strength Training System™* workout will give you the option of a 1 hour 2-3 days per week program or a 30 minute workout done 4 days per week for those individuals who only have an hour on their lunch break or who are pressed for time.

Q: How should I breathe during each exercise?

    A: Breathing is an art!

    A: Breathing can either make or break you during your *Dynamic C2C Strength Training System™ workout*. It is your lifeline and is even more important in your ability to perform an exercise than the actual strength of your muscles. Think of a high performance sports car. Though it has a powerful engine, if it isn't getting enough oxygen, it looses power and performance. Your body is the same way.

    A: Breath in as the muscle you are working is lengthening or stretching and blow out when the muscle you are working is shortening.

    A. When using dumbbells (most of the time) remember to breathe "out" as the dumbbell goes up or away from the floor and "in" as the dumbbell goes down. When using a cable system it is usually the opposite.

Q: How should I spread out my strength training days?

    A: Especially if you are a beginner, unless you are doing the 30/30 program 4 days per week, give yourself 1-2 days between your C2C strength training days on the 2-3 day regime. (Don't forget about your cardio!)

    A: Look at your schedule. You may have to play around with it. Few people have the same schedule with the same time commitments and responsibilities. The following is a list of days that have worked with our clients over the years on the 2-3 day regime: (remember the 3rd day of training is optional)

- ❖ 3 days per week
    - ♣ Monday, Wednesday, Friday
    - ♣ Monday, Thursday, Saturday
    - ♣ Monday, Wednesday, Saturday
    - ♣ Tuesday, Thursday, Saturday
    - ♣ Tuesday, Thursday, Sunday (Sunday is a good day of rest)
- ❖ 2 days per week
    - ♣ Monday, Thursday
    - ♣ Monday, Friday
    - ♣ Tuesday, Thursday
    - ♣ Tuesday, Friday
    - ♣ Tuesday, Saturday
- ❖ 30/30 program - 4 days per week regime
    - ♣ As an example in your 4 day regime I have used Monday, Tuesday, Thursday, Friday. The following scenarios also work according to your schedule:
    - ♣ Monday, Wednesday, Friday, Saturday
    - ♣ Monday, Tuesday, Friday, Saturday
    - ♣ Tuesday, Wednesday, Friday, Saturday

Q: What if I strain something while working out?

A: You are more likely to strain something while working in your yard than during your *C2C strength training session* because you are focused more on technique during your session. But in the event that something does happen, along with consulting your physician if it is bad enough, live by this acronym:

I like RICE, or I RICE (Ibuprophen, rest, ice, compression, elevation)

- ❖ **I** = Ibuprophen – An anti-inflammatory should be used for swelling. Consult your physician to learn how much you need and what you can use.
- ❖ **R** = Rest - An injured area of your body needs rest. How much is determined by the severity of the injury. Consult your physician on the length of time the area needs to rest.
- ❖ **I** = Ice – Ice is critical within the first 24 hours of an injury. The quicker you ice the quicker the recovery. After 48 hours alternate ice and heat but always do ice first. An ice pack should consist of 2/3 ice, 1/3 water. Crushed is best. The water will ensure no gaps or pockets in the ice will leave parts of your body unattended. The best is an ice massage. Take a paper cup and fill with water and freeze. Once frozen, tear away cup with a little left on the bottom. Apply directly on the injured area and apply pressure while massaging area with circular motions and figure eights. Be sure to ice the entire area and go several inches in every direction beyond the injured area. The ice pack can be done for 20 minutes. The ice massage shouldn't go longer than 12 minutes each time. 2-3 times per day is recommended until swelling is under control. Badly sprained ankles should be iced in a bucket of 2/3 ice, 1/3 water submerged halfway up the calf.

- ❖ **C** = Compression – Once you have iced the injured area it is good to apply pressure by rapping.
- ❖ **E** = Elevation – Elevating the injured area will help keep the blood from pooling in the injured area and will help swelling stay down.

The C2C 2-3 Program™ guidelines

The *C2C 2-3 Program*™ is designed for individuals who may only be able to strength train or make it to the gym 2-3 days per week.

Those of you who commute may also have an hour to two hours drive time every day which makes it difficult to find the time to effectively workout before or after work.

Those of you who have multiple children also have a difficult time. You have 15 places to be at the same time. Soccer, baseball, drama, dance, football, basketball, track, volleyball, cheerleading, debate, parent-teacher conferences, homework and projects, and the hundreds of other events make parenting hard. Many of you do these things AND work! Learning how to maximize your training efforts in a short amount of time is crucial. Most of you who are in college also work full or part time, study, and even may be raising a family. For those of you who fit the above profiles the *C2C 2-3 Program*™ is perfect for you. Because of the types of exercises I am teaching you, virtually the entire program can be done at home or in your facility of choice with minimal equipment!

Note: If you have never worked with an exercise ball before I recommend taking 3 days of doing nothing but playing on the ball. Spend your hour practicing rolling up and rolling down into you bridge position over and over until it feels natural. Once you get the hang of it then you can add weights to your hands and follow your training regime.

1. You will strength train 2-3 days per week for 60 minutes (3rd day is optional)
2. You will do cardiovascular exercise 30-45 minutes in the morning or evening on those days you strength train, 45 minutes to 1 hour on those days you do not strength train.
3. These are the guidelines for how to follow the C2C 2-3 workout.

   ➢ Sets = 1 ½ minutes
   ➢ Circuits = 7 ½ minutes
   ➢ Rest time = 2 ½ minutes (stretch time)
   ➢ How it is broken down - If you have 5 exercises in a circuit and each set takes 1 ½ minutes that is 7 ½ minutes to finish 1 round of your circuit. Add the 2 ½ minute rest/stretch interval and that makes 10 minutes. Because you will work up to doing each circuit 3 times it will take you 30 minutes to finish your training.
   ➢ With time you will be able to structure your sets and circuits according to these time guidelines. Some exercises take longer because you are doing one side at a time. Just do your best to stay in the time guidelines.

Monday morning before breakfast – 30-45 minutes cardio
Monday day – Strength training - Circuit 1 (first 30 minutes) - eat before you go!

Begin with Warm-up then start circuit 1

Exercise	Muscles	set 1	set 2	set 3	Breathing
Ball dumbbell chest press	chest, legs, core	15 reps	15 reps	15 reps	Breathe out on up phase, in on down phase
Cable pull-downs or Pull-ups	back, legs	15 reps	15 reps	15 reps	Breathe out on down phase, in on up phase / Breathe out on down phase, in on up phase
Squats	quads, glutes	20 reps	20 reps	20 reps	Breathe out on up phase, in on down phase
Ball hamstring curls	hamstrings, core	20 reps	20 reps	20 reps	Breathe out on in phase, in on away phase
Plank	core	1 min	1 min	1 min	Breathe fluently
Stretch during rest time	2 ½ min rest				

Monday Circuit 2 (second 30 minutes)

Exercise	Muscles	set 1	set 2	set 3	Breathing
Ball dumbbell chest fly	chest, legs, core	15 reps	15 reps	15 reps	Breathe out on up phase, in on down phase
Ball dumbbell pullovers or Dumbbell rows	back, legs, core	20 reps	20 reps	20 reps	Breathe out on up phase, in on down phase / Breathe out on up phase, in on down phase
Reverse lunges	quads, glutes	15/side	15/side	15/side	Breathe out on up phase, in on down phase
Straight legged dead lift	hamstrings, back	15 reps	15 reps	15 reps	Breathe out on up phase, in on down phase
Side plank (both sides)	oblique's	45 sec.	45 sec.	45 sec.	Breathe fluently
Stretch during rest time	2 ½ min rest				

Tuesday morning before breakfast

Begin with Warm-up then start cardio

Cardiovascular Exercise – 45 minutes to 1 hour (Treadmill, Elliptical, or Stationary Bike (best for beginners)

Wednesday morning before breakfast – 30-45 minutes cardio
Wednesday day – Strength training - Circuit 1 (first 30 minutes) - eat before you go!

Begin with Warm-up then start circuit 1

Exercise	Muscles	set 1	set 2	set 3	Breathing
Standing dumbbell shoulder press	shoulders	15 reps	15 reps	15 reps	Breathe out on up phase, in on down phase
Single leg biceps curls	biceps, hips, core	15 reps	15 reps	15 reps	Breathe out on up phase, in on down phase
Triceps extensions on ball	triceps, legs, core	15 reps	15 reps	15 reps	Breathe out on up phase, in on down phase
Standing calf raises	calves	20 reps	20 reps	20 reps	Breathe out on up phase, in on down phase
Bent knee leg raises	low abs	30 reps	30 reps	30 reps	Breathe out on up phase, in on down phase
Stretch during rest time	2 ½ min rest				

Wednesday Circuit 2 (second 30 minutes)

Exercise	Muscles	set 1	set 2	set 3	Breathing
Dumbbell side raises	shoulders	15 reps	15 reps	15 reps	Breathe out on up phase, in on down phase
Single leg hammer curls	biceps, hip, core	15 reps	15 reps	15 reps	Breathe out on up phase, in on down phase
Triceps bench/chair dips	triceps, core	15 reps	15 reps	15 reps	Breathe out on up phase, in on down phase
Seated calf raises	calves	20 reps	20 reps	20 reps	Breathe out on up phase, in on down phase
Ball crunch with twist	core, oblique's	50 reps	50 reps	50 reps	Breathe out on up phase, in on down phase
Stretch during rest time	2 ½ min rest				

Thursday morning before breakfast

Begin with Warm-up then start cardio

Cardiovascular Exercise – 45 minutes to 1 hour (Treadmill, Elliptical, or Stationary Bike (best for beginners)

Friday morning before breakfast – 30-45 minutes cardio
Friday day - Strength training - Circuit 1 (first 30 minutes) - eat before you go!

Begin with Warm-up then start circuit 1

Exercise	Muscles	set 1	set 2	set 3	Breathing
Ball dumbbell chest press	chest, legs, core	15 reps	15 reps	15 reps	Breathe out on up phase, in on down phase
Cable pull-downs or Pull-ups	back, legs	15 reps	15 reps	15 reps	Breathe out on down phase, in on up phase / Breathe out on up phase, in on down phase
Squats	quads, glutes	20 reps	20 reps	20 reps	Breathe out on up phase, in on down phase
Ball hamstring curls	hamstrings, core	20 reps	20 reps	20 reps	Breathe out on in phase, in on away phase
Plank	core	1 min	1 min	1 min	Breathe fluently
Stretch during rest time	2 ½ min rest				

Friday Circuit 2 (second 30 minutes)

Exercise	Muscles	set 1	set 2	set 3	Breathing
Standing dumbbell shoulder press	shoulders	15 reps	15 reps	15 reps	Breathe out on up phase, in on down phase
Single leg biceps curls	biceps, hips, core	15 reps	15 reps	15 reps	Breathe out on up phase, in on down phase
Triceps extensions on ball	triceps, legs, core	15 reps	15 reps	15 reps	Breathe out on up phase, in on down phase
Standing calf raises	calves	20 reps	20 reps	20 reps	Breathe out on up phase, in on down phase
Bent knee leg raises	low abs	30 reps	30 reps	30 reps	Breathe out on up phase, in on down phase
Stretch during rest time	2 ½ min rest				

Saturday morning before breakfast

Begin with Warm-up then start cardio

Cardiovascular Exercise – 45 minutes to 1 hour (Treadmill, Elliptical, or Stationary Bike (best for beginners)

Sunday
REST

30/30 Program™ guidelines

The 30/30 program™ is designed for individuals who only have a small window of which to train. Many of you only have an hour or less lunch-break of which this time is used for the following:

1.   Get to the gym if your work doesn't have one,
2.   Change into workout clothes,
3.   Warm-up,
4.   Exercise,
5.   Stretch,
6.   Shower,
7.   Change back into work clothes,
8.   Eat lunch,
9.   And get back to work.

Those of you who commute may also have an hour to two hours drive time every day which makes it difficult to find the time to effectively workout before or after work.

Those of you who have multiple children also have a difficult time. You have 15 places to be at the same time. Soccer, baseball, drama, dance, football, basketball, track, volleyball, cheerleading, debate, parent-teacher conferences, homework and projects, and the hundreds of other events make parenting hard. Many of you do these things AND work! Learning how to maximize your training efforts in a short amount of time is crucial. For those of you who fit the above profiles the *30/30 Program*™ is perfect for you. Because of the types of exercises I am teaching you, virtually the entire program can be done at home or in your facility of choice with minimal equipment!

1.   You will strength train only 30 minutes four days per week.
2.   You will do cardiovascular exercise 30 minutes in the morning, evening or directly after your strength training session on those days you strength train. Adhere to your cardio guidelines found earlier in this book for the other days, based on your goals.
3.   I have set up your program on a Monday, Tuesday, Thursday, Friday regime. You can change the days around if you need to. For example: Monday, Wednesday, Friday, Saturday, or Tuesday, Wednesday, Saturday, Sunday. Remember, I recommend one day of doing absolutely nothing in regards to exercise. You need at least one day off.
4.   Due to the dynamics of the *30/30 Program*™, it will work for the beginner, intermediate, or advanced person.
5.   The same time principles apply to the *30/30 Program*™ that applied to the previous program.

   ➢   Sets = 1 ½ minutes
   ➢   Circuits = 7 ½ minutes
   ➢   Rest time = 2 ½ minutes (stretch time)

> ➤ How it is broken down - If you have 5 exercises in a circuit and each set takes 1 ½ minutes that is 7 ½ minutes to finish 1 round of your circuit. Add the 2 ½ minute rest/stretch interval and that makes 10 minutes. Because you will work up to doing each circuit 3 times it will take you 30 minutes to finish your training.
> ➤ With time you will be able to structure your sets and circuits according to these time guidelines. Some exercises take longer because you are doing one side at a time. Just do your best to stay in the time guidelines.

Monday
Begin with Warm-up then start circuit

Exercise	Muscles	set 1	set 2	set 3	Breathing
Ball dumbbell chest press	chest, legs, core	15 reps	15 reps	15 reps	Breathe out on up phase, in on down phase
Cable pull-downs or Pull-ups	back, legs	15 reps	15 reps	15 reps	Breathe out on down phase, in on up phase / Breathe out on up phase, in on down phase
Squats	quads, glutes	20 reps	20 reps	20 reps	Breathe out on up phase, in on down phase
Ball hamstring curls	hamstrings, core	20 reps	20 reps	20 reps	Breathe out on in phase, in on away phase
Plank	core	1 min	1 min	1 min	Breathe fluently
Stretch during rest time	2 ½ min rest				

After 30 minute strength training is completed do 30 minutes Cardiovascular Exercise (Treadmill, Elliptical, or Stationary Bike (best for beginners)

Tuesday
Begin with Warm-up then start circuit

Exercise	Muscles	set 1	set 2	set 3	Breathing
Standing dumbbell shoulder press	shoulders	15 reps	15 reps	15 reps	Breathe out on up phase, in on down phase
Single leg biceps curls	biceps, hips, core	15 reps	15 reps	15 reps	Breathe out on up phase, in on down phase
Triceps extensions on ball	triceps, legs, core	15 reps	15 reps	15 reps	Breathe out on up phase, in on down phase
Standing calf raises	calves	20 reps	20 reps	20 reps	Breathe out on up phase, in on down phase
Bent knee leg raises	low abs	30 reps	30 reps	30 reps	Breathe out on up phase, in on down phase
Stretch during rest time	2 ½ min rest				

After 30 minute strength training is completed do 30 minutes Cardiovascular Exercise (Treadmill, Elliptical, or Stationary Bike (best for beginners)

Wednesday before breakfast
Begin with Warm-up then start cardio

Cardiovascular Exercise – 45 minutes to 1 hour (Treadmill, Elliptical, or Stationary Bike (best for beginners)

Thursday
Begin with Warm-up then start circuit

Exercise	Muscles	set 1	set 2	set 3	Breathing
Ball dumbbell chest fly	chest, legs, core	15 reps	15 reps	15 reps	Breathe out on up phase, in on down phase
Ball dumbbell pullovers or Dumbbell rows	back, legs, core	20 reps	20 reps	20 reps	Breathe out on up phase, in on down phase / Breathe out on up phase, in on down phase
Reverse lunges	quads, glutes	15/side	15/side	15/side	Breathe out on up phase, in on down phase
Straight legged dead lift	hamstrings, back	15 reps	15 reps	15 reps	Breathe out on up phase, in on down phase
Side plank (both sides)	oblique's	45 sec.	45 sec.	45 sec.	Breathe fluently
Stretch during rest time	2 ½ min rest				

After 30 minute strength training is completed do 30 minutes Cardiovascular Exercise (Treadmill, Elliptical, or Stationary Bike (best for beginners)

Friday

Exercise	Muscles	set 1	set 2	set 3	Breathing
Dumbbell side raises	shoulders	15 reps	15 reps	15 reps	Breathe out on up phase, in on down phase
Single leg hammer curls	biceps, hip, core	15 reps	15 reps	15 reps	Breathe out on up phase, in on down phase
Triceps bench/chair dips	triceps, core	15 reps	15 reps	15 reps	Breathe out on up phase, in on down phase
Seated calf raises	calves	20 reps	20 reps	20 reps	Breathe out on up phase, in on down phase
Ball crunch with twist	core, oblique's	50 reps	50 reps	50 reps	Breathe out on up phase, in on down phase
Stretch during rest time	2 ½ min rest				

After 30 minute strength training is completed do 30 minutes Cardiovascular Exercise (Treadmill, Elliptical, or Stationary Bike (best for beginners)

Saturday before breakfast
Begin with Warm-up then start cardio

Cardiovascular Exercise – 45 minutes to 1 hour (Treadmill, Elliptical, or Stationary Bike (best for beginners)

Sunday
REST

Myths

5 common myths in fitness

MYTH #1: "Resistance training or weight lifting and supplements that promote lean muscle gain causes women to get bulky and look like a man?"

TRUTH: Absolutely Not! Women have beautiful muscles. God intended you to use your muscles and glorify Him with them. It is hard enough to get guys bulky even if that is their goal and they have 10 times the testosterone than women. Never, ever be afraid of your muscles. The majority of body builders, male and female, you see on television and in the magazines that look all bulked up are on illegal anabolic steroids and growth hormones and are not in any way a true representation of fitness and health. The reasons many women feel bulky is because as they tone up and develop their lean muscle tissue they don't eat right and do their cardio effectively and don't lose their body fat. When you lean down or lose your body fat to a healthy and fit level you will no longer feel bulky, but will enjoy a beautifully sculptured, functional, athletic, feminine looking body; just the way God intended it to be!

MYTH #2: "To be a real man I have to be buff and bulky. Being buff and bulky is also what I need for women to find me attractive."

TRUTH: Absolutely Not! God wants all men to be in good health with lean and tone bodies but the bulked up look is not what makes you a man at all and is NOT what women ultimately want in a man. What makes you a true man is your love and surrender to Jesus Christ. I have talked with numerous women throughout my career and have found that most are more interested in how a man treats her with respect, honor, integrity and the gentleness of Jesus. A woman wants and deserves security and a Spiritual covering by a Godly man more than anything. Sure you are to be healthy for the woman in your life but if the reason she is with you is because of the size of your biceps, you may want to not only find a new girl, but you need to deal with your insecurity of what truly makes you a man, Jesus Christ. This also applies in reverse to women.

MYTH #3: "I may lose a few pounds but I am so overweight and have so far to go that I will never have a lean, tone body so why bother? It is just way too overwhelming."

TRUTH: Your body can be tone and healthy regardless of how big you currently are. Excuse the cliché but Rome wasn't built in a day! When climbing a mountain it takes one foot in front of the other. It may take a while. When you exercise to be healthy and glorify God with your body on a daily basis the natural result of this is a lean healthy body. Watch where you put your focus. Is it on the result and how f-a-a-a-a-r you have to go or is it on your intention of serving God and others with a healthy lifestyle? Use your daily journaling to God to help you stay in the present and take one step at a time during this journey of life-change regarding your health and well-being. You can and will get the body you desire. It is just a matter of time, patience and perseverance all of which God will give you as you do the work.

MYTH #4: "I am going to have to eat chicken and broccoli for the rest of my life."

TRUTH: Though you don't have to eat chicken and broccoli every day and do have a variety of foods to choose from, the more you surrender to your health and honor your covenant with God to be healthy the less you will feel deprived of certain foods.

Being too strict on certain foods is one way to burn out. You have been provided a comprehensive meal plan in this book that gives you a variety of different foods to choose from. Once you lean down you can moderately work certain foods back into your diet like breads and pastas, cheese and many others. These can even be implemented into your leaning phase nutritional requirements if used sparingly. But remember you are teaching your body how detrimental too many carbohydrates and fats can be. Our grocery stores are jam packed with carbohydrates everywhere you look. There are a lot of things in this world you have access to, but that doesn't mean it is in God's will for you to participate in them!

MYTH #5: "I have no idea where to start and know nothing of exercise and nutrition."

TRUTH: There is so much information out there and it is easy to get overwhelmed, even for us in the industry who are experts. That is why we all must always stick to the basics of good nutrition and exercise. Most of the Courage to Change Program was written by answering the basic questions of clients over the years. I have weeded out the unnecessary details that don't pertain to the basics of good health. Take one step at a time.

www.courage2change.org

"Go and be the Captain of your life. Take charge and take up your sword. Let God show you each moment how to live with courage, discipline, enthusiasm and a relentless Christ-like attitude.

Rise to the occasion, the occasion being life and seize the day, be heard, let out a roar and make yourself strong enough in the Lord to repel any poison that dares touch your skin!

Be encouraged and enjoy the beautiful healthy body God has given you!

I love all of you!"

......Brian Wellbrock

12 week Captain's Log daily accountability journal

LAYING the FOUNDATION

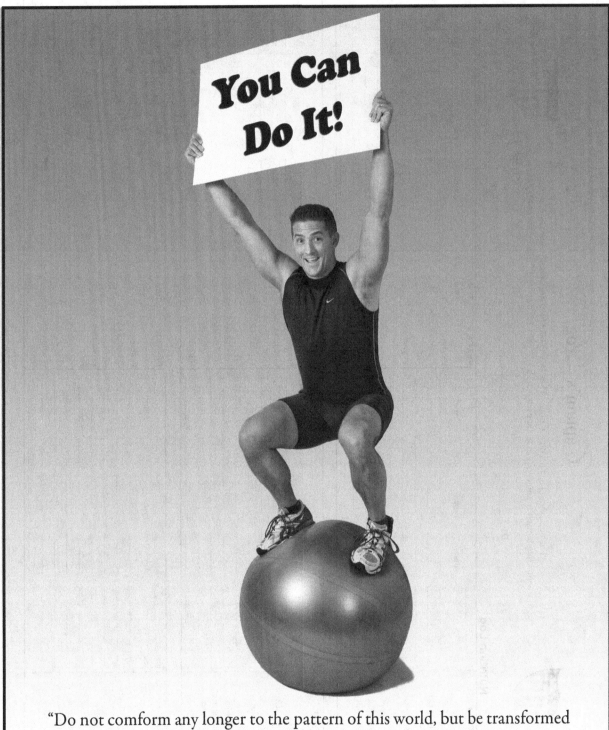

"Do not comform any longer to the pattern of this world, but be transformed by the renewing of your mind." (Romans 12:2)

WEEK ONE

Captain's Log

"Each one should test his own actions. Then he can take pride in himself without comparing himself to somebody else, for each one should carry his own load." (Galatians 6:40)

Day: _____   Date: ____ / ____ / ____

Nutrition Log

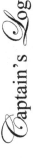

BREAKFAST   Time: _____

	Type	Amt:		Type	Amt:
Protein	1.			2.	
Complex Carbs	1.			2.	
Fruit	1.			2.	
Vegetables	1.			2.	
Fat	1.			2.	
Liquid/drink	1.			2.	
Meal Replace.	1.			2.	
Condiments	1.			2.	
Other	1.			2.	

LUNCH   Time: _____

	Type	Amt:		Type	Amt:
Protein	1.			2.	
Complex Carbs	1.			2.	
Fruit	1.			2.	
Vegetables	1.			2.	
Fat	1.			2.	
Liquid/drink	1.			2.	
Meal Replace.	1.			2.	
Condiments	1.			2.	
Other	1.			2.	

SNACK 3   Time: _____

	Type	Amt:		Type	Amt:
Protein	1.			2.	
Complex Carbs	1.			2.	
Fruit	1.			2.	
Vegetables	1.			2.	
Fat	1.			2.	
Liquid/drink	1.			2.	
Meal Replace.	1.			2.	
Condiments	1.			2.	
Other	1.			2.	

SNACK 1   Time: _____

	Type	Amt:		Type	Amt:
Protein	1.			2.	
Complex Carbs	1.			2.	
Fruit	1.			2.	
Vegetables	1.			2.	
Fat	1.			2.	
Liquid/drink	1.			2.	
Meal Replace.	1.			2.	
Condiments	1.			2.	
Other	1.			2.	

SNACK 2   Time: _____

	Type	Amt:		Type	Amt:
Protein	1.			2.	
Complex Carbs	1.			2.	
Fruit	1.			2.	
Vegetables	1.			2.	
Fat	1.			2.	
Liquid/drink	1.			2.	
Meal Replace.	1.			2.	
Condiments	1.			2.	
Other	1.			2.	

DINNER   Time: _____

	Type	Amt:		Type	Amt:
Protein	1.			2.	
Complex Carbs	1.			2.	
Fruit	1.			2.	
Vegetables	1.			2.	
Fat	1.			2.	
Liquid/drink	1.			2.	
Meal Replace.	1.			2.	
Condiments	1.			2.	
Other	1.			2.	

Resistance Training

Time of day: _____
Warmed up   Yes _____   No _____

Name of exercise 1: _____
Weight: _____   Reps: _____
Set 1: _____
Set 2: _____
Muscles worked: _____
Set 3: _____
Set 4: _____
Stretched?   Yes _____   No _____

Name of exercise 3: _____
Weight: _____   Reps: _____
Set 1: _____
Set 2: _____
Muscles worked: _____
Set 3: _____
Set 4: _____
Stretched?   Yes _____   No _____

Name of exercise 5: _____
Weight: _____   Reps: _____
Set 1: _____
Set 2: _____
Muscles worked: _____
Set 3: _____
Set 4: _____
Stretched?   Yes _____   No _____

Name of exercise 7: _____
Weight: _____   Reps: _____
Set 1: _____
Set 2: _____
Muscles worked: _____
Set 3: _____
Set 4: _____
Stretched?   Yes _____   No _____

Name of exercise 9: _____
Weight: _____   Reps: _____
Set 1: _____
Set 2: _____
Muscles worked: _____
Set 3: _____
Set 4: _____
Stretched?   Yes _____   No _____

Name of exercise 2: _____
Weight: _____   Reps: _____
Set 1: _____
Set 2: _____
Muscles worked: _____
Set 3: _____
Set 4: _____
Stretched?   Yes _____   No _____

Name of exercise 4: _____
Weight: _____   Reps: _____
Set 1: _____
Set 2: _____
Muscles worked: _____
Set 3: _____
Set 4: _____
Stretched?   Yes _____   No _____

Name of exercise 6: _____
Weight: _____   Reps: _____
Set 1: _____
Set 2: _____
Muscles worked: _____
Set 3: _____
Set 4: _____
Stretched?   Yes _____   No _____

Name of exercise 8: _____
Weight: _____   Reps: _____
Set 1: _____
Set 2: _____
Muscles worked: _____
Set 3: _____
Set 4: _____
Stretched?   Yes _____   No _____

Name of exercise 10: _____
Weight: _____   Reps: _____
Set 1: _____
Set 2: _____
Muscles worked: _____
Set 3: _____
Set 4: _____
Stretched?   Yes _____   No _____

Cardiovascular Training

Warmed up   Yes _____   No _____

Time of day:	For how long?	Heart Rate
Type 1:		
Type 2:		
Type 3:		
Type 4:		

Stretched?   Yes _____   No _____

Evening Reflection

Did I put my faith in Action today?	Yes _____	No _____
I prayed for somone today	Yes _____	No _____
I read my Bible today	Yes _____	No _____
I helped someone in need today	Yes _____	No _____
I got 6 1/2 to 8 hours of sleep last night	Yes _____	No _____
I know I ate right today	Yes _____	No _____
I ate breakfast today	Yes _____	No _____
I ate starches after 4:00 p.m. today	Yes _____	No _____
I ate at least 4 meals today	Yes _____	No _____
I drank at least a gallon of water today	Yes _____	No _____
I had Courage to Change today	Yes _____	No _____

Tonight I forgive… _____

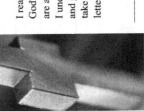

Captain's Log Statement of Faith

I realize that my actions don't earn my way into God's love or earn my way to heaven but that they are a reflection of my love affair with Jesus! I understand that by taking care of myself I honor and glorify God. I matter to God and the actions I take toward good health are daily written love letters telling God, "Thank you for my life"!

_____
Signature

"I press on toward the goal to win the prize for which God has called me heavenward in Christ Jesus."
Philippians 3:14

Captain's Log

Day: _____   Date: ____ / ____ / ____

Nutrition Log

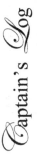
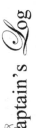

BREAKFAST   Time: _____

	Type 1.	Amt:	Type 2.	Amt:
Protein				
Complex Carbs				
Fruit				
Vegetables				
Fat				
Liquid/drink				
Meal Replace.				
Condiments				
Other				

LUNCH   Time: _____

	Type 1.	Amt:	Type 2.	Amt:
Protein				
Complex Carbs				
Fruit				
Vegetables				
Fat				
Liquid/drink				
Meal Replace.				
Condiments				
Other				

SNACK 3   Time: _____

	Type 1.	Amt:	Type 2.	Amt:
Protein				
Complex Carbs				
Fruit				
Vegetables				
Fat				
Liquid/drink				
Meal Replace.				
Condiments				
Other				

SNACK 1   Time: _____

	Type 1.	Amt:	Type 2.	Amt:
Protein				
Complex Carbs				
Fruit				
Vegetables				
Fat				
Liquid/drink				
Meal Replace.				
Condiments				
Other				

SNACK 2   Time: _____

	Type 1.	Amt:	Type 2.	Amt:
Protein				
Complex Carbs				
Fruit				
Vegetables				
Fat				
Liquid/drink				
Meal Replace.				
Condiments				
Other				

DINNER   Time: _____

	Type 1.	Amt:	Type 2.	Amt:
Protein				
Complex Carbs				
Fruit				
Vegetables				
Fat				
Liquid/drink				
Meal Replace.				
Condiments				
Other				

Cardiovascular Training

Warmed up   Yes _____   No _____

Time of day: _____

	For how long?	Heart Rate
Type 1:	_____	_____
Type 2:	_____	_____
Type 3:	_____	_____
Type 4:	_____	_____

Stretched?   Yes _____   No _____

Evening Reflection

Did I put my faith in Action today?   Yes _____   No _____

I prayed for somone today   Yes _____   No _____

I read my Bible today   Yes _____   No _____

I helped someone in need today   Yes _____   No _____

I got 6 1/2 to 8 hours of sleep last night   Yes _____   No _____

I know I ate right today   Yes _____   No _____

I ate breakfast today   Yes _____   No _____

I ate starches after 4:00 p.m. today   Yes _____   No _____

I ate at least 4 meals today   Yes _____   No _____

I drank at least a gallon of water today   Yes _____   No _____

I had Courage to Change today   Yes _____   No _____

Tonight I forgive…

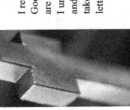

Captain's Log Statement of Faith

I realize that my actions don't earn my way into God's love or earn my way to heaven but that they are a reflection of my love affair with Jesus! I understand that by taking care of myself I honor and glorify God. I matter to God and the actions I take toward good health are daily written love letters telling God, "Thank you for my life"!

_____
Signature

Resistance Training

Time of day: _____

Warmed up   Yes _____   No _____

Name of exercise 1:

	Weight:	Reps:
Set 1:	_____	_____
Set 2:	_____	_____
Set 3:	_____	_____
Set 4:	_____	_____

Muscles worked:

Stretched?   Yes _____   No _____

Name of exercise 2:

	Weight:	Reps:
Set 1:	_____	_____
Set 2:	_____	_____
Set 3:	_____	_____
Set 4:	_____	_____

Muscles worked:

Stretched?   Yes _____   No _____

Name of exercise 3:

	Weight:	Reps:
Set 1:	_____	_____
Set 2:	_____	_____
Set 3:	_____	_____
Set 4:	_____	_____

Muscles worked:

Stretched?   Yes _____   No _____

Name of exercise 4:

	Weight:	Reps:
Set 1:	_____	_____
Set 2:	_____	_____
Set 3:	_____	_____
Set 4:	_____	_____

Muscles worked:

Stretched?   Yes _____   No _____

Name of exercise 5:

	Weight:	Reps:
Set 1:	_____	_____
Set 2:	_____	_____
Set 3:	_____	_____
Set 4:	_____	_____

Muscles worked:

Stretched?   Yes _____   No _____

Name of exercise 6:

	Weight:	Reps:
Set 1:	_____	_____
Set 2:	_____	_____
Set 3:	_____	_____
Set 4:	_____	_____

Muscles worked:

Stretched?   Yes _____   No _____

Name of exercise 7:

	Weight:	Reps:
Set 1:	_____	_____
Set 2:	_____	_____
Set 3:	_____	_____
Set 4:	_____	_____

Muscles worked:

Stretched?   Yes _____   No _____

Name of exercise 8:

	Weight:	Reps:
Set 1:	_____	_____
Set 2:	_____	_____
Set 3:	_____	_____
Set 4:	_____	_____

Muscles worked:

Stretched?   Yes _____   No _____

Name of exercise 9:

	Weight:	Reps:
Set 1:	_____	_____
Set 2:	_____	_____
Set 3:	_____	_____
Set 4:	_____	_____

Muscles worked:

Stretched?   Yes _____   No _____

Name of exercise 10:

	Weight:	Reps:
Set 1:	_____	_____
Set 2:	_____	_____
Set 3:	_____	_____
Set 4:	_____	_____

Muscles worked:

Stretched?   Yes _____   No _____

"I press on toward the goal to win the prize for which God has called me heavenward in Christ Jesus."
Philippians 3:14

Captain's Log

"Each one should test his own actions. Then he can take pride in himself without comparing himself to somebody else, for each one should carry his own load." (Galatians 6:40)

Day: _____   Date: _____ / _____ / _____

Nutrition Log

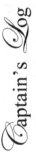
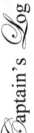

BREAKFAST Time: _____

	Type	Amt:		Type	Amt:
Protein	1.			2.	
Complex Carbs	1.			2.	
Fruit	1.			2.	
Vegetables	1.			2.	
Fat	1.			2.	
Liquid/drink	1.			2.	
Meal Replace.	1.			2.	
Condiments	1.			2.	
Other	1.			2.	

LUNCH Time: _____

	Type	Amt:		Type	Amt:
Protein	1.			2.	
Complex Carbs	1.			2.	
Fruit	1.			2.	
Vegetables	1.			2.	
Fat	1.			2.	
Liquid/drink	1.			2.	
Meal Replace.	1.			2.	
Condiments	1.			2.	
Other	1.			2.	

SNACK 3 Time: _____

	Type	Amt:		Type	Amt:
Protein	1.			2.	
Complex Carbs	1.			2.	
Fruit	1.			2.	
Vegetables	1.			2.	
Fat	1.			2.	
Liquid/drink	1.			2.	
Meal Replace.	1.			2.	
Condiments	1.			2.	
Other	1.			2.	

SNACK 1 Time: _____

	Type	Amt:		Type	Amt:
Protein	1.			2.	
Complex Carbs	1.			2.	
Fruit	1.			2.	
Vegetables	1.			2.	
Fat	1.			2.	
Liquid/drink	1.			2.	
Meal Replace.	1.			2.	
Condiments	1.			2.	
Other	1.			2.	

SNACK 2 Time: _____

	Type	Amt:		Type	Amt:
Protein	1.			2.	
Complex Carbs	1.			2.	
Fruit	1.			2.	
Vegetables	1.			2.	
Fat	1.			2.	
Liquid/drink	1.			2.	
Meal Replace.	1.			2.	
Condiments	1.			2.	
Other	1.			2.	

DINNER Time: _____

	Type	Amt:		Type	Amt:
Protein	1.			2.	
Complex Carbs	1.			2.	
Fruit	1.			2.	
Vegetables	1.			2.	
Fat	1.			2.	
Liquid/drink	1.			2.	
Meal Replace.	1.			2.	
Condiments	1.			2.	
Other	1.			2.	

Resistance Training

Time of day: _____

Warmed up   Yes _____   No _____

Name of exercise 1: _____   Weight: _____   Reps: _____

Set 1: _____
Set 2: _____
Muscles worked: _____   Set 3: _____
_____   Set 4: _____

Stretched?   Yes _____   No _____

Name of exercise 3: _____   Weight: _____   Reps: _____

Set 1: _____
Set 2: _____
Muscles worked: _____   Set 3: _____
_____   Set 4: _____

Stretched?   Yes _____   No _____

Name of exercise 5: _____   Weight: _____   Reps: _____

Set 1: _____
Set 2: _____
Muscles worked: _____   Set 3: _____
_____   Set 4: _____

Stretched?   Yes _____   No _____

Name of exercise 7: _____   Weight: _____   Reps: _____

Set 1: _____
Set 2: _____
Muscles worked: _____   Set 3: _____
_____   Set 4: _____

Stretched?   Yes _____   No _____

Name of exercise 9: _____   Weight: _____   Reps: _____

Set 1: _____
Set 2: _____
Muscles worked: _____   Set 3: _____
_____   Set 4: _____

Stretched?   Yes _____   No _____

Name of exercise 2: _____   Weight: _____   Reps: _____

Set 1: _____
Set 2: _____
Muscles worked: _____   Set 3: _____
_____   Set 4: _____

Stretched?   Yes _____   No _____

Name of exercise 4: _____   Weight: _____   Reps: _____

Set 1: _____
Set 2: _____
Muscles worked: _____   Set 3: _____
_____   Set 4: _____

Stretched?   Yes _____   No _____

Name of exercise 6: _____   Weight: _____   Reps: _____

Set 1: _____
Set 2: _____
Muscles worked: _____   Set 3: _____
_____   Set 4: _____

Stretched?   Yes _____   No _____

Name of exercise 8: _____   Weight: _____   Reps: _____

Set 1: _____
Set 2: _____
Muscles worked: _____   Set 3: _____
_____   Set 4: _____

Stretched?   Yes _____   No _____

Name of exercise 10: _____   Weight: _____   Reps: _____

Set 1: _____
Set 2: _____
Muscles worked: _____   Set 3: _____
_____   Set 4: _____

Stretched?   Yes _____   No _____

Cardiovascular Training

Warmed up   Yes _____   No _____

Time of day: _____   For how long?   Heart Rate

Type 1: _____
Type 2: _____
Type 3: _____
Type 4: _____

Stretched?   Yes _____   No _____

Evening Reflection

Did I put my faith in Action today?   Yes _____   No _____
I prayed for somone today   Yes _____   No _____
I read my Bible today   Yes _____   No _____
I helped someone in need today   Yes _____   No _____
I got 6 1/2 to 8 hours of sleep last night   Yes _____   No _____
I know I ate right today   Yes _____   No _____
I ate breakfast today   Yes _____   No _____
I ate starches after 4:00 p.m. today   Yes _____   No _____
I ate at least 4 meals today   Yes _____   No _____
I drank at least a gallon of water today   Yes _____   No _____
I had Courage to Change today   Yes _____   No _____
Tonight I forgive…. _____

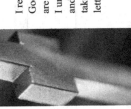

Captain's Log Statement of Faith

I realize that my actions don't earn my way into God's love or earn my way to heaven but that they are a reflection of my love affair with Jesus! I understand that by taking care of myself I honor and glorify God. I matter to God and the actions I take toward good health are daily written love letters telling God, "Thank you for my life"!

_____
Signature

"I press on toward the goal to win the prize for which God has called me heavenward in Christ Jesus."
Philippians 3:14

Captain's Log

Day: _____   Date: ____ / ____ / ____

Nutrition Log

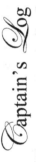

BREAKFAST   Time: _____

	Type	Amt:	Type	Amt:
Protein	1.		2.	
Complex Carbs	1.		2.	
Fruit	1.		2.	
Vegetables	1.		2.	
Fat	1.		2.	
Liquid/drink	1.		2.	
Meal Replace.	1.		2.	
Condiments	1.		2.	
Other	1.		2.	

LUNCH   Time: _____

	Type	Amt:	Type	Amt:
Protein	1.		2.	
Complex Carbs	1.		2.	
Fruit	1.		2.	
Vegetables	1.		2.	
Fat	1.		2.	
Liquid/drink	1.		2.	
Meal Replace.	1.		2.	
Condiments	1.		2.	
Other	1.		2.	

SNACK 3   Time: _____

	Type	Amt:	Type	Amt:
Protein	1.		2.	
Complex Carbs	1.		2.	
Fruit	1.		2.	
Vegetables	1.		2.	
Fat	1.		2.	
Liquid/drink	1.		2.	
Meal Replace.	1.		2.	
Condiments	1.		2.	
Other	1.		2.	

SNACK 1   Time: _____

	Type	Amt:	Type	Amt:
Protein	1.		2.	
Complex Carbs	1.		2.	
Fruit	1.		2.	
Vegetables	1.		2.	
Fat	1.		2.	
Liquid/drink	1.		2.	
Meal Replace.	1.		2.	
Condiments	1.		2.	
Other	1.		2.	

SNACK 2   Time: _____

	Type	Amt:	Type	Amt:
Protein	1.		2.	
Complex Carbs	1.		2.	
Fruit	1.		2.	
Vegetables	1.		2.	
Fat	1.		2.	
Liquid/drink	1.		2.	
Meal Replace.	1.		2.	
Condiments	1.		2.	
Other	1.		2.	

DINNER   Time: _____

	Type	Amt:	Type	Amt:
Protein	1.		2.	
Complex Carbs	1.		2.	
Fruit	1.		2.	
Vegetables	1.		2.	
Fat	1.		2.	
Liquid/drink	1.		2.	
Meal Replace.	1.		2.	
Condiments	1.		2.	
Other	1.		2.	

Cardiovascular Training

Time of day: _____

Warmed up   Yes _____   No _____

Time of day:	For how long?	Heart Rate
Type 1:		
Type 2:		
Type 3:		
Type 4:		

Stretched?   Yes _____   No _____

Evening Reflection

Did I put my faith in Action today?	Yes _____	No _____
I prayed for somone today	Yes _____	No _____
I read my Bible today	Yes _____	No _____
I helped someone in need today	Yes _____	No _____
I got 6 1/2 to 8 hours of sleep last night	Yes _____	No _____
I know I ate right today	Yes _____	No _____
I ate breakfast today	Yes _____	No _____
I ate starches after 4:00 p.m. today	Yes _____	No _____
I ate at least 4 meals today	Yes _____	No _____
I drank at least a gallon of water today	Yes _____	No _____
I had Courage to Change today	Yes _____	No _____
Tonight I forgive…		

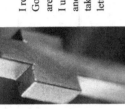

Captain's Log Statement of Faith

I realize that my actions don't earn my way into God's love or earn my way to heaven but that they are a reflection of my love affair with Jesus! I understand that by taking care of myself I honor and glorify God. I matter to God and the actions I take toward good health are daily written love letters telling God, "Thank you for my life"!

_____
Signature

Resistance Training

Time of day: _____

Warmed up   Yes _____   No _____

Name of exercise 1:

	Weight:	Reps:
Set 1:		
Set 2:		
Set 3:		
Set 4:		

Muscles worked: _____

Stretched?   Yes _____   No _____

Name of exercise 2:

	Weight:	Reps:
Set 1:		
Set 2:		
Set 3:		
Set 4:		

Muscles worked: _____

Stretched?   Yes _____   No _____

Name of exercise 3:

	Weight:	Reps:
Set 1:		
Set 2:		
Set 3:		
Set 4:		

Muscles worked: _____

Stretched?   Yes _____   No _____

Name of exercise 4:

	Weight:	Reps:
Set 1:		
Set 2:		
Set 3:		
Set 4:		

Muscles worked: _____

Stretched?   Yes _____   No _____

Name of exercise 5:

	Weight:	Reps:
Set 1:		
Set 2:		
Set 3:		
Set 4:		

Muscles worked: _____

Stretched?   Yes _____   No _____

Name of exercise 6:

	Weight:	Reps:
Set 1:		
Set 2:		
Set 3:		
Set 4:		

Muscles worked: _____

Stretched?   Yes _____   No _____

Name of exercise 7:

	Weight:	Reps:
Set 1:		
Set 2:		
Set 3:		
Set 4:		

Muscles worked: _____

Stretched?   Yes _____   No _____

Name of exercise 8:

	Weight:	Reps:
Set 1:		
Set 2:		
Set 3:		
Set 4:		

Muscles worked: _____

Stretched?   Yes _____   No _____

Name of exercise 9:

	Weight:	Reps:
Set 1:		
Set 2:		
Set 3:		
Set 4:		

Muscles worked: _____

Stretched?   Yes _____   No _____

Name of exercise 10:

	Weight:	Reps:
Set 1:		
Set 2:		
Set 3:		
Set 4:		

Muscles worked: _____

Stretched?   Yes _____   No _____

"I press on toward the goal to win the prize for which God has called me heavenward in Christ Jesus."
Philippians 3:14

Captain's Log

Day: _____   Date: _____ / _____ / _____

Nutrition Log

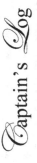
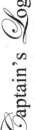

BREAKFAST   Time: _____

	Type 1	Amt:	Type 2	Amt:
Protein				
Complex Carbs				
Fruit				
Vegetables				
Fat				
Liquid/drink				
Meal Replace.				
Condiments				
Other				

LUNCH   Time: _____

	Type 1	Amt:	Type 2	Amt:
Protein				
Complex Carbs				
Fruit				
Vegetables				
Fat				
Liquid/drink				
Meal Replace.				
Condiments				
Other				

SNACK 3   Time: _____

	Type 1	Amt:	Type 2	Amt:
Protein				
Complex Carbs				
Fruit				
Vegetables				
Fat				
Liquid/drink				
Meal Replace.				
Condiments				
Other				

SNACK 1   Time: _____

	Type 1	Amt:	Type 2	Amt:
Protein				
Complex Carbs				
Fruit				
Vegetables				
Fat				
Liquid/drink				
Meal Replace.				
Condiments				
Other				

SNACK 2   Time: _____

	Type 1	Amt:	Type 2	Amt:
Protein				
Complex Carbs				
Fruit				
Vegetables				
Fat				
Liquid/drink				
Meal Replace.				
Condiments				
Other				

DINNER   Time: _____

	Type 1	Amt:	Type 2	Amt:
Protein				
Complex Carbs				
Fruit				
Vegetables				
Fat				
Liquid/drink				
Meal Replace.				
Condiments				
Other				

Cardiovascular Training

Warmed up   Yes _____   No _____

Time of day: _____	For how long?	Heart Rate
Type 1: _____	_____	_____
Type 2: _____	_____	_____
Type 3: _____	_____	_____
Type 4: _____	_____	_____
Stretched? Yes _____ No _____		

Evening Reflection

Did I put my faith in Action today?	Yes _____	No _____
I prayed for somone today	Yes _____	No _____
I read my Bible today	Yes _____	No _____
I helped someone in need today	Yes _____	No _____
I got 6 1/2 to 8 hours of sleep last night	Yes _____	No _____
I know I ate right today	Yes _____	No _____
I ate breakfast today	Yes _____	No _____
I ate starches after 4:00 p.m. today	Yes _____	No _____
I ate at least 4 meals today	Yes _____	No _____
I drank at least a gallon of water today	Yes _____	No _____
I had Courage to Change today	Yes _____	No _____
Tonight I forgive….		

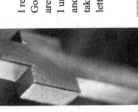

Captain's Log Statement of Faith

I realize that my actions don't earn my way into God's love or earn my way to heaven but that they are a reflection of my love affair with Jesus! I understand that by taking care of myself I honor and glorify God. I matter to God and the actions I take toward good health are daily written love letters telling God, "Thank you for my life"!

_____   **Signature**

Resistance Training

Time of day: _____

Warmed up   Yes _____   No _____

Name of exercise 1: _____   Weight: _____   Reps: _____

Set 1: _____
Set 2: _____
Set 3: _____
Set 4: _____

Muscles worked: _____

Stretched?   Yes _____   No _____

Name of exercise 2: _____   Weight: _____   Reps: _____

Set 1: _____
Set 2: _____
Set 3: _____
Set 4: _____

Muscles worked: _____

Stretched?   Yes _____   No _____

Name of exercise 3: _____   Weight: _____   Reps: _____

Set 1: _____
Set 2: _____
Set 3: _____
Set 4: _____

Muscles worked: _____

Stretched?   Yes _____   No _____

Name of exercise 4: _____   Weight: _____   Reps: _____

Set 1: _____
Set 2: _____
Set 3: _____
Set 4: _____

Muscles worked: _____

Stretched?   Yes _____   No _____

Name of exercise 5: _____   Weight: _____   Reps: _____

Set 1: _____
Set 2: _____
Set 3: _____
Set 4: _____

Muscles worked: _____

Stretched?   Yes _____   No _____

Name of exercise 6: _____   Weight: _____   Reps: _____

Set 1: _____
Set 2: _____
Set 3: _____
Set 4: _____

Muscles worked: _____

Stretched?   Yes _____   No _____

Name of exercise 7: _____   Weight: _____   Reps: _____

Set 1: _____
Set 2: _____
Set 3: _____
Set 4: _____

Muscles worked: _____

Stretched?   Yes _____   No _____

Name of exercise 8: _____   Weight: _____   Reps: _____

Set 1: _____
Set 2: _____
Set 3: _____
Set 4: _____

Muscles worked: _____

Stretched?   Yes _____   No _____

Name of exercise 9: _____   Weight: _____   Reps: _____

Set 1: _____
Set 2: _____
Set 3: _____
Set 4: _____

Muscles worked: _____

Stretched?   Yes _____   No _____

Name of exercise 10: _____   Weight: _____   Reps: _____

Set 1: _____
Set 2: _____
Set 3: _____
Set 4: _____

Muscles worked: _____

Stretched?   Yes _____   No _____

"I press on toward the goal to win the prize for which God has called me heavenward in Christ Jesus."
Philippians 3:14

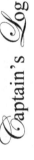

Captain's Log

"Each one should test his own actions. Then he can take pride in himself without comparing himself to somebody else, for each one should carry his own load." (Galatians 6:40)

Day: _____   Date: ____/____/____

Nutrition Log

BREAKFAST   Time: _____

	Amt:	Type		Amt:
Protein	1.	2.		
Complex Carbs	1.	2.		
Fruit	1.	2.		
Vegetables	1.	2.		
Fat	1.	2.		
Liquid/drink	1.	2.		
Meal Replace.	1.	2.		
Condiments	1.	2.		
Other	1.	2.		

SNACK 1   Time: _____

	Type		Amt:	Type	Amt:
Protein	1.			2.	
Complex Carbs	1.			2.	
Fruit	1.			2.	
Vegetables	1.			2.	
Fat	1.			2.	
Liquid/drink	1.			2.	
Meal Replace.	1.			2.	
Condiments	1.			2.	
Other	1.			2.	

LUNCH   Time: _____

	Amt:	Type		Amt:
Protein	1.	2.		
Complex Carbs	1.	2.		
Fruit	1.	2.		
Vegetables	1.	2.		
Fat	1.	2.		
Liquid/drink	1.	2.		
Meal Replace.	1.	2.		
Condiments	1.	2.		
Other	1.	2.		

SNACK 2   Time: _____

	Type		Amt:	Type	Amt:
Protein	1.			2.	
Complex Carbs	1.			2.	
Fruit	1.			2.	
Vegetables	1.			2.	
Fat	1.			2.	
Liquid/drink	1.			2.	
Meal Replace.	1.			2.	
Condiments	1.			2.	
Other	1.			2.	

SNACK 3   Time: _____

	Type		Amt:	Type	Amt:
Protein	1.			2.	
Complex Carbs	1.			2.	
Fruit	1.			2.	
Vegetables	1.			2.	
Fat	1.			2.	
Liquid/drink	1.			2.	
Meal Replace.	1.			2.	
Condiments	1.			2.	
Other	1.			2.	

DINNER   Time: _____

	Type		Amt:	Type	Amt:
Protein	1.			2.	
Complex Carbs	1.			2.	
Fruit	1.			2.	
Vegetables	1.			2.	
Fat	1.			2.	
Liquid/drink	1.			2.	
Meal Replace.	1.			2.	
Condiments	1.			2.	
Other	1.			2.	

Cardiovascular Training

Warmed up   Yes _____   No _____

Time of day: _____	For how long?	Heart Rate
Type 1: _____	_____	_____
Type 2: _____	_____	_____
Type 3: _____	_____	_____
Type 4: _____	_____	_____
Stretched?	Yes _____	No _____

Evening Reflection

Did I put my faith in Action today?	Yes _____	No _____
I prayed for somone today	Yes _____	No _____
I read my Bible today	Yes _____	No _____
I helped someone in need today	Yes _____	No _____
I got 6 1/2 to 8 hours of sleep last night	Yes _____	No _____
I know I ate right today	Yes _____	No _____
I ate breakfast today	Yes _____	No _____
I ate starches after 4:00 p.m. today	Yes _____	No _____
I ate at least 4 meals today	Yes _____	No _____
I drank at least a gallon of water today	Yes _____	No _____
I had Courage to Change today	Yes _____	No _____
Tonight I forgive…		

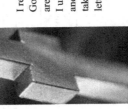

Captain's Log Statement of Faith

I realize that my actions don't earn my way into God's love or earn my way to heaven but that they are a reflection of my love affair with Jesus! I understand that by taking care of myself I honor and glorify God. I matter to God and the actions I take toward good health are daily written love letters telling God, "Thank you for my life"!

_____
Signature

Resistance Training

Time of day: _____

Warmed up   Yes _____   No _____

Name of exercise 1: _____	Weight:	Reps:
	Set 1: _____	_____
	Set 2: _____	_____
Muscles worked: _____	Set 3: _____	_____
_____	Set 4: _____	_____
Stretched? Yes _____	No _____	

Name of exercise 2: _____	Weight:	Reps:
	Set 1: _____	_____
	Set 2: _____	_____
Muscles worked: _____	Set 3: _____	_____
_____	Set 4: _____	_____
Stretched? Yes _____	No _____	

Name of exercise 3: _____	Weight:	Reps:
	Set 1: _____	_____
	Set 2: _____	_____
Muscles worked: _____	Set 3: _____	_____
_____	Set 4: _____	_____
Stretched? Yes _____	No _____	

Name of exercise 4: _____	Weight:	Reps:
	Set 1: _____	_____
	Set 2: _____	_____
Muscles worked: _____	Set 3: _____	_____
_____	Set 4: _____	_____
Stretched? Yes _____	No _____	

Name of exercise 5: _____	Weight:	Reps:
	Set 1: _____	_____
	Set 2: _____	_____
Muscles worked: _____	Set 3: _____	_____
_____	Set 4: _____	_____
Stretched? Yes _____	No _____	

Name of exercise 6: _____	Weight:	Reps:
	Set 1: _____	_____
	Set 2: _____	_____
Muscles worked: _____	Set 3: _____	_____
_____	Set 4: _____	_____
Stretched? Yes _____	No _____	

Name of exercise 7: _____	Weight:	Reps:
	Set 1: _____	_____
	Set 2: _____	_____
Muscles worked: _____	Set 3: _____	_____
_____	Set 4: _____	_____
Stretched? Yes _____	No _____	

Name of exercise 8: _____	Weight:	Reps:
	Set 1: _____	_____
	Set 2: _____	_____
Muscles worked: _____	Set 3: _____	_____
_____	Set 4: _____	_____
Stretched? Yes _____	No _____	

Name of exercise 9: _____	Weight:	Reps:
	Set 1: _____	_____
	Set 2: _____	_____
Muscles worked: _____	Set 3: _____	_____
_____	Set 4: _____	_____
Stretched? Yes _____	No _____	

Name of exercise 10: _____	Weight:	Reps:
	Set 1: _____	_____
	Set 2: _____	_____
Muscles worked: _____	Set 3: _____	_____
_____	Set 4: _____	_____
Stretched? Yes _____	No _____	

"I press on toward the goal to win the prize for which God has called me heavenward in Christ Jesus."
Philippians 3:14

Captain's Log

"Each one should test his own actions. Then he can take pride in himself without comparing himself to somebody else, for each one should carry his own load." (Galatians 6:40)

Day: _____ Date: _____ / _____ / _____

Nutrition Log

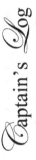
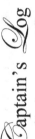

BREAKFAST

Time: _____

	Type	Amt:	Type	Amt:
Protein	1.		2.	
Complex Carbs	1.		2.	
Fruit	1.		2.	
Vegetables	1.		2.	
Fat	1.		2.	
Liquid/drink	1.		2.	
Meal Replace.	1.		2.	
Condiments	1.		2.	
Other	1.		2.	

LUNCH

Time: _____

	Type	Amt:	Type	Amt:
Protein	1.		2.	
Complex Carbs	1.		2.	
Fruit	1.		2.	
Vegetables	1.		2.	
Fat	1.		2.	
Liquid/drink	1.		2.	
Meal Replace.	1.		2.	
Condiments	1.		2.	
Other	1.		2.	

SNACK 3

Time: _____

	Type	Amt:	Type	Amt:
Protein	1.		2.	
Complex Carbs	1.		2.	
Fruit	1.		2.	
Vegetables	1.		2.	
Fat	1.		2.	
Liquid/drink	1.		2.	
Meal Replace.	1.		2.	
Condiments	1.		2.	
Other	1.		2.	

SNACK 1

Time: _____

	Type	Amt:	Type	Amt:
Protein	1.		2.	
Complex Carbs	1.		2.	
Fruit	1.		2.	
Vegetables	1.		2.	
Fat	1.		2.	
Liquid/drink	1.		2.	
Meal Replace.	1.		2.	
Condiments	1.		2.	
Other	1.		2.	

SNACK 2

Time: _____

	Type	Amt:	Type	Amt:
Protein	1.		2.	
Complex Carbs	1.		2.	
Fruit	1.		2.	
Vegetables	1.		2.	
Fat	1.		2.	
Liquid/drink	1.		2.	
Meal Replace.	1.		2.	
Condiments	1.		2.	
Other	1.		2.	

DINNER

Time: _____

	Type	Amt:	Type	Amt:
Protein	1.		2.	
Complex Carbs	1.		2.	
Fruit	1.		2.	
Vegetables	1.		2.	
Fat	1.		2.	
Liquid/drink	1.		2.	
Meal Replace.	1.		2.	
Condiments	1.		2.	
Other	1.		2.	

Resistance Training

Time of day: _____
Warmed up   Yes _____   No _____

Name of exercise 1:
_____
_____

	Weight:	Reps:
Set 1:	_____	_____
Set 2:	_____	_____
Set 3:	_____	_____
Set 4:	_____	_____

Muscles worked:
_____
_____

Stretched?   Yes _____   No _____

Name of exercise 3:
_____
_____

	Weight:	Reps:
Set 1:	_____	_____
Set 2:	_____	_____
Set 3:	_____	_____
Set 4:	_____	_____

Muscles worked:
_____
_____

Stretched?   Yes _____   No _____

Name of exercise 5:
_____
_____

	Weight:	Reps:
Set 1:	_____	_____
Set 2:	_____	_____
Set 3:	_____	_____
Set 4:	_____	_____

Muscles worked:
_____
_____

Stretched?   Yes _____   No _____

Name of exercise 7:
_____
_____

	Weight:	Reps:
Set 1:	_____	_____
Set 2:	_____	_____
Set 3:	_____	_____
Set 4:	_____	_____

Muscles worked:
_____
_____

Stretched?   Yes _____   No _____

Name of exercise 9:
_____
_____

	Weight:	Reps:
Set 1:	_____	_____
Set 2:	_____	_____
Set 3:	_____	_____
Set 4:	_____	_____

Muscles worked:
_____
_____

Stretched?   Yes _____   No _____

Cardiovascular Training

Warmed up   Yes _____   No _____

Time of day: _____	For how long?	Heart Rate
Type 1: _____	_____	_____
Type 2: _____	_____	_____
Type 3: _____	_____	_____
Type 4: _____	_____	_____

Stretched?   Yes _____   No _____

Name of exercise 2:
_____
_____

	Weight:	Reps:
Set 1:	_____	_____
Set 2:	_____	_____
Set 3:	_____	_____
Set 4:	_____	_____

Muscles worked:
_____
_____

Stretched?   Yes _____   No _____

Name of exercise 4:
_____
_____

	Weight:	Reps:
Set 1:	_____	_____
Set 2:	_____	_____
Set 3:	_____	_____
Set 4:	_____	_____

Muscles worked:
_____
_____

Stretched?   Yes _____   No _____

Name of exercise 6:
_____
_____

	Weight:	Reps:
Set 1:	_____	_____
Set 2:	_____	_____
Set 3:	_____	_____
Set 4:	_____	_____

Muscles worked:
_____
_____

Stretched?   Yes _____   No _____

Name of exercise 8:
_____
_____

	Weight:	Reps:
Set 1:	_____	_____
Set 2:	_____	_____
Set 3:	_____	_____
Set 4:	_____	_____

Muscles worked:
_____
_____

Stretched?   Yes _____   No _____

Name of exercise 10:
_____
_____

	Weight:	Reps:
Set 1:	_____	_____
Set 2:	_____	_____
Set 3:	_____	_____
Set 4:	_____	_____

Muscles worked:
_____
_____

Stretched?   Yes _____   No _____

Evening Reflection

Did I put my faith in Action today?	Yes _____	No _____
I prayed for somone today	Yes _____	No _____
I read my Bible today	Yes _____	No _____
I helped someone in need today	Yes _____	No _____
I got 6 1/2 to 8 hours of sleep last night	Yes _____	No _____
I know I ate right today	Yes _____	No _____
I ate breakfast today	Yes _____	No _____
I ate starches after 4:00 p.m. today	Yes _____	No _____
I ate at least 4 meals today	Yes _____	No _____
I drank at least a gallon of water today	Yes _____	No _____
I had Courage to Change today	Yes _____	No _____

Tonight I forgive… _____

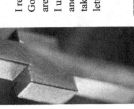

Captain's Log Statement of Faith

I realize that my actions don't earn my way into God's love or earn my way to heaven but that they are a reflection of my love affair with Jesus! I understand that by taking care of myself I honor and glorify God. I matter to God and the actions I take toward good health are daily written love letters telling God, "Thank you for my life"!

_____
Signature

"I press on toward the goal to win the prize for which God has called me heavenward in Christ Jesus."
Philippians 3:14

COMMITMENT & FORGIVENESS

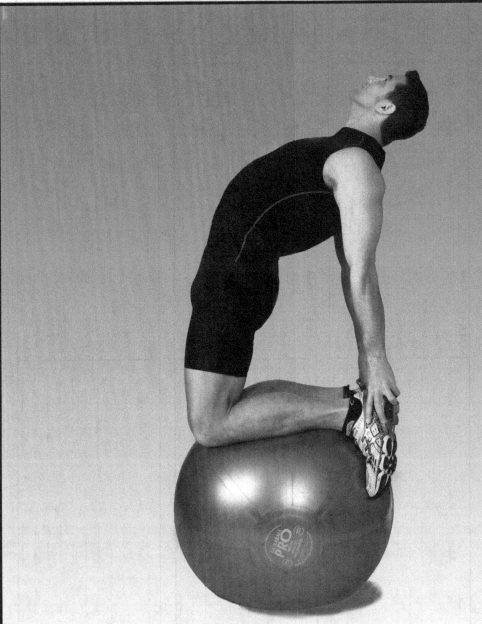

"But your hearts must be fully committed to the LORD our God, to live by his decrees and obey his commands, as at this time." (1 Kings 8:61)
"Bear with each other and forgive whatever grievances you may have against one another. Forgive as the Lord forgave you. And over all these virtues put on love, which binds them all together in perfect unity." (Colossians 3:13-14)

WEEK TWO

Captain's Log

Day: _____   Date: _____ / _____ / _____

Nutrition Log

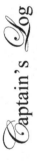

BREAKFAST   Time: _____

	Type	Amt:		Type	Amt:
Protein	1.			2.	
Complex Carbs	1.			2.	
Fruit	1.			2.	
Vegetables	1.			2.	
Fat	1.			2.	
Liquid/drink	1.			2.	
Meal Replace.	1.			2.	
Condiments	1.			2.	
Other	1.			2.	

LUNCH   Time: _____

	Type	Amt:		Type	Amt:
Protein	1.			2.	
Complex Carbs	1.			2.	
Fruit	1.			2.	
Vegetables	1.			2.	
Fat	1.			2.	
Liquid/drink	1.			2.	
Meal Replace.	1.			2.	
Condiments	1.			2.	
Other	1.			2.	

SNACK 3   Time: _____

	Type	Amt:		Type	Amt:
Protein	1.			2.	
Complex Carbs	1.			2.	
Fruit	1.			2.	
Vegetables	1.			2.	
Fat	1.			2.	
Liquid/drink	1.			2.	
Meal Replace.	1.			2.	
Condiments	1.			2.	
Other	1.			2.	

SNACK 1   Time: _____

	Type	Amt:		Type	Amt:
Protein	1.			2.	
Complex Carbs	1.			2.	
Fruit	1.			2.	
Vegetables	1.			2.	
Fat	1.			2.	
Liquid/drink	1.			2.	
Meal Replace.	1.			2.	
Condiments	1.			2.	
Other	1.			2.	

SNACK 2   Time: _____

	Type	Amt:		Type	Amt:
Protein	1.			2.	
Complex Carbs	1.			2.	
Fruit	1.			2.	
Vegetables	1.			2.	
Fat	1.			2.	
Liquid/drink	1.			2.	
Meal Replace.	1.			2.	
Condiments	1.			2.	
Other	1.			2.	

DINNER   Time: _____

	Type	Amt:		Type	Amt:
Protein	1.			2.	
Complex Carbs	1.			2.	
Fruit	1.			2.	
Vegetables	1.			2.	
Fat	1.			2.	
Liquid/drink	1.			2.	
Meal Replace.	1.			2.	
Condiments	1.			2.	
Other	1.			2.	

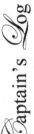

Cardiovascular Training

Warmed up   Yes_____   No_____

Time of day: _____

	For how long?	Heart Rate
Type 1:	_____	_____
Type 2:	_____	_____
Type 3:	_____	_____
Type 4:	_____	_____

Stretched?   Yes_____   No_____

Evening Reflection

Did I put my faith in Action today?	Yes_____	No_____
I prayed for somone today	Yes_____	No_____
I read my Bible today	Yes_____	No_____
I helped someone in need today	Yes_____	No_____
I got 6 1/2 to 8 hours of sleep last night	Yes_____	No_____
I know I ate right today	Yes_____	No_____
I ate breakfast today	Yes_____	No_____
I ate starches after 4:00 p.m. today	Yes_____	No_____
I ate at least 4 meals today	Yes_____	No_____
I drank at least a gallon of water today	Yes_____	No_____
I had Courage to Change today	Yes_____	No_____
Tonight I forgive…		

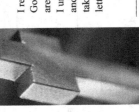

Captain's Log Statement of Faith

I realize that my actions don't earn my way into God's love or earn my way to heaven but that they are a reflection of my love affair with Jesus! I understand that by taking care of myself I honor and glorify God. I matter to God and the actions I take toward good health are daily written love letters telling God, "Thank you for my life"!

_____
Signature

Resistance Training

Time of day: _____   Warmed up   Yes_____   No_____

Name of exercise 1:

	Weight:	Reps:
Set 1:	_____	_____
Set 2:	_____	_____
Set 3:	_____	_____
Set 4:	_____	_____

Muscles worked: _____

Stretched?   Yes_____   No_____

Name of exercise 2:

	Weight:	Reps:
Set 1:	_____	_____
Set 2:	_____	_____
Set 3:	_____	_____
Set 4:	_____	_____

Muscles worked: _____

Stretched?   Yes_____   No_____

Name of exercise 3:

	Weight:	Reps:
Set 1:	_____	_____
Set 2:	_____	_____
Set 3:	_____	_____
Set 4:	_____	_____

Muscles worked: _____

Stretched?   Yes_____   No_____

Name of exercise 4:

	Weight:	Reps:
Set 1:	_____	_____
Set 2:	_____	_____
Set 3:	_____	_____
Set 4:	_____	_____

Muscles worked: _____

Stretched?   Yes_____   No_____

Name of exercise 5:

	Weight:	Reps:
Set 1:	_____	_____
Set 2:	_____	_____
Set 3:	_____	_____
Set 4:	_____	_____

Muscles worked: _____

Stretched?   Yes_____   No_____

Name of exercise 6:

	Weight:	Reps:
Set 1:	_____	_____
Set 2:	_____	_____
Set 3:	_____	_____
Set 4:	_____	_____

Muscles worked: _____

Stretched?   Yes_____   No_____

Name of exercise 7:

	Weight:	Reps:
Set 1:	_____	_____
Set 2:	_____	_____
Set 3:	_____	_____
Set 4:	_____	_____

Muscles worked: _____

Stretched?   Yes_____   No_____

Name of exercise 8:

	Weight:	Reps:
Set 1:	_____	_____
Set 2:	_____	_____
Set 3:	_____	_____
Set 4:	_____	_____

Muscles worked: _____

Stretched?   Yes_____   No_____

Name of exercise 9:

	Weight:	Reps:
Set 1:	_____	_____
Set 2:	_____	_____
Set 3:	_____	_____
Set 4:	_____	_____

Muscles worked: _____

Stretched?   Yes_____   No_____

Name of exercise 10:

	Weight:	Reps:
Set 1:	_____	_____
Set 2:	_____	_____
Set 3:	_____	_____
Set 4:	_____	_____

Muscles worked: _____

Stretched?   Yes_____   No_____

"I press on toward the goal to win the prize for which God has called me heavenward in Christ Jesus."
Philippians 3:14

Captain's Log

"Each one should test his own actions. Then he can take pride in himself without comparing himself to somebody else, for each one should carry his own load." (Galatians 6:40)

Day: _____   Date: _____ / _____ / _____

Nutrition Log

BREAKFAST   Time: _____

	Type	Amt:		Type	Amt:
Protein	1. ___ 2. ___				
Complex Carbs	1. ___ 2. ___				
Fruit	1. ___ 2. ___				
Vegetables	1. ___ 2. ___				
Fat	1. ___ 2. ___				
Liquid/drink	1. ___ 2. ___				
Meal Replace.	1. ___ 2. ___				
Condiments	1. ___ 2. ___				
Other	1. ___ 2. ___				

LUNCH   Time: _____

	Type	Amt:
Protein	1. ___ 2. ___	
Complex Carbs	1. ___ 2. ___	
Fruit	1. ___ 2. ___	
Vegetables	1. ___ 2. ___	
Fat	1. ___ 2. ___	
Liquid/drink	1. ___ 2. ___	
Meal Replace.	1. ___ 2. ___	
Condiments	1. ___ 2. ___	
Other	1. ___ 2. ___	

SNACK 3   Time: _____

	Type	Amt:
Protein	1. ___ 2. ___	
Complex Carbs	1. ___ 2. ___	
Fruit	1. ___ 2. ___	
Vegetables	1. ___ 2. ___	
Fat	1. ___ 2. ___	
Liquid/drink	1. ___ 2. ___	
Meal Replace.	1. ___ 2. ___	
Condiments	1. ___ 2. ___	
Other	1. ___ 2. ___	

SNACK 1   Time: _____

	Type	Amt:
Protein	1. ___ 2. ___	
Complex Carbs	1. ___ 2. ___	
Fruit	1. ___ 2. ___	
Vegetables	1. ___ 2. ___	
Fat	1. ___ 2. ___	
Liquid/drink	1. ___ 2. ___	
Meal Replace.	1. ___ 2. ___	
Condiments	1. ___ 2. ___	
Other	1. ___ 2. ___	

SNACK 2   Time: _____

	Type	Amt:
Protein	1. ___ 2. ___	
Complex Carbs	1. ___ 2. ___	
Fruit	1. ___ 2. ___	
Vegetables	1. ___ 2. ___	
Fat	1. ___ 2. ___	
Liquid/drink	1. ___ 2. ___	
Meal Replace.	1. ___ 2. ___	
Condiments	1. ___ 2. ___	
Other	1. ___ 2. ___	

DINNER   Time: _____

	Type	Amt:
Protein	1. ___ 2. ___	
Complex Carbs	1. ___ 2. ___	
Fruit	1. ___ 2. ___	
Vegetables	1. ___ 2. ___	
Fat	1. ___ 2. ___	
Liquid/drink	1. ___ 2. ___	
Meal Replace.	1. ___ 2. ___	
Condiments	1. ___ 2. ___	
Other	1. ___ 2. ___	

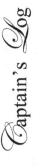
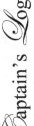

Resistance Training

Time of day: _____
Warmed up: Yes _____ No _____

Name of exercise 1: _____
Weight: _____ Reps: _____
Set 1: _____
Set 2: _____
Set 3: _____
Set 4: _____
Muscles worked: _____
Stretched? Yes _____ No _____

Name of exercise 3: _____
Weight: _____ Reps: _____
Set 1: _____
Set 2: _____
Set 3: _____
Set 4: _____
Muscles worked: _____
Stretched? Yes _____ No _____

Name of exercise 5: _____
Weight: _____ Reps: _____
Set 1: _____
Set 2: _____
Set 3: _____
Set 4: _____
Muscles worked: _____
Stretched? Yes _____ No _____

Name of exercise 7: _____
Weight: _____ Reps: _____
Set 1: _____
Set 2: _____
Set 3: _____
Set 4: _____
Muscles worked: _____
Stretched? Yes _____ No _____

Name of exercise 9: _____
Weight: _____ Reps: _____
Set 1: _____
Set 2: _____
Set 3: _____
Set 4: _____
Muscles worked: _____
Stretched? Yes _____ No _____

Name of exercise 2: _____
Weight: _____ Reps: _____
Set 1: _____
Set 2: _____
Set 3: _____
Set 4: _____
Muscles worked: _____
Stretched? Yes _____ No _____

Name of exercise 4: _____
Weight: _____ Reps: _____
Set 1: _____
Set 2: _____
Set 3: _____
Set 4: _____
Muscles worked: _____
Stretched? Yes _____ No _____

Name of exercise 6: _____
Weight: _____ Reps: _____
Set 1: _____
Set 2: _____
Set 3: _____
Set 4: _____
Muscles worked: _____
Stretched? Yes _____ No _____

Name of exercise 8: _____
Weight: _____ Reps: _____
Set 1: _____
Set 2: _____
Set 3: _____
Set 4: _____
Muscles worked: _____
Stretched? Yes _____ No _____

Name of exercise 10: _____
Weight: _____ Reps: _____
Set 1: _____
Set 2: _____
Set 3: _____
Set 4: _____
Muscles worked: _____
Stretched? Yes _____ No _____

Cardiovascular Training

Warmed up: Yes _____ No _____

Time of day: _____
For how long? _____ Heart Rate _____
Type 1: _____
Type 2: _____
Type 3: _____
Type 4: _____
Stretched? Yes _____ No _____

Evening Reflection

Did I put my faith in Action today?	Yes _____	No _____
I prayed for somone today	Yes _____	No _____
I read my Bible today	Yes _____	No _____
I helped someone in need today	Yes _____	No _____
I got 6 1/2 to 8 hours of sleep last night	Yes _____	No _____
I know I ate right today	Yes _____	No _____
I ate breakfast today	Yes _____	No _____
I ate starches after 4:00 p.m. today	Yes _____	No _____
I ate at least 4 meals today	Yes _____	No _____
I drank at least a gallon of water today	Yes _____	No _____
I had Courage to Change today	Yes _____	No _____
Tonight I forgive… _____		

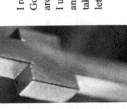

Captain's Log Statement of Faith

I realize that my actions don't earn my way into God's love or earn my way to heaven but that they are a reflection of my love affair with Jesus! I understand that by taking care of myself I honor and glorify God. I matter to God and the actions I take toward good health are daily written love letters telling God, "Thank you for my life"!

_____
Signature

"I press on toward the goal to win the prize for which God has called me heavenward in Christ Jesus."
Philippians 3:14

Captain's Log

"Each one should test his own actions. Then he can take pride in himself without comparing himself to somebody else, for each one should carry his own load." (Galatians 6:40)

Day: _____   Date: _____ / _____ / _____

Nutrition Log

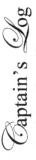

BREAKFAST Time: _____

	Type	Amt:	Type	Amt:
Protein	1._____	_____	2._____	_____
Complex Carbs	1._____	_____	2._____	_____
Fruit	1._____	_____	2._____	_____
Vegetables	1._____	_____	2._____	_____
Fat	1._____	_____	2._____	_____
Liquid/drink	1._____	_____	2._____	_____
Meal Replace.	1._____	_____	2._____	_____
Condiments	1._____	_____	2._____	_____
Other	1._____	_____	2._____	_____

LUNCH Time: _____

	Type	Amt:	Type	Amt:
Protein	1._____	_____	2._____	_____
Complex Carbs	1._____	_____	2._____	_____
Fruit	1._____	_____	2._____	_____
Vegetables	1._____	_____	2._____	_____
Fat	1._____	_____	2._____	_____
Liquid/drink	1._____	_____	2._____	_____
Meal Replace.	1._____	_____	2._____	_____
Condiments	1._____	_____	2._____	_____
Other	1._____	_____	2._____	_____

SNACK 3 Time: _____

	Type	Amt:	Type	Amt:
Protein	1._____	_____	2._____	_____
Complex Carbs	1._____	_____	2._____	_____
Fruit	1._____	_____	2._____	_____
Vegetables	1._____	_____	2._____	_____
Fat	1._____	_____	2._____	_____
Liquid/drink	1._____	_____	2._____	_____
Meal Replace.	1._____	_____	2._____	_____
Condiments	1._____	_____	2._____	_____
Other	1._____	_____	2._____	_____

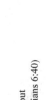

SNACK 1 Time: _____

	Type	Amt:	Type	Amt:
Protein	1._____	_____	2._____	_____
Complex Carbs	1._____	_____	2._____	_____
Fruit	1._____	_____	2._____	_____
Vegetables	1._____	_____	2._____	_____
Fat	1._____	_____	2._____	_____
Liquid/drink	1._____	_____	2._____	_____
Meal Replace.	1._____	_____	2._____	_____
Condiments	1._____	_____	2._____	_____
Other	1._____	_____	2._____	_____

SNACK 2 Time: _____

	Type	Amt:	Type	Amt:
Protein	1._____	_____	2._____	_____
Complex Carbs	1._____	_____	2._____	_____
Fruit	1._____	_____	2._____	_____
Vegetables	1._____	_____	2._____	_____
Fat	1._____	_____	2._____	_____
Liquid/drink	1._____	_____	2._____	_____
Meal Replace.	1._____	_____	2._____	_____
Condiments	1._____	_____	2._____	_____
Other	1._____	_____	2._____	_____

DINNER Time: _____

	Type	Amt:	Type	Amt:
Protein	1._____	_____	2._____	_____
Complex Carbs	1._____	_____	2._____	_____
Fruit	1._____	_____	2._____	_____
Vegetables	1._____	_____	2._____	_____
Fat	1._____	_____	2._____	_____
Liquid/drink	1._____	_____	2._____	_____
Meal Replace.	1._____	_____	2._____	_____
Condiments	1._____	_____	2._____	_____
Other	1._____	_____	2._____	_____

Resistance Training

Time of day: _____

Warmed up   Yes _____   No _____

Name of exercise 1: _____

	Weight:	Reps:
Set 1:		
Set 2:		
Set 3:		
Set 4:		

Muscles worked: _____

Stretched?   Yes _____   No _____

Name of exercise 3: _____

	Weight:	Reps:
Set 1:		
Set 2:		
Set 3:		
Set 4:		

Muscles worked: _____

Stretched?   Yes _____   No _____

Name of exercise 5: _____

	Weight:	Reps:
Set 1:		
Set 2:		
Set 3:		
Set 4:		

Muscles worked: _____

Stretched?   Yes _____   No _____

Name of exercise 7: _____

	Weight:	Reps:
Set 1:		
Set 2:		
Set 3:		
Set 4:		

Muscles worked: _____

Stretched?   Yes _____   No _____

Name of exercise 9: _____

	Weight:	Reps:
Set 1:		
Set 2:		
Set 3:		
Set 4:		

Muscles worked: _____

Stretched?   Yes _____   No _____

Name of exercise 2: _____

	Weight:	Reps:
Set 1:		
Set 2:		
Set 3:		
Set 4:		

Muscles worked: _____

Stretched?   Yes _____   No _____

Name of exercise 4: _____

	Weight:	Reps:
Set 1:		
Set 2:		
Set 3:		
Set 4:		

Muscles worked: _____

Stretched?   Yes _____   No _____

Name of exercise 6: _____

	Weight:	Reps:
Set 1:		
Set 2:		
Set 3:		
Set 4:		

Muscles worked: _____

Stretched?   Yes _____   No _____

Name of exercise 8: _____

	Weight:	Reps:
Set 1:		
Set 2:		
Set 3:		
Set 4:		

Muscles worked: _____

Stretched?   Yes _____   No _____

Name of exercise 10: _____

	Weight:	Reps:
Set 1:		
Set 2:		
Set 3:		
Set 4:		

Muscles worked: _____

Stretched?   Yes _____   No _____

Cardiovascular Training

Warmed up   Yes _____   No _____

Time of day: _____

	For how long?	Heart Rate
Type 1:		
Type 2:		
Type 3:		
Type 4:		

Stretched?   Yes _____   No _____

Evening Reflection

Did I put my faith in Action today?	Yes _____	No _____
I prayed for somone today	Yes _____	No _____
I read my Bible today	Yes _____	No _____
I helped someone in need today	Yes _____	No _____
I got 6 1/2 to 8 hours of sleep last night	Yes _____	No _____
I know I ate right today	Yes _____	No _____
I ate breakfast today	Yes _____	No _____
I ate starches after 4:00 p.m. today	Yes _____	No _____
I ate at least 4 meals today	Yes _____	No _____
I drank at least a gallon of water today	Yes _____	No _____
I had Courage to Change today	Yes _____	No _____

Tonight I forgive… _____

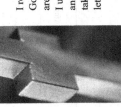

Captain's Log Statement of Faith

I realize that my actions don't earn my way into God's love or earn my way to heaven but that they are a reflection of my love affair with Jesus! I understand that by taking care of myself I honor and glorify God. I matter to God and the actions I take toward good health are daily written love letters telling God, "Thank you for my life"!

_____
Signature

"I press on toward the goal to win the prize for which God has called me heavenward in Christ Jesus."

Philippians 3:14

Captain's Log

"Each one should test his own actions. Then he can take pride in himself without comparing himself to somebody else, for each one should carry his own load." (Galatians 6:40)

Day: _____   Date: _____ / _____ / _____

Nutrition Log

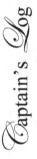
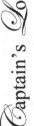

BREAKFAST   Time: _____

	Type	Amt:		Type	Amt:
Protein	1.			2.	
Complex Carbs	1.			2.	
Fruit	1.			2.	
Vegetables	1.			2.	
Fat	1.			2.	
Liquid/drink	1.			2.	
Meal Replace.	1.			2.	
Condiments	1.			2.	
Other	1.			2.	

SNACK 1   Time: _____

	Type	Amt:		Type	Amt:
Protein	1.			2.	
Complex Carbs	1.			2.	
Fruit	1.			2.	
Vegetables	1.			2.	
Fat	1.			2.	
Liquid/drink	1.			2.	
Meal Replace.	1.			2.	
Condiments	1.			2.	
Other	1.			2.	

LUNCH   Time: _____

	Type	Amt:		Type	Amt:
Protein	1.			2.	
Complex Carbs	1.			2.	
Fruit	1.			2.	
Vegetables	1.			2.	
Fat	1.			2.	
Liquid/drink	1.			2.	
Meal Replace.	1.			2.	
Condiments	1.			2.	
Other	1.			2.	

SNACK 2   Time: _____

	Type	Amt:		Type	Amt:
Protein	1.			2.	
Complex Carbs	1.			2.	
Fruit	1.			2.	
Vegetables	1.			2.	
Fat	1.			2.	
Liquid/drink	1.			2.	
Meal Replace.	1.			2.	
Condiments	1.			2.	
Other	1.			2.	

SNACK 3   Time: _____

	Type	Amt:		Type	Amt:
Protein	1.			2.	
Complex Carbs	1.			2.	
Fruit	1.			2.	
Vegetables	1.			2.	
Fat	1.			2.	
Liquid/drink	1.			2.	
Meal Replace.	1.			2.	
Condiments	1.			2.	
Other	1.			2.	

DINNER   Time: _____

	Type	Amt:		Type	Amt:
Protein	1.			2.	
Complex Carbs	1.			2.	
Fruit	1.			2.	
Vegetables	1.			2.	
Fat	1.			2.	
Liquid/drink	1.			2.	
Meal Replace.	1.			2.	
Condiments	1.			2.	
Other	1.			2.	

Resistance Training

Time of day: _____
Warmed up   Yes _____   No _____

Name of exercise 1: _____   Weight: _____   Reps: _____
_____   Set 1: _____
_____   Set 2: _____
Muscles worked: _____   Set 3: _____
_____   Set 4: _____
Stretched?   Yes _____   No _____

Name of exercise 3: _____   Weight: _____   Reps: _____
_____   Set 1: _____
_____   Set 2: _____
Muscles worked: _____   Set 3: _____
_____   Set 4: _____
Stretched?   Yes _____   No _____

Name of exercise 5: _____   Weight: _____   Reps: _____
_____   Set 1: _____
_____   Set 2: _____
Muscles worked: _____   Set 3: _____
_____   Set 4: _____
Stretched?   Yes _____   No _____

Name of exercise 7: _____   Weight: _____   Reps: _____
_____   Set 1: _____
_____   Set 2: _____
Muscles worked: _____   Set 3: _____
_____   Set 4: _____
Stretched?   Yes _____   No _____

Name of exercise 9: _____   Weight: _____   Reps: _____
_____   Set 1: _____
_____   Set 2: _____
Muscles worked: _____   Set 3: _____
_____   Set 4: _____
Stretched?   Yes _____   No _____

Cardiovascular Training

Warmed up   Yes _____   No _____

Time of day: _____	For how long?	Heart Rate
Type 1: _____	_____	_____
Type 2: _____	_____	_____
Type 3: _____	_____	_____
Type 4: _____	_____	_____
Stretched? Yes _____ No _____		

Evening Reflection

Did I put my faith in Action today?	Yes _____	No _____
I prayed for somone today	Yes _____	No _____
I read my Bible today	Yes _____	No _____
I helped someone in need today	Yes _____	No _____
I got 6 1/2 to 8 hours of sleep last night	Yes _____	No _____
I know I ate right today	Yes _____	No _____
I ate breakfast today	Yes _____	No _____
I ate starches after 4:00 p.m. today	Yes _____	No _____
I ate at least 4 meals today	Yes _____	No _____
I drank at least a gallon of water today	Yes _____	No _____
I had Courage to Change today	Yes _____	No _____
Tonight I forgive…		

Name of exercise 2: _____   Weight: _____   Reps: _____
_____   Set 1: _____
_____   Set 2: _____
Muscles worked: _____   Set 3: _____
_____   Set 4: _____
Stretched?   Yes _____   No _____

Name of exercise 4: _____   Weight: _____   Reps: _____
_____   Set 1: _____
_____   Set 2: _____
Muscles worked: _____   Set 3: _____
_____   Set 4: _____
Stretched?   Yes _____   No _____

Name of exercise 6: _____   Weight: _____   Reps: _____
_____   Set 1: _____
_____   Set 2: _____
Muscles worked: _____   Set 3: _____
_____   Set 4: _____
Stretched?   Yes _____   No _____

Name of exercise 8: _____   Weight: _____   Reps: _____
_____   Set 1: _____
_____   Set 2: _____
Muscles worked: _____   Set 3: _____
_____   Set 4: _____
Stretched?   Yes _____   No _____

Name of exercise 10: _____   Weight: _____   Reps: _____
_____   Set 1: _____
_____   Set 2: _____
Muscles worked: _____   Set 3: _____
_____   Set 4: _____
Stretched?   Yes _____   No _____

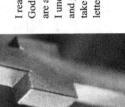

Captain's Log Statement of Faith

I realize that my actions don't earn my way into God's love or earn my way to heaven but that they are a reflection of my love affair with Jesus! I understand that by taking care of myself I honor and glorify God. I matter to God and the actions I take toward good health are daily written love letters telling God, "Thank you for my life"!

_____
Signature

"I press on toward the goal to win the prize for which God has called me heavenward in Christ Jesus."
Philippians 3:14

Captain's Log

"Each one should test his own actions. Then he can take pride in himself without comparing himself to somebody else, for each one should carry his own load." (Galatians 6:40)

Day: _____ Date: _____ / _____ / _____

Nutrition Log

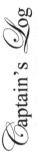
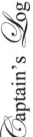

BREAKFAST Time: _____

	Type 1.	Amt:	Type 2.	Amt:
Protein				
Complex Carbs				
Fruit				
Vegetables				
Fat				
Liquid/drink				
Meal Replace.				
Condiments				
Other				

SNACK 1 Time: _____

	Type 1.	Amt:	Type 2.	Amt:
Protein				
Complex Carbs				
Fruit				
Vegetables				
Fat				
Liquid/drink				
Meal Replace.				
Condiments				
Other				

LUNCH Time: _____

	Type 1.	Amt:	Type 2.	Amt:
Protein				
Complex Carbs				
Fruit				
Vegetables				
Fat				
Liquid/drink				
Meal Replace.				
Condiments				
Other				

SNACK 2 Time: _____

	Type 1.	Amt:	Type 2.	Amt:
Protein				
Complex Carbs				
Fruit				
Vegetables				
Fat				
Liquid/drink				
Meal Replace.				
Condiments				
Other				

SNACK 3 Time: _____

	Type 1.	Amt:	Type 2.	Amt:
Protein				
Complex Carbs				
Fruit				
Vegetables				
Fat				
Liquid/drink				
Meal Replace.				
Condiments				
Other				

DINNER Time: _____

	Type 1.	Amt:	Type 2.	Amt:
Protein				
Complex Carbs				
Fruit				
Vegetables				
Fat				
Liquid/drink				
Meal Replace.				
Condiments				
Other				

Cardiovascular Training

Warmed up   Yes _____   No _____

Time of day: _____	For how long?	Heart Rate
Type 1:		
Type 2:		
Type 3:		
Type 4:		

Stretched?   Yes _____   No _____

Evening Reflection

Did I put my faith in Action today?	Yes _____	No _____
I prayed for somone today	Yes _____	No _____
I read my Bible today	Yes _____	No _____
I helped someone in need today	Yes _____	No _____
I got 6 1/2 to 8 hours of sleep last night	Yes _____	No _____
I know I ate right today	Yes _____	No _____
I ate breakfast today	Yes _____	No _____
I ate starches after 4:00 p.m. today	Yes _____	No _____
I ate at least 4 meals today	Yes _____	No _____
I drank at least a gallon of water today	Yes _____	No _____
I had Courage to Change today	Yes _____	No _____

Tonight I forgive…

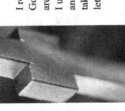

Captain's Log Statement of Faith

I realize that my actions don't earn my way into God's love or earn my way to heaven but that they are a reflection of my love affair with Jesus! I understand that by taking care of myself I honor and glorify God. I matter to God and the actions I take toward good health are daily written love letters telling God, "Thank you for my life"!

_____
Signature

Resistance Training

Time of day: _____

Warmed up   Yes _____   No _____

Name of exercise 1: _____

	Weight:	Reps:
Set 1:		
Set 2:		
Set 3:		
Set 4:		

Muscles worked: _____

Stretched?   Yes _____   No _____

Name of exercise 2: _____

	Weight:	Reps:
Set 1:		
Set 2:		
Set 3:		
Set 4:		

Muscles worked: _____

Stretched?   Yes _____   No _____

Name of exercise 3: _____

	Weight:	Reps:
Set 1:		
Set 2:		
Set 3:		
Set 4:		

Muscles worked: _____

Stretched?   Yes _____   No _____

Name of exercise 4: _____

	Weight:	Reps:
Set 1:		
Set 2:		
Set 3:		
Set 4:		

Muscles worked: _____

Stretched?   Yes _____   No _____

Name of exercise 5: _____

	Weight:	Reps:
Set 1:		
Set 2:		
Set 3:		
Set 4:		

Muscles worked: _____

Stretched?   Yes _____   No _____

Name of exercise 6: _____

	Weight:	Reps:
Set 1:		
Set 2:		
Set 3:		
Set 4:		

Muscles worked: _____

Stretched?   Yes _____   No _____

Name of exercise 7: _____

	Weight:	Reps:
Set 1:		
Set 2:		
Set 3:		
Set 4:		

Muscles worked: _____

Stretched?   Yes _____   No _____

Name of exercise 8: _____

	Weight:	Reps:
Set 1:		
Set 2:		
Set 3:		
Set 4:		

Muscles worked: _____

Stretched?   Yes _____   No _____

Name of exercise 9: _____

	Weight:	Reps:
Set 1:		
Set 2:		
Set 3:		
Set 4:		

Muscles worked: _____

Stretched?   Yes _____   No _____

Name of exercise 10: _____

	Weight:	Reps:
Set 1:		
Set 2:		
Set 3:		
Set 4:		

Muscles worked: _____

Stretched?   Yes _____   No _____

"I press on toward the goal to win the prize for which God has called me heavenward in Christ Jesus."
Philippians 3:14

Captain's Log

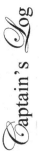
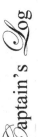

"Each one should test his own actions. Then he can take pride in himself without comparing himself to somebody else, for each one should carry his own load." (Galatians 6:40)

Day: _____   Date: _____ / _____ / _____

Nutrition Log

BREAKFAST	Time: _____		
	Type	Amt:	Type	Amt:
Protein	1. _____		2. _____
Complex Carbs	1. _____		2. _____
Fruit	1. _____		2. _____
Vegetables	1. _____		2. _____
Fat	1. _____		2. _____
Liquid/drink	1. _____		2. _____
Meal Replace.	1. _____		2. _____
Condiments	1. _____		2. _____
Other	1. _____		2. _____

SNACK 1	Time: _____		
	Type	Amt:	Type	Amt:
Protein	1. _____		2. _____
Complex Carbs	1. _____		2. _____
Fruit	1. _____		2. _____
Vegetables	1. _____		2. _____
Fat	1. _____		2. _____
Liquid/drink	1. _____		2. _____
Meal Replace.	1. _____		2. _____
Condiments	1. _____		2. _____
Other	1. _____		2. _____

LUNCH	Time: _____		
	Type	Amt:	Type	Amt:
Protein	1. _____		2. _____
Complex Carbs	1. _____		2. _____
Fruit	1. _____		2. _____
Vegetables	1. _____		2. _____
Fat	1. _____		2. _____
Liquid/drink	1. _____		2. _____
Meal Replace.	1. _____		2. _____
Condiments	1. _____		2. _____
Other	1. _____		2. _____

SNACK 2	Time: _____		
	Type	Amt:	Type	Amt:
Protein	1. _____		2. _____
Complex Carbs	1. _____		2. _____
Fruit	1. _____		2. _____
Vegetables	1. _____		2. _____
Fat	1. _____		2. _____
Liquid/drink	1. _____		2. _____
Meal Replace.	1. _____		2. _____
Condiments	1. _____		2. _____
Other	1. _____		2. _____

SNACK 3	Time: _____		
	Type	Amt:	Type	Amt:
Protein	1. _____		2. _____
Complex Carbs	1. _____		2. _____
Fruit	1. _____		2. _____
Vegetables	1. _____		2. _____
Fat	1. _____		2. _____
Liquid/drink	1. _____		2. _____
Meal Replace.	1. _____		2. _____
Condiments	1. _____		2. _____
Other	1. _____		2. _____

DINNER	Time: _____		
	Type	Amt:	Type	Amt:
Protein	1. _____		2. _____
Complex Carbs	1. _____		2. _____
Fruit	1. _____		2. _____
Vegetables	1. _____		2. _____
Fat	1. _____		2. _____
Liquid/drink	1. _____		2. _____
Meal Replace.	1. _____		2. _____
Condiments	1. _____		2. _____
Other	1. _____		2. _____

Cardiovascular Training

Warmed up   Yes _____   No _____

Time of day: _____	For how long?	Heart Rate
Type 1: _____	_____	_____
Type 2: _____	_____	_____
Type 3: _____	_____	_____
Type 4: _____	_____	_____
Stretched? Yes _____ No _____		

Evening Reflection

Did I put my faith in Action today?	Yes _____	No _____
I prayed for somone today	Yes _____	No _____
I read my Bible today	Yes _____	No _____
I helped someone in need today	Yes _____	No _____
I got 6 1/2 to 8 hours of sleep last night	Yes _____	No _____
I know I ate right today	Yes _____	No _____
I ate breakfast today	Yes _____	No _____
I ate starches after 4:00 p.m. today	Yes _____	No _____
I ate at least 4 meals today	Yes _____	No _____
I drank at least a gallon of water today	Yes _____	No _____
I had Courage to Change today	Yes _____	No _____
Tonight I forgive…		

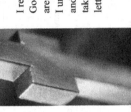

Captain's Log Statement of Faith

I realize that my actions don't earn my way into God's love or earn my way to heaven but that they are a reflection of my love affair with Jesus! I understand that by taking care of myself I honor and glorify God. I matter to God and the actions I take toward good health are daily written love letters telling God, "Thank you for my life"!

_____
Signature

Resistance Training

Time of day: _____

Warmed up   Yes _____   No _____

Name of exercise 1: _____	Weight:	Reps:
	Set 1: _____	_____
	Set 2: _____	_____
Muscles worked: _____	Set 3: _____	_____
	Set 4: _____	_____
Stretched? Yes _____	No _____	

Name of exercise 2: _____	Weight:	Reps:
	Set 1: _____	_____
	Set 2: _____	_____
Muscles worked: _____	Set 3: _____	_____
	Set 4: _____	_____
Stretched? Yes _____	No _____	

Name of exercise 3: _____	Weight:	Reps:
	Set 1: _____	_____
	Set 2: _____	_____
Muscles worked: _____	Set 3: _____	_____
	Set 4: _____	_____
Stretched? Yes _____	No _____	

Name of exercise 4: _____	Weight:	Reps:
	Set 1: _____	_____
	Set 2: _____	_____
Muscles worked: _____	Set 3: _____	_____
	Set 4: _____	_____
Stretched? Yes _____	No _____	

Name of exercise 5: _____	Weight:	Reps:
	Set 1: _____	_____
	Set 2: _____	_____
Muscles worked: _____	Set 3: _____	_____
	Set 4: _____	_____
Stretched? Yes _____	No _____	

Name of exercise 6: _____	Weight:	Reps:
	Set 1: _____	_____
	Set 2: _____	_____
Muscles worked: _____	Set 3: _____	_____
	Set 4: _____	_____
Stretched? Yes _____	No _____	

Name of exercise 7: _____	Weight:	Reps:
	Set 1: _____	_____
	Set 2: _____	_____
Muscles worked: _____	Set 3: _____	_____
	Set 4: _____	_____
Stretched? Yes _____	No _____	

Name of exercise 8: _____	Weight:	Reps:
	Set 1: _____	_____
	Set 2: _____	_____
Muscles worked: _____	Set 3: _____	_____
	Set 4: _____	_____
Stretched? Yes _____	No _____	

Name of exercise 9: _____	Weight:	Reps:
	Set 1: _____	_____
	Set 2: _____	_____
Muscles worked: _____	Set 3: _____	_____
	Set 4: _____	_____
Stretched? Yes _____	No _____	

Name of exercise 10: _____	Weight:	Reps:
	Set 1: _____	_____
	Set 2: _____	_____
Muscles worked: _____	Set 3: _____	_____
	Set 4: _____	_____
Stretched? Yes _____	No _____	

"I press on toward the goal to win the prize for which God has called me heavenward in Christ Jesus."
Philippians 3:14

Captain's Log

"Each one should test his own actions. Then he can take pride in himself without comparing himself to somebody else, for each one should carry his own load." (Galatians 6:40)

Day: _____   Date: _____ / _____ / _____

Nutrition Log

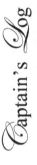
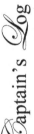

BREAKFAST   Time: _____

	Type (1.)	Amt:	Type (2.)	Amt:
Protein	1.		2.	
Complex Carbs	1.		2.	
Fruit	1.		2.	
Vegetables	1.		2.	
Fat	1.		2.	
Liquid/drink	1.		2.	
Meal Replace.	1.		2.	
Condiments	1.		2.	
Other	1.		2.	

LUNCH   Time: _____

	Type (1.)	Amt:	Type (2.)	Amt:
Protein	1.		2.	
Complex Carbs	1.		2.	
Fruit	1.		2.	
Vegetables	1.		2.	
Fat	1.		2.	
Liquid/drink	1.		2.	
Meal Replace.	1.		2.	
Condiments	1.		2.	
Other	1.		2.	

SNACK 3   Time: _____

	Type (1.)	Amt:	Type (2.)	Amt:
Protein	1.		2.	
Complex Carbs	1.		2.	
Fruit	1.		2.	
Vegetables	1.		2.	
Fat	1.		2.	
Liquid/drink	1.		2.	
Meal Replace.	1.		2.	
Condiments	1.		2.	
Other	1.		2.	

SNACK 1   Time: _____

	Type (1.)	Amt:	Type (2.)	Amt:
Protein	1.		2.	
Complex Carbs	1.		2.	
Fruit	1.		2.	
Vegetables	1.		2.	
Fat	1.		2.	
Liquid/drink	1.		2.	
Meal Replace.	1.		2.	
Condiments	1.		2.	
Other	1.		2.	

SNACK 2   Time: _____

	Type (1.)	Amt:	Type (2.)	Amt:
Protein	1.		2.	
Complex Carbs	1.		2.	
Fruit	1.		2.	
Vegetables	1.		2.	
Fat	1.		2.	
Liquid/drink	1.		2.	
Meal Replace.	1.		2.	
Condiments	1.		2.	
Other	1.		2.	

DINNER   Time: _____

	Type (1.)	Amt:	Type (2.)	Amt:
Protein	1.		2.	
Complex Carbs	1.		2.	
Fruit	1.		2.	
Vegetables	1.		2.	
Fat	1.		2.	
Liquid/drink	1.		2.	
Meal Replace.	1.		2.	
Condiments	1.		2.	
Other	1.		2.	

Resistance Training

Time of day: _____

Warmed up   Yes _____   No _____

Name of exercise 1:
_____
Muscles worked:
_____
Stretched?   Yes _____   No _____

	Weight:	Reps:
Set 1:	_____	_____
Set 2:	_____	_____
Set 3:	_____	_____
Set 4:	_____	_____

Name of exercise 2:
_____
Muscles worked:
_____
Stretched?   Yes _____   No _____

	Weight:	Reps:
Set 1:	_____	_____
Set 2:	_____	_____
Set 3:	_____	_____
Set 4:	_____	_____

Name of exercise 3:
_____
Muscles worked:
_____
Stretched?   Yes _____   No _____

	Weight:	Reps:
Set 1:	_____	_____
Set 2:	_____	_____
Set 3:	_____	_____
Set 4:	_____	_____

Name of exercise 4:
_____
Muscles worked:
_____
Stretched?   Yes _____   No _____

	Weight:	Reps:
Set 1:	_____	_____
Set 2:	_____	_____
Set 3:	_____	_____
Set 4:	_____	_____

Name of exercise 5:
_____
Muscles worked:
_____
Stretched?   Yes _____   No _____

	Weight:	Reps:
Set 1:	_____	_____
Set 2:	_____	_____
Set 3:	_____	_____
Set 4:	_____	_____

Name of exercise 6:
_____
Muscles worked:
_____
Stretched?   Yes _____   No _____

	Weight:	Reps:
Set 1:	_____	_____
Set 2:	_____	_____
Set 3:	_____	_____
Set 4:	_____	_____

Name of exercise 7:
_____
Muscles worked:
_____
Stretched?   Yes _____   No _____

	Weight:	Reps:
Set 1:	_____	_____
Set 2:	_____	_____
Set 3:	_____	_____
Set 4:	_____	_____

Name of exercise 8:
_____
Muscles worked:
_____
Stretched?   Yes _____   No _____

	Weight:	Reps:
Set 1:	_____	_____
Set 2:	_____	_____
Set 3:	_____	_____
Set 4:	_____	_____

Name of exercise 9:
_____
Muscles worked:
_____
Stretched?   Yes _____   No _____

	Weight:	Reps:
Set 1:	_____	_____
Set 2:	_____	_____
Set 3:	_____	_____
Set 4:	_____	_____

Name of exercise 10:
_____
Muscles worked:
_____
Stretched?   Yes _____   No _____

	Weight:	Reps:
Set 1:	_____	_____
Set 2:	_____	_____
Set 3:	_____	_____
Set 4:	_____	_____

Cardiovascular Training

Warmed up   Yes _____   No _____

Time of day: _____

	For how long?	Heart Rate
Type 1:	_____	_____
Type 2:	_____	_____
Type 3:	_____	_____
Type 4:	_____	_____

Stretched?   Yes _____   No _____

Evening Reflection

Did I put my faith in Action today?	Yes _____	No _____
I prayed for somone today	Yes _____	No _____
I read my Bible today	Yes _____	No _____
I helped someone in need today	Yes _____	No _____
I got 6 1/2 to 8 hours of sleep last night	Yes _____	No _____
I know I ate right today	Yes _____	No _____
I ate breakfast today	Yes _____	No _____
I ate starches after 4:00 p.m. today	Yes _____	No _____
I ate at least 4 meals today	Yes _____	No _____
I drank at least a gallon of water today	Yes _____	No _____
I had Courage to Change today	Yes _____	No _____
Tonight I forgive…		

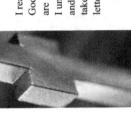

Captain's Log Statement of Faith

I realize that my actions don't earn my way into God's love or earn my way to heaven but that they are a reflection of my love affair with Jesus! I understand that by taking care of myself I honor and glorify God. I matter to God and the actions I take toward good health are daily written love letters telling God, "Thank you for my life"!

_____
Signature

"I press on toward the goal to win the prize for which God has called me heavenward in Christ Jesus."
Philippians 3:14

SETTING, REACHING and SURPASSING

YOUR GOALS and DREAMS

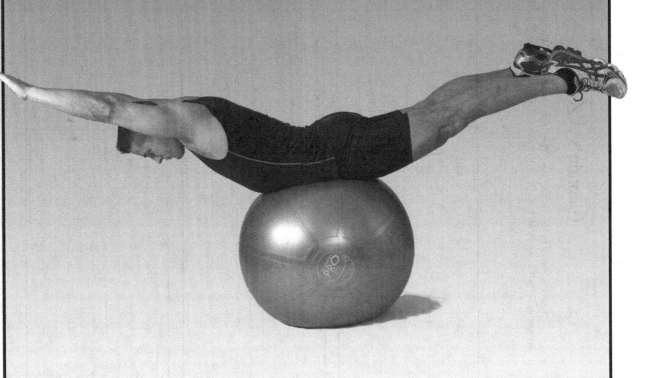

"Where there is no vision, the people perish." (Proverbs 29:18)

WEEK THREE

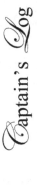

Captain's Log

"Each one should test his own actions. Then he can take pride in himself without comparing himself to somebody else, for each one should carry his own load." (Galatians 6:40)

Day: _____   Date: ____ / ____ / ____

Nutrition Log

BREAKFAST   Time: _____

	Type	Amt:		Type	Amt:
Protein	1. ____	____	2. ____	____
Complex Carbs	1. ____	____	2. ____	____
Fruit	1. ____	____	2. ____	____
Vegetables	1. ____	____	2. ____	____
Fat	1. ____	____	2. ____	____
Liquid/drink	1. ____	____	2. ____	____
Meal Replace.	1. ____	____	2. ____	____
Condiments	1. ____	____	2. ____	____
Other	1. ____	____	2. ____	____

LUNCH   Time: _____

	Type	Amt:		Type	Amt:
Protein	1. ____	____	2. ____	____
Complex Carbs	1. ____	____	2. ____	____
Fruit	1. ____	____	2. ____	____
Vegetables	1. ____	____	2. ____	____
Fat	1. ____	____	2. ____	____
Liquid/drink	1. ____	____	2. ____	____
Meal Replace.	1. ____	____	2. ____	____
Condiments	1. ____	____	2. ____	____
Other	1. ____	____	2. ____	____

SNACK 3   Time: _____

	Type	Amt:		Type	Amt:
Protein	1. ____	____	2. ____	____
Complex Carbs	1. ____	____	2. ____	____
Fruit	1. ____	____	2. ____	____
Vegetables	1. ____	____	2. ____	____
Fat	1. ____	____	2. ____	____
Liquid/drink	1. ____	____	2. ____	____
Meal Replace.	1. ____	____	2. ____	____
Condiments	1. ____	____	2. ____	____
Other	1. ____	____	2. ____	____

SNACK 1   Time: _____

	Type	Amt:		Type	Amt:
Protein	1. ____	____	2. ____	____
Complex Carbs	1. ____	____	2. ____	____
Fruit	1. ____	____	2. ____	____
Vegetables	1. ____	____	2. ____	____
Fat	1. ____	____	2. ____	____
Liquid/drink	1. ____	____	2. ____	____
Meal Replace.	1. ____	____	2. ____	____
Condiments	1. ____	____	2. ____	____
Other	1. ____	____	2. ____	____

SNACK 2   Time: _____

	Type	Amt:		Type	Amt:
Protein	1. ____	____	2. ____	____
Complex Carbs	1. ____	____	2. ____	____
Fruit	1. ____	____	2. ____	____
Vegetables	1. ____	____	2. ____	____
Fat	1. ____	____	2. ____	____
Liquid/drink	1. ____	____	2. ____	____
Meal Replace.	1. ____	____	2. ____	____
Condiments	1. ____	____	2. ____	____
Other	1. ____	____	2. ____	____

DINNER   Time: _____

	Type	Amt:		Type	Amt:
Protein	1. ____	____	2. ____	____
Complex Carbs	1. ____	____	2. ____	____
Fruit	1. ____	____	2. ____	____
Vegetables	1. ____	____	2. ____	____
Fat	1. ____	____	2. ____	____
Liquid/drink	1. ____	____	2. ____	____
Meal Replace.	1. ____	____	2. ____	____
Condiments	1. ____	____	2. ____	____
Other	1. ____	____	2. ____	____

Cardiovascular Training

Warmed up   Yes _____   No _____

Time of day: _____	For how long?	Heart Rate
Type 1:	_____	_____
Type 2:	_____	_____
Type 3:	_____	_____
Type 4:	_____	_____
Stretched? Yes _____ No _____		

Evening Reflection

Did I put my faith in Action today?	Yes _____	No _____
I prayed for somone today	Yes _____	No _____
I read my Bible today	Yes _____	No _____
I helped someone in need today	Yes _____	No _____
I got 6 1/2 to 8 hours of sleep last night	Yes _____	No _____
I know I ate right today	Yes _____	No _____
I ate breakfast today	Yes _____	No _____
I ate starches after 4:00 p.m. today	Yes _____	No _____
I ate at least 4 meals today	Yes _____	No _____
I drank at least a gallon of water today	Yes _____	No _____
I had Courage to Change today	Yes _____	No _____
Tonight I forgive....		

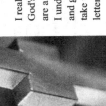

Captain's Log Statement of Faith

I realize that my actions don't earn my way into God's love or earn my way to heaven but that they are a reflection of my love affair with Jesus! I understand that by taking care of myself I honor and glorify God. I matter to God and the actions I take toward good health are daily written love letters telling God, "Thank you for my life"!

_____
Signature

"I press on toward the goal to win the prize for which God has called me heavenward in Christ Jesus."
Philippians 3:14

Resistance Training

Time of day: _____
Warmed up   Yes _____   No _____

Name of exercise 1:	Weight:	Reps:
	Set 1:	_____
	Set 2:	_____
Muscles worked:	Set 3:	_____
	Set 4:	_____
Stretched? Yes _____ No _____		

Name of exercise 2:	Weight:	Reps:
	Set 1:	_____
	Set 2:	_____
Muscles worked:	Set 3:	_____
	Set 4:	_____
Stretched? Yes _____ No _____		

Name of exercise 3:	Weight:	Reps:
	Set 1:	_____
	Set 2:	_____
Muscles worked:	Set 3:	_____
	Set 4:	_____
Stretched? Yes _____ No _____		

Name of exercise 4:	Weight:	Reps:
	Set 1:	_____
	Set 2:	_____
Muscles worked:	Set 3:	_____
	Set 4:	_____
Stretched? Yes _____ No _____		

Name of exercise 5:	Weight:	Reps:
	Set 1:	_____
	Set 2:	_____
Muscles worked:	Set 3:	_____
	Set 4:	_____
Stretched? Yes _____ No _____		

Name of exercise 6:	Weight:	Reps:
	Set 1:	_____
	Set 2:	_____
Muscles worked:	Set 3:	_____
	Set 4:	_____
Stretched? Yes _____ No _____		

Name of exercise 7:	Weight:	Reps:
	Set 1:	_____
	Set 2:	_____
Muscles worked:	Set 3:	_____
	Set 4:	_____
Stretched? Yes _____ No _____		

Name of exercise 8:	Weight:	Reps:
	Set 1:	_____
	Set 2:	_____
Muscles worked:	Set 3:	_____
	Set 4:	_____
Stretched? Yes _____ No _____		

Name of exercise 9:	Weight:	Reps:
	Set 1:	_____
	Set 2:	_____
Muscles worked:	Set 3:	_____
	Set 4:	_____
Stretched? Yes _____ No _____		

Name of exercise 10:	Weight:	Reps:
	Set 1:	_____
	Set 2:	_____
Muscles worked:	Set 3:	_____
	Set 4:	_____
Stretched? Yes _____ No _____		

Captain's Log

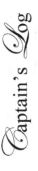

Day: _____   Date: _____ / _____ / _____

Nutrition Log

BREAKFAST   Time: _____

	Type	Amt:
Protein	1. _____ 2. _____	_____
Complex Carbs	1. _____ 2. _____	_____
Fruit	1. _____ 2. _____	_____
Vegetables	1. _____ 2. _____	_____
Fat	1. _____ 2. _____	_____
Liquid/drink	1. _____ 2. _____	_____
Meal Replace.	1. _____ 2. _____	_____
Condiments	1. _____ 2. _____	_____
Other	1. _____ 2. _____	_____

SNACK 1   Time: _____

	Type	Amt:
Protein	1. _____ 2. _____	_____
Complex Carbs	1. _____ 2. _____	_____
Fruit	1. _____ 2. _____	_____
Vegetables	1. _____ 2. _____	_____
Fat	1. _____ 2. _____	_____
Liquid/drink	1. _____ 2. _____	_____
Meal Replace.	1. _____ 2. _____	_____
Condiments	1. _____ 2. _____	_____
Other	1. _____ 2. _____	_____

LUNCH   Time: _____

	Type	Amt:
Protein	1. _____ 2. _____	_____
Complex Carbs	1. _____ 2. _____	_____
Fruit	1. _____ 2. _____	_____
Vegetables	1. _____ 2. _____	_____
Fat	1. _____ 2. _____	_____
Liquid/drink	1. _____ 2. _____	_____
Meal Replace.	1. _____ 2. _____	_____
Condiments	1. _____ 2. _____	_____
Other	1. _____ 2. _____	_____

SNACK 2   Time: _____

	Type	Amt:
Protein	1. _____ 2. _____	_____
Complex Carbs	1. _____ 2. _____	_____
Fruit	1. _____ 2. _____	_____
Vegetables	1. _____ 2. _____	_____
Fat	1. _____ 2. _____	_____
Liquid/drink	1. _____ 2. _____	_____
Meal Replace.	1. _____ 2. _____	_____
Condiments	1. _____ 2. _____	_____
Other	1. _____ 2. _____	_____

SNACK 3   Time: _____

	Type	Amt:
Protein	1. _____ 2. _____	_____
Complex Carbs	1. _____ 2. _____	_____
Fruit	1. _____ 2. _____	_____
Vegetables	1. _____ 2. _____	_____
Fat	1. _____ 2. _____	_____
Liquid/drink	1. _____ 2. _____	_____
Meal Replace.	1. _____ 2. _____	_____
Condiments	1. _____ 2. _____	_____
Other	1. _____ 2. _____	_____

DINNER   Time: _____

	Type	Amt:
Protein	1. _____ 2. _____	_____
Complex Carbs	1. _____ 2. _____	_____
Fruit	1. _____ 2. _____	_____
Vegetables	1. _____ 2. _____	_____
Fat	1. _____ 2. _____	_____
Liquid/drink	1. _____ 2. _____	_____
Meal Replace.	1. _____ 2. _____	_____
Condiments	1. _____ 2. _____	_____
Other	1. _____ 2. _____	_____

Cardiovascular Training

Warmed up   Yes _____   No _____

Time of day: _____		For how long?	Heart Rate
Type 1:		_____	_____
Type 2:		_____	_____
Type 3:		_____	_____
Type 4:		_____	_____
Stretched? Yes _____ No _____			

Evening Reflection

Did I put my faith in Action today?	Yes _____	No _____
I prayed for somone today	Yes _____	No _____
I read my Bible today	Yes _____	No _____
I helped someone in need today	Yes _____	No _____
I got 6 1/2 to 8 hours of sleep last night	Yes _____	No _____
I know I ate right today	Yes _____	No _____
I ate breakfast today	Yes _____	No _____
I ate starches after 4:00 p.m. today	Yes _____	No _____
I ate at least 4 meals today	Yes _____	No _____
I drank at least a gallon of water today	Yes _____	No _____
I had Courage to Change today	Yes _____	No _____
Tonight I forgive…		

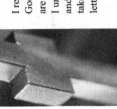

Captain's Log Statement of Faith

I realize that my actions don't earn my way into God's love or earn my way to heaven but that they are a reflection of my love affair with Jesus! I understand that by taking care of myself I honor and glorify God. I matter to God and the actions I take toward good health are daily written love letters telling God, "Thank you for my life"!

_____   **Signature**

Resistance Training

Time of day: _____

Warmed up   Yes _____   No _____

Name of exercise 1: _____

	Weight:	Reps:
Set 1:	_____	_____
Set 2:	_____	_____
Set 3:	_____	_____
Set 4:	_____	_____

Muscles worked: _____

Stretched?   Yes _____   No _____

Name of exercise 3: _____

	Weight:	Reps:
Set 1:	_____	_____
Set 2:	_____	_____
Set 3:	_____	_____
Set 4:	_____	_____

Muscles worked: _____

Stretched?   Yes _____   No _____

Name of exercise 5: _____

	Weight:	Reps:
Set 1:	_____	_____
Set 2:	_____	_____
Set 3:	_____	_____
Set 4:	_____	_____

Muscles worked: _____

Stretched?   Yes _____   No _____

Name of exercise 7: _____

	Weight:	Reps:
Set 1:	_____	_____
Set 2:	_____	_____
Set 3:	_____	_____
Set 4:	_____	_____

Muscles worked: _____

Stretched?   Yes _____   No _____

Name of exercise 9: _____

	Weight:	Reps:
Set 1:	_____	_____
Set 2:	_____	_____
Set 3:	_____	_____
Set 4:	_____	_____

Muscles worked: _____

Stretched?   Yes _____   No _____

Name of exercise 2: _____

	Weight:	Reps:
Set 1:	_____	_____
Set 2:	_____	_____
Set 3:	_____	_____
Set 4:	_____	_____

Muscles worked: _____

Stretched?   Yes _____   No _____

Name of exercise 4: _____

	Weight:	Reps:
Set 1:	_____	_____
Set 2:	_____	_____
Set 3:	_____	_____
Set 4:	_____	_____

Muscles worked: _____

Stretched?   Yes _____   No _____

Name of exercise 6: _____

	Weight:	Reps:
Set 1:	_____	_____
Set 2:	_____	_____
Set 3:	_____	_____
Set 4:	_____	_____

Muscles worked: _____

Stretched?   Yes _____   No _____

Name of exercise 8: _____

	Weight:	Reps:
Set 1:	_____	_____
Set 2:	_____	_____
Set 3:	_____	_____
Set 4:	_____	_____

Muscles worked: _____

Stretched?   Yes _____   No _____

Name of exercise 10: _____

	Weight:	Reps:
Set 1:	_____	_____
Set 2:	_____	_____
Set 3:	_____	_____
Set 4:	_____	_____

Muscles worked: _____

Stretched?   Yes _____   No _____

"I press on toward the goal to win the prize for which God has called me heavenward in Christ Jesus."
Philippians 3:14

Captain's Log

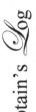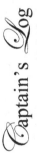

"Each one should test his own actions. Then he can take pride in himself without comparing himself to somebody else, for each one should carry his own load." (Galatians 6:40)

Day: _____ Date: _____ / _____ / _____

Nutrition Log

BREAKFAST Time: _____

	Amt:		Type	Amt:
Protein		1. _____	2. _____	
Complex Carbs		1. _____	2. _____	
Fruit		1. _____	2. _____	
Vegetables		1. _____	2. _____	
Fat		1. _____	2. _____	
Liquid/drink		1. _____	2. _____	
Meal Replace.		1. _____	2. _____	
Condiments		1. _____	2. _____	
Other		1. _____	2. _____	

LUNCH Time: _____

	Amt:		Type	Amt:
Protein		1. _____	2. _____	
Complex Carbs		1. _____	2. _____	
Fruit		1. _____	2. _____	
Vegetables		1. _____	2. _____	
Fat		1. _____	2. _____	
Liquid/drink		1. _____	2. _____	
Meal Replace.		1. _____	2. _____	
Condiments		1. _____	2. _____	
Other		1. _____	2. _____	

SNACK 3 Time: _____

	Amt:		Type	Amt:
Protein		1. _____	2. _____	
Complex Carbs		1. _____	2. _____	
Fruit		1. _____	2. _____	
Vegetables		1. _____	2. _____	
Fat		1. _____	2. _____	
Liquid/drink		1. _____	2. _____	
Meal Replace.		1. _____	2. _____	
Condiments		1. _____	2. _____	
Other		1. _____	2. _____	

SNACK 1 Time: _____

		Type	Amt:		Type	Amt:
Protein		1. _____			2. _____	
Complex Carbs		1. _____			2. _____	
Fruit		1. _____			2. _____	
Vegetables		1. _____			2. _____	
Fat		1. _____			2. _____	
Liquid/drink		1. _____			2. _____	
Meal Replace.		1. _____			2. _____	
Condiments		1. _____			2. _____	
Other		1. _____			2. _____	

SNACK 2 Time: _____

		Type	Amt:		Type	Amt:
Protein		1. _____			2. _____	
Complex Carbs		1. _____			2. _____	
Fruit		1. _____			2. _____	
Vegetables		1. _____			2. _____	
Fat		1. _____			2. _____	
Liquid/drink		1. _____			2. _____	
Meal Replace.		1. _____			2. _____	
Condiments		1. _____			2. _____	
Other		1. _____			2. _____	

DINNER Time: _____

		Type	Amt:		Type	Amt:
Protein		1. _____			2. _____	
Complex Carbs		1. _____			2. _____	
Fruit		1. _____			2. _____	
Vegetables		1. _____			2. _____	
Fat		1. _____			2. _____	
Liquid/drink		1. _____			2. _____	
Meal Replace.		1. _____			2. _____	
Condiments		1. _____			2. _____	
Other		1. _____			2. _____	

Resistance Training

Time of day: _____

Warmed up   Yes _____   No _____

Name of exercise 1: _____

	Weight:	Reps:
Set 1:		
Set 2:		
Set 3:		
Set 4:		

Muscles worked: _____

Stretched?   Yes _____   No _____

Name of exercise 3: _____

	Weight:	Reps:
Set 1:		
Set 2:		
Set 3:		
Set 4:		

Muscles worked: _____

Stretched?   Yes _____   No _____

Name of exercise 5: _____

	Weight:	Reps:
Set 1:		
Set 2:		
Set 3:		
Set 4:		

Muscles worked: _____

Stretched?   Yes _____   No _____

Name of exercise 7: _____

	Weight:	Reps:
Set 1:		
Set 2:		
Set 3:		
Set 4:		

Muscles worked: _____

Stretched?   Yes _____   No _____

Name of exercise 9: _____

	Weight:	Reps:
Set 1:		
Set 2:		
Set 3:		
Set 4:		

Muscles worked: _____

Stretched?   Yes _____   No _____

Name of exercise 2: _____

	Weight:	Reps:
Set 1:		
Set 2:		
Set 3:		
Set 4:		

Muscles worked: _____

Stretched?   Yes _____   No _____

Name of exercise 4: _____

	Weight:	Reps:
Set 1:		
Set 2:		
Set 3:		
Set 4:		

Muscles worked: _____

Stretched?   Yes _____   No _____

Name of exercise 6: _____

	Weight:	Reps:
Set 1:		
Set 2:		
Set 3:		
Set 4:		

Muscles worked: _____

Stretched?   Yes _____   No _____

Name of exercise 8: _____

	Weight:	Reps:
Set 1:		
Set 2:		
Set 3:		
Set 4:		

Muscles worked: _____

Stretched?   Yes _____   No _____

Name of exercise 10: _____

	Weight:	Reps:
Set 1:		
Set 2:		
Set 3:		
Set 4:		

Muscles worked: _____

Stretched?   Yes _____   No _____

Cardiovascular Training

Warmed up   Yes _____   No _____

Time of day: _____

	For how long?	Heart Rate
Type 1:		
Type 2:		
Type 3:		
Type 4:		

Stretched?   Yes _____   No _____

Evening Reflection

Did I put my faith in Action today?	Yes _____	No _____
I prayed for somone today	Yes _____	No _____
I read my Bible today	Yes _____	No _____
I helped someone in need today	Yes _____	No _____
I got 6 1/2 to 8 hours of sleep last night	Yes _____	No _____
I know I ate right today	Yes _____	No _____
I ate breakfast today	Yes _____	No _____
I ate starches after 4:00 p.m. today	Yes _____	No _____
I ate at least 4 meals today	Yes _____	No _____
I drank at least a gallon of water today	Yes _____	No _____
I had Courage to Change today	Yes _____	No _____
Tonight I forgive…		

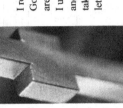

Captain's Log Statement of Faith

I realize that my actions don't earn my way into God's love or earn my way to heaven but that they are a reflection of my love affair with Jesus! I understand that by taking care of myself I honor and glorify God. I matter to God and the actions I take toward good health are daily written love letters telling God, "Thank you for my life"!

_____
Signature

"I press on toward the goal to win the prize for which God has called me heavenward in Christ Jesus."
Philippians 3:14

Captain's Log

"Each one should test his own actions. Then he can take pride in himself without comparing himself to somebody else, for each one should carry his own load." (Galatians 6:40)

Day: _____   Date: _____ / _____ / _____

Nutrition Log

BREAKFAST Time: _____

	Type	Amt:		Type	Amt:
Protein	1.			2.	
Complex Carbs	1.			2.	
Fruit	1.			2.	
Vegetables	1.			2.	
Fat	1.			2.	
Liquid/drink	1.			2.	
Meal Replace.	1.			2.	
Condiments	1.			2.	
Other	1.			2.	

SNACK 1 Time: _____

	Type	Amt:		Type	Amt:
Protein	1.			2.	
Complex Carbs	1.			2.	
Fruit	1.			2.	
Vegetables	1.			2.	
Fat	1.			2.	
Liquid/drink	1.			2.	
Meal Replace.	1.			2.	
Condiments	1.			2.	
Other	1.			2.	

LUNCH Time: _____

	Type	Amt:		Type	Amt:
Protein	1.			2.	
Complex Carbs	1.			2.	
Fruit	1.			2.	
Vegetables	1.			2.	
Fat	1.			2.	
Liquid/drink	1.			2.	
Meal Replace.	1.			2.	
Condiments	1.			2.	
Other	1.			2.	

SNACK 2 Time: _____

	Type	Amt:		Type	Amt:
Protein	1.			2.	
Complex Carbs	1.			2.	
Fruit	1.			2.	
Vegetables	1.			2.	
Fat	1.			2.	
Liquid/drink	1.			2.	
Meal Replace.	1.			2.	
Condiments	1.			2.	
Other	1.			2.	

SNACK 3 Time: _____

	Type	Amt:		Type	Amt:
Protein	1.			2.	
Complex Carbs	1.			2.	
Fruit	1.			2.	
Vegetables	1.			2.	
Fat	1.			2.	
Liquid/drink	1.			2.	
Meal Replace.	1.			2.	
Condiments	1.			2.	
Other	1.			2.	

DINNER Time: _____

	Type	Amt:		Type	Amt:
Protein	1.			2.	
Complex Carbs	1.			2.	
Fruit	1.			2.	
Vegetables	1.			2.	
Fat	1.			2.	
Liquid/drink	1.			2.	
Meal Replace.	1.			2.	
Condiments	1.			2.	
Other	1.			2.	

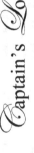
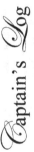

Cardiovascular Training

Warmed up   Yes _____   No _____

Time of day: _____	For how long?	Heart Rate
Type 1:	_____	_____
Type 2:	_____	_____
Type 3:	_____	_____
Type 4:	_____	_____

Stretched?   Yes _____   No _____

Evening Reflection

Did I put my faith in Action today?	Yes _____	No _____
I prayed for somone today	Yes _____	No _____
I read my Bible today	Yes _____	No _____
I helped someone in need today	Yes _____	No _____
I got 6 1/2 to 8 hours of sleep last night	Yes _____	No _____
I know I ate right today	Yes _____	No _____
I ate breakfast today	Yes _____	No _____
I ate starches after 4:00 p.m. today	Yes _____	No _____
I ate at least 4 meals today	Yes _____	No _____
I drank at least a gallon of water today	Yes _____	No _____
I had Courage to Change today	Yes _____	No _____
Tonight I forgive...		

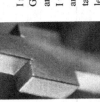

Captain's Log Statement of Faith

I realize that my actions don't earn my way into God's love or earn my way to heaven but that they are a reflection of my love affair with Jesus! I understand that by taking care of myself I honor and glorify God. I matter to God and the actions I take toward good health are daily written love letters telling God, "Thank you for my life"!

_____
Signature

Resistance Training

Time of day: _____

Warmed up   Yes _____   No _____

Name of exercise 1:

	Weight:	Reps:
Set 1:	_____	_____
Set 2:	_____	_____
Set 3:	_____	_____
Set 4:	_____	_____

Muscles worked: _____

Stretched?   Yes _____   No _____

Name of exercise 2:

	Weight:	Reps:
Set 1:	_____	_____
Set 2:	_____	_____
Set 3:	_____	_____
Set 4:	_____	_____

Muscles worked: _____

Stretched?   Yes _____   No _____

Name of exercise 3:

	Weight:	Reps:
Set 1:	_____	_____
Set 2:	_____	_____
Set 3:	_____	_____
Set 4:	_____	_____

Muscles worked: _____

Stretched?   Yes _____   No _____

Name of exercise 4:

	Weight:	Reps:
Set 1:	_____	_____
Set 2:	_____	_____
Set 3:	_____	_____
Set 4:	_____	_____

Muscles worked: _____

Stretched?   Yes _____   No _____

Name of exercise 5:

	Weight:	Reps:
Set 1:	_____	_____
Set 2:	_____	_____
Set 3:	_____	_____
Set 4:	_____	_____

Muscles worked: _____

Stretched?   Yes _____   No _____

Name of exercise 6:

	Weight:	Reps:
Set 1:	_____	_____
Set 2:	_____	_____
Set 3:	_____	_____
Set 4:	_____	_____

Muscles worked: _____

Stretched?   Yes _____   No _____

Name of exercise 7:

	Weight:	Reps:
Set 1:	_____	_____
Set 2:	_____	_____
Set 3:	_____	_____
Set 4:	_____	_____

Muscles worked: _____

Stretched?   Yes _____   No _____

Name of exercise 8:

	Weight:	Reps:
Set 1:	_____	_____
Set 2:	_____	_____
Set 3:	_____	_____
Set 4:	_____	_____

Muscles worked: _____

Stretched?   Yes _____   No _____

Name of exercise 9:

	Weight:	Reps:
Set 1:	_____	_____
Set 2:	_____	_____
Set 3:	_____	_____
Set 4:	_____	_____

Muscles worked: _____

Stretched?   Yes _____   No _____

Name of exercise 10:

	Weight:	Reps:
Set 1:	_____	_____
Set 2:	_____	_____
Set 3:	_____	_____
Set 4:	_____	_____

Muscles worked: _____

Stretched?   Yes _____   No _____

"I press on toward the goal to win the prize for which God has called me heavenward in Christ Jesus."
Philippians 3:14

Captain's Log

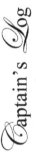

"Each one should test his own actions. Then he can take pride in himself without comparing himself to somebody else, for each one should carry his own load." (Galatians 6:40)

Day: _____   Date: _____ / _____ / _____

Nutrition Log

BREAKFAST	Time: _____					Type	Amt:
	Type	Amt:					
Protein	1. _____	_____				2. _____	_____
Complex Carbs	1. _____	_____				2. _____	_____
Fruit	1. _____	_____				2. _____	_____
Vegetables	1. _____	_____				2. _____	_____
Fat	1. _____	_____				2. _____	_____
Liquid/drink	1. _____	_____				2. _____	_____
Meal Replace.	1. _____	_____				2. _____	_____
Condiments	1. _____	_____				2. _____	_____
Other	1. _____	_____				2. _____	_____

SNACK 1	Time: _____					Type	Amt:
	Type	Amt:					
Protein	1. _____	_____				2. _____	_____
Complex Carbs	1. _____	_____				2. _____	_____
Fruit	1. _____	_____				2. _____	_____
Vegetables	1. _____	_____				2. _____	_____
Fat	1. _____	_____				2. _____	_____
Liquid/drink	1. _____	_____				2. _____	_____
Meal Replace.	1. _____	_____				2. _____	_____
Condiments	1. _____	_____				2. _____	_____
Other	1. _____	_____				2. _____	_____

LUNCH	Time: _____					Type	Amt:
	Type	Amt:					
Protein	1. _____	_____				2. _____	_____
Complex Carbs	1. _____	_____				2. _____	_____
Fruit	1. _____	_____				2. _____	_____
Vegetables	1. _____	_____				2. _____	_____
Fat	1. _____	_____				2. _____	_____
Liquid/drink	1. _____	_____				2. _____	_____
Meal Replace.	1. _____	_____				2. _____	_____
Condiments	1. _____	_____				2. _____	_____
Other	1. _____	_____				2. _____	_____

SNACK 2	Time: _____					Type	Amt:
	Type	Amt:					
Protein	1. _____	_____				2. _____	_____
Complex Carbs	1. _____	_____				2. _____	_____
Fruit	1. _____	_____				2. _____	_____
Vegetables	1. _____	_____				2. _____	_____
Fat	1. _____	_____				2. _____	_____
Liquid/drink	1. _____	_____				2. _____	_____
Meal Replace.	1. _____	_____				2. _____	_____
Condiments	1. _____	_____				2. _____	_____
Other	1. _____	_____				2. _____	_____

SNACK 3	Time: _____					Type	Amt:
	Type	Amt:					
Protein	1. _____	_____				2. _____	_____
Complex Carbs	1. _____	_____				2. _____	_____
Fruit	1. _____	_____				2. _____	_____
Vegetables	1. _____	_____				2. _____	_____
Fat	1. _____	_____				2. _____	_____
Liquid/drink	1. _____	_____				2. _____	_____
Meal Replace.	1. _____	_____				2. _____	_____
Condiments	1. _____	_____				2. _____	_____
Other	1. _____	_____				2. _____	_____

DINNER	Time: _____					Type	Amt:
	Type	Amt:					
Protein	1. _____	_____				2. _____	_____
Complex Carbs	1. _____	_____				2. _____	_____
Fruit	1. _____	_____				2. _____	_____
Vegetables	1. _____	_____				2. _____	_____
Fat	1. _____	_____				2. _____	_____
Liquid/drink	1. _____	_____				2. _____	_____
Meal Replace.	1. _____	_____				2. _____	_____
Condiments	1. _____	_____				2. _____	_____
Other	1. _____	_____				2. _____	_____

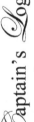

Resistance Training

Time of day: _____

Warmed up   Yes _____   No _____

Name of exercise 1:	Weight:	Reps:
_____	Set 1: _____	
_____	Set 2: _____	
Muscles worked:	Set 3: _____	
_____	Set 4: _____	
Stretched? Yes _____	No _____	

Name of exercise 3:	Weight:	Reps:
_____	Set 1: _____	
_____	Set 2: _____	
Muscles worked:	Set 3: _____	
_____	Set 4: _____	
Stretched? Yes _____	No _____	

Name of exercise 5:	Weight:	Reps:
_____	Set 1: _____	
_____	Set 2: _____	
Muscles worked:	Set 3: _____	
_____	Set 4: _____	
Stretched? Yes _____	No _____	

Name of exercise 7:	Weight:	Reps:
_____	Set 1: _____	
_____	Set 2: _____	
Muscles worked:	Set 3: _____	
_____	Set 4: _____	
Stretched? Yes _____	No _____	

Name of exercise 9:	Weight:	Reps:
_____	Set 1: _____	
_____	Set 2: _____	
Muscles worked:	Set 3: _____	
_____	Set 4: _____	
Stretched? Yes _____	No _____	

Cardiovascular Training

Warmed up   Yes _____   No _____

Time of day: _____	For how long?	Heart Rate
Type 1:	_____	_____
Type 2:	_____	_____
Type 3:	_____	_____
Type 4:	_____	_____
Stretched? Yes _____ No _____		

Evening Reflection

Did I put my faith in Action today?	Yes _____	No _____
I prayed for somone today	Yes _____	No _____
I read my Bible today	Yes _____	No _____
I helped someone in need today	Yes _____	No _____
I got 6 1/2 to 8 hours of sleep last night	Yes _____	No _____
I know I ate right today	Yes _____	No _____
I ate breakfast today	Yes _____	No _____
I ate starches after 4:00 p.m. today	Yes _____	No _____
I ate at least 4 meals today	Yes _____	No _____
I drank at least a gallon of water today	Yes _____	No _____
I had Courage to Change today	Yes _____	No _____
Tonight I forgive…. _____		

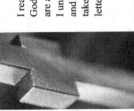

Name of exercise 2:
	Weight:	Reps:
_____	Set 1: _____	
_____	Set 2: _____	
Muscles worked:	Set 3: _____	
_____	Set 4: _____	
Stretched? Yes _____	No _____	

Name of exercise 4:
	Weight:	Reps:
_____	Set 1: _____	
_____	Set 2: _____	
Muscles worked:	Set 3: _____	
_____	Set 4: _____	
Stretched? Yes _____	No _____	

Name of exercise 6:
	Weight:	Reps:
_____	Set 1: _____	
_____	Set 2: _____	
Muscles worked:	Set 3: _____	
_____	Set 4: _____	
Stretched? Yes _____	No _____	

Name of exercise 8:
	Weight:	Reps:
_____	Set 1: _____	
_____	Set 2: _____	
Muscles worked:	Set 3: _____	
_____	Set 4: _____	
Stretched? Yes _____	No _____	

Name of exercise 10:
	Weight:	Reps:
_____	Set 1: _____	
_____	Set 2: _____	
Muscles worked:	Set 3: _____	
_____	Set 4: _____	
Stretched? Yes _____	No _____	

Captain's Log Statement of Faith

I realize that my actions don't earn my way into God's love or earn my way to heaven but that they are a reflection of my love affair with Jesus! I understand that by taking care of myself I honor and glorify God. I matter to God and the actions I take toward good health are daily written love letters telling God, "Thank you for my life"!

_____
Signature

"I press on toward the goal to win the prize for which God has called me heavenward in Christ Jesus."
Philippians 3:14

Captain's Log

"Each one should test his own actions. Then he can take pride in himself without comparing himself to somebody else, for each one should carry his own load." (Galatians 6:40)

Day:________________________ Date:______/______/______

Nutrition Log

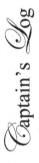

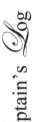

BREAKFAST	Time:__________			
	Type	Amt:	Type	Amt:
Protein	1.________	______	2.________	______
Complex Carbs	1.________	______	2.________	______
Fruit	1.________	______	2.________	______
Vegetables	1.________	______	2.________	______
Fat	1.________	______	2.________	______
Liquid/drink	1.________	______	2.________	______
Meal Replace.	1.________	______	2.________	______
Condiments	1.________	______	2.________	______
Other	1.________	______	2.________	______

SNACK 1	Time:__________			
	Type	Amt:	Type	Amt:
Protein	1.________	______	2.________	______
Complex Carbs	1.________	______	2.________	______
Fruit	1.________	______	2.________	______
Vegetables	1.________	______	2.________	______
Fat	1.________	______	2.________	______
Liquid/drink	1.________	______	2.________	______
Meal Replace.	1.________	______	2.________	______
Condiments	1.________	______	2.________	______
Other	1.________	______	2.________	______

LUNCH	Time:__________			
	Type	Amt:	Type	Amt:
Protein	1.________	______	2.________	______
Complex Carbs	1.________	______	2.________	______
Fruit	1.________	______	2.________	______
Vegetables	1.________	______	2.________	______
Fat	1.________	______	2.________	______
Liquid/drink	1.________	______	2.________	______
Meal Replace.	1.________	______	2.________	______
Condiments	1.________	______	2.________	______
Other	1.________	______	2.________	______

SNACK 2	Time:__________			
	Type	Amt:	Type	Amt:
Protein	1.________	______	2.________	______
Complex Carbs	1.________	______	2.________	______
Fruit	1.________	______	2.________	______
Vegetables	1.________	______	2.________	______
Fat	1.________	______	2.________	______
Liquid/drink	1.________	______	2.________	______
Meal Replace.	1.________	______	2.________	______
Condiments	1.________	______	2.________	______
Other	1.________	______	2.________	______

SNACK 3	Time:__________			
	Type	Amt:	Type	Amt:
Protein	1.________	______	2.________	______
Complex Carbs	1.________	______	2.________	______
Fruit	1.________	______	2.________	______
Vegetables	1.________	______	2.________	______
Fat	1.________	______	2.________	______
Liquid/drink	1.________	______	2.________	______
Meal Replace.	1.________	______	2.________	______
Condiments	1.________	______	2.________	______
Other	1.________	______	2.________	______

DINNER	Time:__________			
	Type	Amt:	Type	Amt:
Protein	1.________	______	2.________	______
Complex Carbs	1.________	______	2.________	______
Fruit	1.________	______	2.________	______
Vegetables	1.________	______	2.________	______
Fat	1.________	______	2.________	______
Liquid/drink	1.________	______	2.________	______
Meal Replace.	1.________	______	2.________	______
Condiments	1.________	______	2.________	______
Other	1.________	______	2.________	______

Cardiovascular Training

Time of day: _____

Warmed up   Yes _____   No _____

Warmed up   Yes _____   No _____

Time of day: _____	For how long?	Heart Rate
Type 1:	_____	_____
Type 2:	_____	_____
Type 3:	_____	_____
Type 4:	_____	_____
Stretched? Yes _____ No _____		

Evening Reflection

Did I put my faith in Action today?	Yes _____	No _____
I prayed for somone today	Yes _____	No _____
I read my Bible today	Yes _____	No _____
I helped someone in need today	Yes _____	No _____
I got 6 1/2 to 8 hours of sleep last night	Yes _____	No _____
I know I ate right today	Yes _____	No _____
I ate breakfast today	Yes _____	No _____
I ate starches after 4:00 p.m. today	Yes _____	No _____
I ate at least 4 meals today	Yes _____	No _____
I drank at least a gallon of water today	Yes _____	No _____
I had Courage to Change today	Yes _____	No _____
Tonight I forgive… _____		

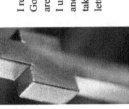

Captain's Log Statement of Faith

I realize that my actions don't earn my way into God's love or earn my way to heaven but that they are a reflection of my love affair with Jesus! I understand that by taking care of myself I honor and glorify God. I matter to God and the actions I take toward good health are daily written love letters telling God, "Thank you for my life"!

_____   Signature

Resistance Training

Name of exercise 1:
_____

	Weight:	Reps:
Set 1:	_____	_____
Set 2:	_____	_____
Set 3:	_____	_____
Set 4:	_____	_____

Muscles worked: _____

Stretched?   Yes _____   No _____

Name of exercise 2:
_____

	Weight:	Reps:
Set 1:	_____	_____
Set 2:	_____	_____
Set 3:	_____	_____
Set 4:	_____	_____

Muscles worked: _____

Stretched?   Yes _____   No _____

Name of exercise 3:
_____

	Weight:	Reps:
Set 1:	_____	_____
Set 2:	_____	_____
Set 3:	_____	_____
Set 4:	_____	_____

Muscles worked: _____

Stretched?   Yes _____   No _____

Name of exercise 4:
_____

	Weight:	Reps:
Set 1:	_____	_____
Set 2:	_____	_____
Set 3:	_____	_____
Set 4:	_____	_____

Muscles worked: _____

Stretched?   Yes _____   No _____

Name of exercise 5:
_____

	Weight:	Reps:
Set 1:	_____	_____
Set 2:	_____	_____
Set 3:	_____	_____
Set 4:	_____	_____

Muscles worked: _____

Stretched?   Yes _____   No _____

Name of exercise 6:
_____

	Weight:	Reps:
Set 1:	_____	_____
Set 2:	_____	_____
Set 3:	_____	_____
Set 4:	_____	_____

Muscles worked: _____

Stretched?   Yes _____   No _____

Name of exercise 7:
_____

	Weight:	Reps:
Set 1:	_____	_____
Set 2:	_____	_____
Set 3:	_____	_____
Set 4:	_____	_____

Muscles worked: _____

Stretched?   Yes _____   No _____

Name of exercise 8:
_____

	Weight:	Reps:
Set 1:	_____	_____
Set 2:	_____	_____
Set 3:	_____	_____
Set 4:	_____	_____

Muscles worked: _____

Stretched?   Yes _____   No _____

Name of exercise 9:
_____

	Weight:	Reps:
Set 1:	_____	_____
Set 2:	_____	_____
Set 3:	_____	_____
Set 4:	_____	_____

Muscles worked: _____

Stretched?   Yes _____   No _____

Name of exercise 10:
_____

	Weight:	Reps:
Set 1:	_____	_____
Set 2:	_____	_____
Set 3:	_____	_____
Set 4:	_____	_____

Muscles worked: _____

Stretched?   Yes _____   No _____

"I press on toward the goal to win the prize for which God has called me heavenward in Christ Jesus."
Philippians 3:14

Captain's Log

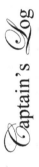
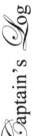

"Each one should test his own actions. Then he can take pride in himself without comparing himself to somebody else, for each one should carry his own load." (Galatians 6:40)

Day: _____   Date: _____ / _____ / _____

Nutrition Log

BREAKFAST Time: _____

	Type	Amt:		Type	Amt:
Protein	1. _____	_____		2. _____	_____
Complex Carbs	1. _____	_____		2. _____	_____
Fruit	1. _____	_____		2. _____	_____
Vegetables	1. _____	_____		2. _____	_____
Fat	1. _____	_____		2. _____	_____
Liquid/drink	1. _____	_____		2. _____	_____
Meal Replace.	1. _____	_____		2. _____	_____
Condiments	1. _____	_____		2. _____	_____
Other	1. _____	_____		2. _____	_____

LUNCH Time: _____

	Type	Amt:		Type	Amt:
Protein	1. _____	_____		2. _____	_____
Complex Carbs	1. _____	_____		2. _____	_____
Fruit	1. _____	_____		2. _____	_____
Vegetables	1. _____	_____		2. _____	_____
Fat	1. _____	_____		2. _____	_____
Liquid/drink	1. _____	_____		2. _____	_____
Meal Replace.	1. _____	_____		2. _____	_____
Condiments	1. _____	_____		2. _____	_____
Other	1. _____	_____		2. _____	_____

SNACK 3 Time: _____

	Type	Amt:		Type	Amt:
Protein	1. _____	_____		2. _____	_____
Complex Carbs	1. _____	_____		2. _____	_____
Fruit	1. _____	_____		2. _____	_____
Vegetables	1. _____	_____		2. _____	_____
Fat	1. _____	_____		2. _____	_____
Liquid/drink	1. _____	_____		2. _____	_____
Meal Replace.	1. _____	_____		2. _____	_____
Condiments	1. _____	_____		2. _____	_____
Other	1. _____	_____		2. _____	_____

SNACK 1 Time: _____

	Type	Amt:		Type	Amt:
Protein	1. _____	_____		2. _____	_____
Complex Carbs	1. _____	_____		2. _____	_____
Fruit	1. _____	_____		2. _____	_____
Vegetables	1. _____	_____		2. _____	_____
Fat	1. _____	_____		2. _____	_____
Liquid/drink	1. _____	_____		2. _____	_____
Meal Replace.	1. _____	_____		2. _____	_____
Condiments	1. _____	_____		2. _____	_____
Other	1. _____	_____		2. _____	_____

SNACK 2 Time: _____

	Type	Amt:		Type	Amt:
Protein	1. _____	_____		2. _____	_____
Complex Carbs	1. _____	_____		2. _____	_____
Fruit	1. _____	_____		2. _____	_____
Vegetables	1. _____	_____		2. _____	_____
Fat	1. _____	_____		2. _____	_____
Liquid/drink	1. _____	_____		2. _____	_____
Meal Replace.	1. _____	_____		2. _____	_____
Condiments	1. _____	_____		2. _____	_____
Other	1. _____	_____		2. _____	_____

DINNER Time: _____

	Type	Amt:		Type	Amt:
Protein	1. _____	_____		2. _____	_____
Complex Carbs	1. _____	_____		2. _____	_____
Fruit	1. _____	_____		2. _____	_____
Vegetables	1. _____	_____		2. _____	_____
Fat	1. _____	_____		2. _____	_____
Liquid/drink	1. _____	_____		2. _____	_____
Meal Replace.	1. _____	_____		2. _____	_____
Condiments	1. _____	_____		2. _____	_____
Other	1. _____	_____		2. _____	_____

Cardiovascular Training

Warmed up   Yes_____   No_____

Time of day:	For how long?	Heart Rate
Type 1: _____	_____	_____
Type 2: _____	_____	_____
Type 3: _____	_____	_____
Type 4: _____	_____	_____

Stretched?   Yes_____   No_____

Evening Reflection

Did I put my faith in Action today?	Yes_____	No_____
I prayed for somone today	Yes_____	No_____
I read my Bible today	Yes_____	No_____
I helped someone in need today	Yes_____	No_____
I got 6 1/2 to 8 hours of sleep last night	Yes_____	No_____
I know I ate right today	Yes_____	No_____
I ate breakfast today	Yes_____	No_____
I ate starches after 4:00 p.m. today	Yes_____	No_____
I ate at least 4 meals today	Yes_____	No_____
I drank at least a gallon of water today	Yes_____	No_____
I had Courage to Change today	Yes_____	No_____
Tonight I forgive…		

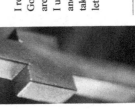

Captain's Log Statement of Faith

I realize that my actions don't earn my way into God's love or earn my way to heaven but that they are a reflection of my love affair with Jesus! I understand that by taking care of myself I honor and glorify God. I matter to God and the actions I take toward good health are daily written love letters telling God, "Thank you for my life"!

_____
Signature

Resistance Training

Time of day: _____

Warmed up   Yes_____   No_____

Name of exercise 1:
_____

	Weight:	Reps:
Set 1:	_____	_____
Set 2:	_____	_____
Set 3:	_____	_____
Set 4:	_____	_____

Muscles worked:
_____

Stretched?   Yes_____   No_____

Name of exercise 3:
_____

	Weight:	Reps:
Set 1:	_____	_____
Set 2:	_____	_____
Set 3:	_____	_____
Set 4:	_____	_____

Muscles worked:
_____

Stretched?   Yes_____   No_____

Name of exercise 5:
_____

	Weight:	Reps:
Set 1:	_____	_____
Set 2:	_____	_____
Set 3:	_____	_____
Set 4:	_____	_____

Muscles worked:
_____

Stretched?   Yes_____   No_____

Name of exercise 7:
_____

	Weight:	Reps:
Set 1:	_____	_____
Set 2:	_____	_____
Set 3:	_____	_____
Set 4:	_____	_____

Muscles worked:
_____

Stretched?   Yes_____   No_____

Name of exercise 9:
_____

	Weight:	Reps:
Set 1:	_____	_____
Set 2:	_____	_____
Set 3:	_____	_____
Set 4:	_____	_____

Muscles worked:
_____

Stretched?   Yes_____   No_____

Name of exercise 2:
_____

	Weight:	Reps:
Set 1:	_____	_____
Set 2:	_____	_____
Set 3:	_____	_____
Set 4:	_____	_____

Muscles worked:
_____

Stretched?   Yes_____   No_____

Name of exercise 4:
_____

	Weight:	Reps:
Set 1:	_____	_____
Set 2:	_____	_____
Set 3:	_____	_____
Set 4:	_____	_____

Muscles worked:
_____

Stretched?   Yes_____   No_____

Name of exercise 6:
_____

	Weight:	Reps:
Set 1:	_____	_____
Set 2:	_____	_____
Set 3:	_____	_____
Set 4:	_____	_____

Muscles worked:
_____

Stretched?   Yes_____   No_____

Name of exercise 8:
_____

	Weight:	Reps:
Set 1:	_____	_____
Set 2:	_____	_____
Set 3:	_____	_____
Set 4:	_____	_____

Muscles worked:
_____

Stretched?   Yes_____   No_____

Name of exercise 10:
_____

	Weight:	Reps:
Set 1:	_____	_____
Set 2:	_____	_____
Set 3:	_____	_____
Set 4:	_____	_____

Muscles worked:
_____

Stretched?   Yes_____   No_____

"I press on toward the goal to win the prize for which God has called me heavenward in Christ Jesus."
Philippians 3:14

LIVING as a DISCIPLE of JESUS CHRIST

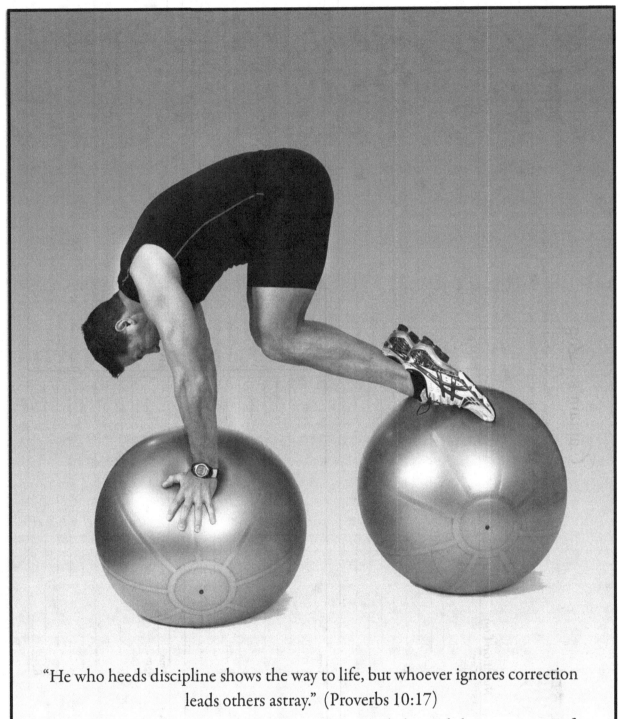

"He who heeds discipline shows the way to life, but whoever ignores correction leads others astray." (Proverbs 10:17)

"For these commands are a lamp, this teaching is a light, and the corrections of discipline are the way to life..." (Proverbs 6:23)

WEEK FOUR

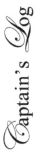

Captain's Log

"Each one should test his own actions. Then he can take pride in himself without comparing himself to somebody else, for each one should carry his own load." (Galatians 6:40)

Day: _____   Date: _____ / _____ / _____

Nutrition Log

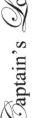

BREAKFAST   Time: _____

	Type	Amt:		Type	Amt:
Protein	1.			2.	
Complex Carbs	1.			2.	
Fruit	1.			2.	
Vegetables	1.			2.	
Fat	1.			2.	
Liquid/drink	1.			2.	
Meal Replace.	1.			2.	
Condiments	1.			2.	
Other	1.			2.	

SNACK 1   Time: _____

	Type	Amt:		Type	Amt:
Protein	1.			2.	
Complex Carbs	1.			2.	
Fruit	1.			2.	
Vegetables	1.			2.	
Fat	1.			2.	
Liquid/drink	1.			2.	
Meal Replace.	1.			2.	
Condiments	1.			2.	
Other	1.			2.	

LUNCH   Time: _____

	Type	Amt:		Type	Amt:
Protein	1.			2.	
Complex Carbs	1.			2.	
Fruit	1.			2.	
Vegetables	1.			2.	
Fat	1.			2.	
Liquid/drink	1.			2.	
Meal Replace.	1.			2.	
Condiments	1.			2.	
Other	1.			2.	

SNACK 2   Time: _____

	Type	Amt:		Type	Amt:
Protein	1.			2.	
Complex Carbs	1.			2.	
Fruit	1.			2.	
Vegetables	1.			2.	
Fat	1.			2.	
Liquid/drink	1.			2.	
Meal Replace.	1.			2.	
Condiments	1.			2.	
Other	1.			2.	

SNACK 3   Time: _____

	Type	Amt:		Type	Amt:
Protein	1.			2.	
Complex Carbs	1.			2.	
Fruit	1.			2.	
Vegetables	1.			2.	
Fat	1.			2.	
Liquid/drink	1.			2.	
Meal Replace.	1.			2.	
Condiments	1.			2.	
Other	1.			2.	

DINNER   Time: _____

	Type	Amt:		Type	Amt:
Protein	1.			2.	
Complex Carbs	1.			2.	
Fruit	1.			2.	
Vegetables	1.			2.	
Fat	1.			2.	
Liquid/drink	1.			2.	
Meal Replace.	1.			2.	
Condiments	1.			2.	
Other	1.			2.	

Resistance Training

Time of day: _____

Warmed up Yes _____ No _____

Name of exercise 1:
_____

	Weight:	Reps:
Set 1:	___	___
Set 2:	___	___
Set 3:	___	___
Set 4:	___	___

Muscles worked: _____

Stretched? Yes _____ No _____

Name of exercise 2:
_____

	Weight:	Reps:
Set 1:	___	___
Set 2:	___	___
Set 3:	___	___
Set 4:	___	___

Muscles worked: _____

Stretched? Yes _____ No _____

Name of exercise 3:
_____

	Weight:	Reps:
Set 1:	___	___
Set 2:	___	___
Set 3:	___	___
Set 4:	___	___

Muscles worked: _____

Stretched? Yes _____ No _____

Name of exercise 4:
_____

	Weight:	Reps:
Set 1:	___	___
Set 2:	___	___
Set 3:	___	___
Set 4:	___	___

Muscles worked: _____

Stretched? Yes _____ No _____

Name of exercise 5:
_____

	Weight:	Reps:
Set 1:	___	___
Set 2:	___	___
Set 3:	___	___
Set 4:	___	___

Muscles worked: _____

Stretched? Yes _____ No _____

Name of exercise 6:
_____

	Weight:	Reps:
Set 1:	___	___
Set 2:	___	___
Set 3:	___	___
Set 4:	___	___

Muscles worked: _____

Stretched? Yes _____ No _____

Name of exercise 7:
_____

	Weight:	Reps:
Set 1:	___	___
Set 2:	___	___
Set 3:	___	___
Set 4:	___	___

Muscles worked: _____

Stretched? Yes _____ No _____

Name of exercise 8:
_____

	Weight:	Reps:
Set 1:	___	___
Set 2:	___	___
Set 3:	___	___
Set 4:	___	___

Muscles worked: _____

Stretched? Yes _____ No _____

Name of exercise 9:
_____

	Weight:	Reps:
Set 1:	___	___
Set 2:	___	___
Set 3:	___	___
Set 4:	___	___

Muscles worked: _____

Stretched? Yes _____ No _____

Name of exercise 10:
_____

	Weight:	Reps:
Set 1:	___	___
Set 2:	___	___
Set 3:	___	___
Set 4:	___	___

Muscles worked: _____

Stretched? Yes _____ No _____

Cardiovascular Training

Warmed up Yes _____ No _____

Time of day:		For how long?	Heart Rate
Type 1:		___	___
Type 2:		___	___
Type 3:		___	___
Type 4:		___	___

Stretched? Yes _____ No _____

Evening Reflection

Did I put my faith in Action today?	Yes ___	No ___
I prayed for somone today	Yes ___	No ___
I read my Bible today	Yes ___	No ___
I helped someone in need today	Yes ___	No ___
I got 6 1/2 to 8 hours of sleep last night	Yes ___	No ___
I know I ate right today	Yes ___	No ___
I ate breakfast today	Yes ___	No ___
I ate starches after 4:00 p.m. today	Yes ___	No ___
I ate at least 4 meals today	Yes ___	No ___
I drank at least a gallon of water today	Yes ___	No ___
I had Courage to Change today	Yes ___	No ___
Tonight I forgive…		

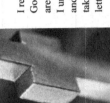

Captain's Log Statement of Faith

I realize that my actions don't earn my way into God's love or earn my way to heaven but that they are a reflection of my love affair with Jesus! I understand that by taking care of myself I honor and glorify God. I matter to God and the actions I take toward good health are daily written love letters telling God, "Thank you for my life"!

_____
Signature

"I press on toward the goal to win the prize for which God has called me heavenward in Christ Jesus."

Philippians 3:14

Captain's Log

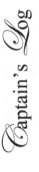

"Each one should test his own actions. Then he can take pride in himself without comparing himself to somebody else, for each one should carry his own load." (Galatians 6:40)

Day: _____   Date: _____ / _____ / _____

Nutrition Log

BREAKFAST   Time: _____

	Type	Amt:	Type	Amt:
Protein	1.		2.	
Complex Carbs	1.		2.	
Fruit	1.		2.	
Vegetables	1.		2.	
Fat	1.		2.	
Liquid/drink	1.		2.	
Meal Replace.	1.		2.	
Condiments	1.		2.	
Other	1.		2.	

SNACK 1   Time: _____

	Type	Amt:	Type	Amt:
Protein	1.		2.	
Complex Carbs	1.		2.	
Fruit	1.		2.	
Vegetables	1.		2.	
Fat	1.		2.	
Liquid/drink	1.		2.	
Meal Replace.	1.		2.	
Condiments	1.		2.	
Other	1.		2.	

LUNCH   Time: _____

	Type	Amt:	Type	Amt:
Protein	1.		2.	
Complex Carbs	1.		2.	
Fruit	1.		2.	
Vegetables	1.		2.	
Fat	1.		2.	
Liquid/drink	1.		2.	
Meal Replace.	1.		2.	
Condiments	1.		2.	
Other	1.		2.	

SNACK 2   Time: _____

	Type	Amt:	Type	Amt:
Protein	1.		2.	
Complex Carbs	1.		2.	
Fruit	1.		2.	
Vegetables	1.		2.	
Fat	1.		2.	
Liquid/drink	1.		2.	
Meal Replace.	1.		2.	
Condiments	1.		2.	
Other	1.		2.	

SNACK 3   Time: _____

	Type	Amt:	Type	Amt:
Protein	1.		2.	
Complex Carbs	1.		2.	
Fruit	1.		2.	
Vegetables	1.		2.	
Fat	1.		2.	
Liquid/drink	1.		2.	
Meal Replace.	1.		2.	
Condiments	1.		2.	
Other	1.		2.	

DINNER   Time: _____

	Type	Amt:	Type	Amt:
Protein	1.		2.	
Complex Carbs	1.		2.	
Fruit	1.		2.	
Vegetables	1.		2.	
Fat	1.		2.	
Liquid/drink	1.		2.	
Meal Replace.	1.		2.	
Condiments	1.		2.	
Other	1.		2.	

Resistance Training

Time of day: _____
Warmed up   Yes _____   No _____

Name of exercise 1:	Weight:	Reps:
	Set 1:	
	Set 2:	
Muscles worked:	Set 3:	
	Set 4:	
Stretched? Yes _____ No _____		

Name of exercise 3:	Weight:	Reps:
	Set 1:	
	Set 2:	
Muscles worked:	Set 3:	
	Set 4:	
Stretched? Yes _____ No _____		

Name of exercise 5:	Weight:	Reps:
	Set 1:	
	Set 2:	
Muscles worked:	Set 3:	
	Set 4:	
Stretched? Yes _____ No _____		

Name of exercise 7:	Weight:	Reps:
	Set 1:	
	Set 2:	
Muscles worked:	Set 3:	
	Set 4:	
Stretched? Yes _____ No _____		

Name of exercise 9:	Weight:	Reps:
	Set 1:	
	Set 2:	
Muscles worked:	Set 3:	
	Set 4:	
Stretched? Yes _____ No _____		

Cardiovascular Training

Warmed up   Yes _____   No _____

Time of day: _____	For how long?	Heart Rate
Type 1:		
Type 2:		
Type 3:		
Type 4:		
Stretched? Yes _____ No _____		

Name of exercise 2:	Weight:	Reps:
	Set 1:	
	Set 2:	
Muscles worked:	Set 3:	
	Set 4:	
Stretched? Yes _____ No _____		

Name of exercise 4:	Weight:	Reps:
	Set 1:	
	Set 2:	
Muscles worked:	Set 3:	
	Set 4:	
Stretched? Yes _____ No _____		

Name of exercise 6:	Weight:	Reps:
	Set 1:	
	Set 2:	
Muscles worked:	Set 3:	
	Set 4:	
Stretched? Yes _____ No _____		

Name of exercise 8:	Weight:	Reps:
	Set 1:	
	Set 2:	
Muscles worked:	Set 3:	
	Set 4:	
Stretched? Yes _____ No _____		

Name of exercise 10:	Weight:	Reps:
	Set 1:	
	Set 2:	
Muscles worked:	Set 3:	
	Set 4:	
Stretched? Yes _____ No _____		

Evening Reflection

Did I put my faith in Action today?	Yes _____	No _____
I prayed for somone today	Yes _____	No _____
I read my Bible today	Yes _____	No _____
I helped someone in need today	Yes _____	No _____
I got 6 1/2 to 8 hours of sleep last night	Yes _____	No _____
I know I ate right today	Yes _____	No _____
I ate breakfast today	Yes _____	No _____
I ate starches after 4:00 p.m. today	Yes _____	No _____
I ate at least 4 meals today	Yes _____	No _____
I drank at least a gallon of water today	Yes _____	No _____
I had Courage to Change today	Yes _____	No _____
Tonight I forgive…		

Captain's Log Statement of Faith

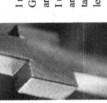

I realize that my actions don't earn my way into God's love or earn my way to heaven but that they are a reflection of my love affair with Jesus! I understand that by taking care of myself I honor and glorify God. I matter to God and the actions I take toward good health are daily written love letters telling God, "Thank you for my life"!

_____ Signature

"I press on toward the goal to win the prize for which God has called me heavenward in Christ Jesus."
Philippians 3:14

Captain's Log

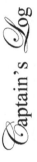 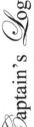

"Each one should test his own actions. Then he can take pride in himself without comparing himself to somebody else, for each one should carry his own load." (Galatians 6:40)

Day: _____   Date: ____ / ____ / ____

Nutrition Log

BREAKFAST Time: _____

	Amt:	Type	Amt:
Protein	____	1. _____	____
Complex Carbs	____	1. _____	____
Fruit	____	1. _____	____
Vegetables	____	1. _____	____
Fat	____	1. _____	____
Liquid/drink	____	1. _____	____
Meal Replace.	____	1. _____	____
Condiments	____	1. _____	____
Other	____	1. _____	____

		Type	
Protein		2. _____	
Complex Carbs		2. _____	
Fruit		2. _____	
Vegetables		2. _____	
Fat		2. _____	
Liquid/drink		2. _____	
Meal Replace.		2. _____	
Condiments		2. _____	
Other		2. _____	

SNACK 1 Time: _____

	Type	Amt:	Type	Amt:
Protein	1. _____	____	2. _____	____
Complex Carbs	1. _____	____	2. _____	____
Fruit	1. _____	____	2. _____	____
Vegetables	1. _____	____	2. _____	____
Fat	1. _____	____	2. _____	____
Liquid/drink	1. _____	____	2. _____	____
Meal Replace.	1. _____	____	2. _____	____
Condiments	1. _____	____	2. _____	____
Other	1. _____	____	2. _____	____

LUNCH Time: _____

	Type	Amt:	Type	Amt:
Protein	1. _____	____	2. _____	____
Complex Carbs	1. _____	____	2. _____	____
Fruit	1. _____	____	2. _____	____
Vegetables	1. _____	____	2. _____	____
Fat	1. _____	____	2. _____	____
Liquid/drink	1. _____	____	2. _____	____
Meal Replace.	1. _____	____	2. _____	____
Condiments	1. _____	____	2. _____	____
Other	1. _____	____	2. _____	____

SNACK 2 Time: _____

	Type	Amt:	Type	Amt:
Protein	1. _____	____	2. _____	____
Complex Carbs	1. _____	____	2. _____	____
Fruit	1. _____	____	2. _____	____
Vegetables	1. _____	____	2. _____	____
Fat	1. _____	____	2. _____	____
Liquid/drink	1. _____	____	2. _____	____
Meal Replace.	1. _____	____	2. _____	____
Condiments	1. _____	____	2. _____	____
Other	1. _____	____	2. _____	____

SNACK 3 Time: _____

	Type	Amt:	Type	Amt:
Protein	1. _____	____	2. _____	____
Complex Carbs	1. _____	____	2. _____	____
Fruit	1. _____	____	2. _____	____
Vegetables	1. _____	____	2. _____	____
Fat	1. _____	____	2. _____	____
Liquid/drink	1. _____	____	2. _____	____
Meal Replace.	1. _____	____	2. _____	____
Condiments	1. _____	____	2. _____	____
Other	1. _____	____	2. _____	____

DINNER Time: _____

	Type	Amt:	Type	Amt:
Protein	1. _____	____	2. _____	____
Complex Carbs	1. _____	____	2. _____	____
Fruit	1. _____	____	2. _____	____
Vegetables	1. _____	____	2. _____	____
Fat	1. _____	____	2. _____	____
Liquid/drink	1. _____	____	2. _____	____
Meal Replace.	1. _____	____	2. _____	____
Condiments	1. _____	____	2. _____	____
Other	1. _____	____	2. _____	____

Cardiovascular Training

Warmed up   Yes_____   No_____

Time of day: _____		For how long?	Heart Rate
Type 1:		_____	_____
Type 2:		_____	_____
Type 3:		_____	_____
Type 4:		_____	_____
Stretched?	Yes_____	No_____	

Evening Reflection

Did I put my faith in Action today?	Yes_____	No_____
I prayed for somone today	Yes_____	No_____
I read my Bible today	Yes_____	No_____
I helped someone in need today	Yes_____	No_____
I got 6 1/2 to 8 hours of sleep last night	Yes_____	No_____
I know I ate right today	Yes_____	No_____
I ate breakfast today	Yes_____	No_____
I ate starches after 4:00 p.m. today	Yes_____	No_____
I ate at least 4 meals today	Yes_____	No_____
I drank at least a gallon of water today	Yes_____	No_____
I had Courage to Change today	Yes_____	No_____
Tonight I forgive... _____		

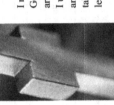

Captain's Log Statement of Faith

I realize that my actions don't earn my way into God's love or earn my way to heaven but that they are a reflection of my love affair with Jesus! I understand that by taking care of myself I honor and glorify God. I matter to God and the actions I take toward good health are daily written love letters telling God, "Thank you for my life"!

_____

Signature

Resistance Training

Time of day: _____

Warmed up   Yes_____   No_____

Name of exercise 1:
_____

	Weight:	Reps:
Set 1:	_____	_____
Set 2:	_____	_____
Set 3:	_____	_____
Set 4:	_____	_____

Muscles worked: _____

Stretched?   Yes_____   No_____

Name of exercise 2:
_____

	Weight:	Reps:
Set 1:	_____	_____
Set 2:	_____	_____
Set 3:	_____	_____
Set 4:	_____	_____

Muscles worked: _____

Stretched?   Yes_____   No_____

Name of exercise 3:
_____

	Weight:	Reps:
Set 1:	_____	_____
Set 2:	_____	_____
Set 3:	_____	_____
Set 4:	_____	_____

Muscles worked: _____

Stretched?   Yes_____   No_____

Name of exercise 4:
_____

	Weight:	Reps:
Set 1:	_____	_____
Set 2:	_____	_____
Set 3:	_____	_____
Set 4:	_____	_____

Muscles worked: _____

Stretched?   Yes_____   No_____

Name of exercise 5:
_____

	Weight:	Reps:
Set 1:	_____	_____
Set 2:	_____	_____
Set 3:	_____	_____
Set 4:	_____	_____

Muscles worked: _____

Stretched?   Yes_____   No_____

Name of exercise 6:
_____

	Weight:	Reps:
Set 1:	_____	_____
Set 2:	_____	_____
Set 3:	_____	_____
Set 4:	_____	_____

Muscles worked: _____

Stretched?   Yes_____   No_____

Name of exercise 7:
_____

	Weight:	Reps:
Set 1:	_____	_____
Set 2:	_____	_____
Set 3:	_____	_____
Set 4:	_____	_____

Muscles worked: _____

Stretched?   Yes_____   No_____

Name of exercise 8:
_____

	Weight:	Reps:
Set 1:	_____	_____
Set 2:	_____	_____
Set 3:	_____	_____
Set 4:	_____	_____

Muscles worked: _____

Stretched?   Yes_____   No_____

Name of exercise 9:
_____

	Weight:	Reps:
Set 1:	_____	_____
Set 2:	_____	_____
Set 3:	_____	_____
Set 4:	_____	_____

Muscles worked: _____

Stretched?   Yes_____   No_____

Name of exercise 10:
_____

	Weight:	Reps:
Set 1:	_____	_____
Set 2:	_____	_____
Set 3:	_____	_____
Set 4:	_____	_____

Muscles worked: _____

Stretched?   Yes_____   No_____

"I press on toward the goal to win the prize for which God has called me heavenward in Christ Jesus."
Philippians 3:14

Captain's Log

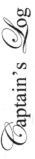
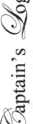

"Each one should test his own actions. Then he can take pride in himself without comparing himself to somebody else, for each one should carry his own load." (Galatians 6:40)

Day: _____ Date: _____ / _____ / _____

Nutrition Log

BREAKFAST Time: _____

	Type	Amt:	Type	Amt:
Protein	1.		2.	
Complex Carbs	1.		2.	
Fruit	1.		2.	
Vegetables	1.		2.	
Fat	1.		2.	
Liquid/drink	1.		2.	
Meal Replace.	1.		2.	
Condiments	1.		2.	
Other	1.		2.	

LUNCH Time: _____

	Type	Amt:	Type	Amt:
Protein	1.		2.	
Complex Carbs	1.		2.	
Fruit	1.		2.	
Vegetables	1.		2.	
Fat	1.		2.	
Liquid/drink	1.		2.	
Meal Replace.	1.		2.	
Condiments	1.		2.	
Other	1.		2.	

SNACK 3 Time: _____

	Type	Amt:	Type	Amt:
Protein	1.		2.	
Complex Carbs	1.		2.	
Fruit	1.		2.	
Vegetables	1.		2.	
Fat	1.		2.	
Liquid/drink	1.		2.	
Meal Replace.	1.		2.	
Condiments	1.		2.	
Other	1.		2.	

SNACK 1 Time: _____

	Type	Amt:	Type	Amt:
Protein	1.		2.	
Complex Carbs	1.		2.	
Fruit	1.		2.	
Vegetables	1.		2.	
Fat	1.		2.	
Liquid/drink	1.		2.	
Meal Replace.	1.		2.	
Condiments	1.		2.	
Other	1.		2.	

SNACK 2 Time: _____

	Type	Amt:	Type	Amt:
Protein	1.		2.	
Complex Carbs	1.		2.	
Fruit	1.		2.	
Vegetables	1.		2.	
Fat	1.		2.	
Liquid/drink	1.		2.	
Meal Replace.	1.		2.	
Condiments	1.		2.	
Other	1.		2.	

DINNER Time: _____

	Type	Amt:	Type	Amt:
Protein	1.		2.	
Complex Carbs	1.		2.	
Fruit	1.		2.	
Vegetables	1.		2.	
Fat	1.		2.	
Liquid/drink	1.		2.	
Meal Replace.	1.		2.	
Condiments	1.		2.	
Other	1.		2.	

Cardiovascular Training

Warmed up   Yes _____   No _____

Time of day: _____	For how long?	Heart Rate
Type 1: _____	_____	_____
Type 2: _____	_____	_____
Type 3: _____	_____	_____
Type 4: _____	_____	_____

Stretched?   Yes _____   No _____

Evening Reflection

Did I put my faith in Action today?	Yes _____	No _____
I prayed for somone today	Yes _____	No _____
I read my Bible today	Yes _____	No _____
I helped someone in need today	Yes _____	No _____
I got 6 1/2 to 8 hours of sleep last night	Yes _____	No _____
I know I ate right today	Yes _____	No _____
I ate breakfast today	Yes _____	No _____
I ate starches after 4:00 p.m. today	Yes _____	No _____
I ate at least 4 meals today	Yes _____	No _____
I drank at least a gallon of water today	Yes _____	No _____
I had Courage to Change today	Yes _____	No _____

Tonight I forgive…_____

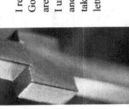

Captain's Log Statement of Faith

I realize that my actions don't earn my way into God's love or earn my way to heaven but that they are a reflection of my love affair with Jesus! I understand that by taking care of myself I honor and glorify God. I matter to God and the actions I take toward good health are daily written love letters telling God, "Thank you for my life"!

_____
Signature

Resistance Training

Time of day: _____
Warmed up   Yes _____   No _____

Name of exercise 1: _____
	Weight:	Reps:
Set 1:	_____	_____
Set 2:	_____	_____
Set 3:	_____	_____
Set 4:	_____	_____

Muscles worked: _____
Stretched?   Yes _____   No _____

Name of exercise 2: _____
	Weight:	Reps:
Set 1:	_____	_____
Set 2:	_____	_____
Set 3:	_____	_____
Set 4:	_____	_____

Muscles worked: _____
Stretched?   Yes _____   No _____

Name of exercise 3: _____
	Weight:	Reps:
Set 1:	_____	_____
Set 2:	_____	_____
Set 3:	_____	_____
Set 4:	_____	_____

Muscles worked: _____
Stretched?   Yes _____   No _____

Name of exercise 4: _____
	Weight:	Reps:
Set 1:	_____	_____
Set 2:	_____	_____
Set 3:	_____	_____
Set 4:	_____	_____

Muscles worked: _____
Stretched?   Yes _____   No _____

Name of exercise 5: _____
	Weight:	Reps:
Set 1:	_____	_____
Set 2:	_____	_____
Set 3:	_____	_____
Set 4:	_____	_____

Muscles worked: _____
Stretched?   Yes _____   No _____

Name of exercise 6: _____
	Weight:	Reps:
Set 1:	_____	_____
Set 2:	_____	_____
Set 3:	_____	_____
Set 4:	_____	_____

Muscles worked: _____
Stretched?   Yes _____   No _____

Name of exercise 7: _____
	Weight:	Reps:
Set 1:	_____	_____
Set 2:	_____	_____
Set 3:	_____	_____
Set 4:	_____	_____

Muscles worked: _____
Stretched?   Yes _____   No _____

Name of exercise 8: _____
	Weight:	Reps:
Set 1:	_____	_____
Set 2:	_____	_____
Set 3:	_____	_____
Set 4:	_____	_____

Muscles worked: _____
Stretched?   Yes _____   No _____

Name of exercise 9: _____
	Weight:	Reps:
Set 1:	_____	_____
Set 2:	_____	_____
Set 3:	_____	_____
Set 4:	_____	_____

Muscles worked: _____
Stretched?   Yes _____   No _____

Name of exercise 10: _____
	Weight:	Reps:
Set 1:	_____	_____
Set 2:	_____	_____
Set 3:	_____	_____
Set 4:	_____	_____

Muscles worked: _____
Stretched?   Yes _____   No _____

"I press on toward the goal to win the prize for which God has called me heavenward in Christ Jesus."
Philippians 3:14

Captain's Log

"Each one should test his own actions. Then he can take pride in himself without comparing himself to somebody else, for each one should carry his own load." (Galatians 6:40)

Day: _____   Date: _____ / _____ / _____

Nutrition Log

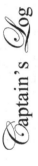

BREAKFAST   Time: _____

	Type	Amt:		Type	Amt:
Protein	1.			2.	
Complex Carbs	1.			2.	
Fruit	1.			2.	
Vegetables	1.			2.	
Fat	1.			2.	
Liquid/drink	1.			2.	
Meal Replace.	1.			2.	
Condiments	1.			2.	
Other	1.			2.	

LUNCH   Time: _____

	Type	Amt:		Type	Amt:
Protein	1.			2.	
Complex Carbs	1.			2.	
Fruit	1.			2.	
Vegetables	1.			2.	
Fat	1.			2.	
Liquid/drink	1.			2.	
Meal Replace.	1.			2.	
Condiments	1.			2.	
Other	1.			2.	

SNACK 3   Time: _____

	Type	Amt:		Type	Amt:
Protein	1.			2.	
Complex Carbs	1.			2.	
Fruit	1.			2.	
Vegetables	1.			2.	
Fat	1.			2.	
Liquid/drink	1.			2.	
Meal Replace.	1.			2.	
Condiments	1.			2.	
Other	1.			2.	

SNACK 1   Time: _____

	Type	Amt:		Type	Amt:
Protein	1.			2.	
Complex Carbs	1.			2.	
Fruit	1.			2.	
Vegetables	1.			2.	
Fat	1.			2.	
Liquid/drink	1.			2.	
Meal Replace.	1.			2.	
Condiments	1.			2.	
Other	1.			2.	

SNACK 2   Time: _____

	Type	Amt:		Type	Amt:
Protein	1.			2.	
Complex Carbs	1.			2.	
Fruit	1.			2.	
Vegetables	1.			2.	
Fat	1.			2.	
Liquid/drink	1.			2.	
Meal Replace.	1.			2.	
Condiments	1.			2.	
Other	1.			2.	

DINNER   Time: _____

	Type	Amt:		Type	Amt:
Protein	1.			2.	
Complex Carbs	1.			2.	
Fruit	1.			2.	
Vegetables	1.			2.	
Fat	1.			2.	
Liquid/drink	1.			2.	
Meal Replace.	1.			2.	
Condiments	1.			2.	
Other	1.			2.	

Cardiovascular Training

Warmed up   Yes_____   No_____

Time of day: _____

	For how long?	Heart Rate
Type 1:	_____	_____
Type 2:	_____	_____
Type 3:	_____	_____
Type 4:	_____	_____

Stretched?   Yes_____   No_____

Evening Reflection

Did I put my faith in Action today?	Yes_____	No_____
I prayed for somone today	Yes_____	No_____
I read my Bible today	Yes_____	No_____
I helped someone in need today	Yes_____	No_____
I got 6 1/2 to 8 hours of sleep last night	Yes_____	No_____
I know I ate right today	Yes_____	No_____
I ate breakfast today	Yes_____	No_____
I ate starches after 4:00 p.m. today	Yes_____	No_____
I ate at least 4 meals today	Yes_____	No_____
I drank at least a gallon of water today	Yes_____	No_____
I had Courage to Change today	Yes_____	No_____
Tonight I forgive...		_____

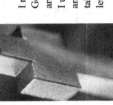

Captain's Log Statement of Faith

I realize that my actions don't earn my way into God's love or earn my way to heaven but that they are a reflection of my love affair with Jesus! I understand that by taking care of myself I honor and glorify God. I matter to God and the actions I take toward good health are daily written love letters telling God, "Thank you for my life"!

_____
Signature

Resistance Training

Time of day: _____

Warmed up   Yes_____   No_____

Name of exercise 1:

	Weight:	Reps:
Set 1:	_____	_____
Set 2:	_____	_____
Set 3:	_____	_____
Set 4:	_____	_____

Muscles worked: _____

Stretched?   Yes_____   No_____

Name of exercise 2:

	Weight:	Reps:
Set 1:	_____	_____
Set 2:	_____	_____
Set 3:	_____	_____
Set 4:	_____	_____

Muscles worked: _____

Stretched?   Yes_____   No_____

Name of exercise 3:

	Weight:	Reps:
Set 1:	_____	_____
Set 2:	_____	_____
Set 3:	_____	_____
Set 4:	_____	_____

Muscles worked: _____

Stretched?   Yes_____   No_____

Name of exercise 4:

	Weight:	Reps:
Set 1:	_____	_____
Set 2:	_____	_____
Set 3:	_____	_____
Set 4:	_____	_____

Muscles worked: _____

Stretched?   Yes_____   No_____

Name of exercise 5:

	Weight:	Reps:
Set 1:	_____	_____
Set 2:	_____	_____
Set 3:	_____	_____
Set 4:	_____	_____

Muscles worked: _____

Stretched?   Yes_____   No_____

Name of exercise 6:

	Weight:	Reps:
Set 1:	_____	_____
Set 2:	_____	_____
Set 3:	_____	_____
Set 4:	_____	_____

Muscles worked: _____

Stretched?   Yes_____   No_____

Name of exercise 7:

	Weight:	Reps:
Set 1:	_____	_____
Set 2:	_____	_____
Set 3:	_____	_____
Set 4:	_____	_____

Muscles worked: _____

Stretched?   Yes_____   No_____

Name of exercise 8:

	Weight:	Reps:
Set 1:	_____	_____
Set 2:	_____	_____
Set 3:	_____	_____
Set 4:	_____	_____

Muscles worked: _____

Stretched?   Yes_____   No_____

Name of exercise 9:

	Weight:	Reps:
Set 1:	_____	_____
Set 2:	_____	_____
Set 3:	_____	_____
Set 4:	_____	_____

Muscles worked: _____

Stretched?   Yes_____   No_____

Name of exercise 10:

	Weight:	Reps:
Set 1:	_____	_____
Set 2:	_____	_____
Set 3:	_____	_____
Set 4:	_____	_____

Muscles worked: _____

Stretched?   Yes_____   No_____

"I press on toward the goal to win the prize for which God has called me heavenward in Christ Jesus."
Philippians 3:14

Captain's Log

"Each one should test his own actions. Then he can take pride in himself without comparing himself to somebody else, for each one should carry his own load." (Galatians 6:40)

Day: _____   Date: _____ / _____ / _____

Nutrition Log

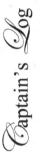

BREAKFAST — Time: _____

	Type	Amt:		Type	Amt:
Protein	1.			2.	
Complex Carbs	1.			2.	
Fruit	1.			2.	
Vegetables	1.			2.	
Fat	1.			2.	
Liquid/drink	1.			2.	
Meal Replace.	1.			2.	
Condiments	1.			2.	
Other	1.			2.	

LUNCH — Time: _____

	Type	Amt:		Type	Amt:
Protein	1.			2.	
Complex Carbs	1.			2.	
Fruit	1.			2.	
Vegetables	1.			2.	
Fat	1.			2.	
Liquid/drink	1.			2.	
Meal Replace.	1.			2.	
Condiments	1.			2.	
Other	1.			2.	

SNACK 3 — Time: _____

	Type	Amt:		Type	Amt:
Protein	1.			2.	
Complex Carbs	1.			2.	
Fruit	1.			2.	
Vegetables	1.			2.	
Fat	1.			2.	
Liquid/drink	1.			2.	
Meal Replace.	1.			2.	
Condiments	1.			2.	
Other	1.			2.	

SNACK 1 — Time: _____

	Type	Amt:		Type	Amt:
Protein	1.			2.	
Complex Carbs	1.			2.	
Fruit	1.			2.	
Vegetables	1.			2.	
Fat	1.			2.	
Liquid/drink	1.			2.	
Meal Replace.	1.			2.	
Condiments	1.			2.	
Other	1.			2.	

SNACK 2 — Time: _____

	Type	Amt:		Type	Amt:
Protein	1.			2.	
Complex Carbs	1.			2.	
Fruit	1.			2.	
Vegetables	1.			2.	
Fat	1.			2.	
Liquid/drink	1.			2.	
Meal Replace.	1.			2.	
Condiments	1.			2.	
Other	1.			2.	

DINNER — Time: _____

	Type	Amt:		Type	Amt:
Protein	1.			2.	
Complex Carbs	1.			2.	
Fruit	1.			2.	
Vegetables	1.			2.	
Fat	1.			2.	
Liquid/drink	1.			2.	
Meal Replace.	1.			2.	
Condiments	1.			2.	
Other	1.			2.	

Resistance Training

Time of day: _____
Warmed up   Yes _____   No _____

Name of exercise 1: _____
Weight: _____   Reps: _____
Set 1: _____
Set 2: _____
Muscles worked: _____
Set 3: _____
Set 4: _____
Stretched?   Yes _____   No _____

Name of exercise 3: _____
Weight: _____   Reps: _____
Set 1: _____
Set 2: _____
Muscles worked: _____
Set 3: _____
Set 4: _____
Stretched?   Yes _____   No _____

Name of exercise 5: _____
Weight: _____   Reps: _____
Set 1: _____
Set 2: _____
Muscles worked: _____
Set 3: _____
Set 4: _____
Stretched?   Yes _____   No _____

Name of exercise 7: _____
Weight: _____   Reps: _____
Set 1: _____
Set 2: _____
Muscles worked: _____
Set 3: _____
Set 4: _____
Stretched?   Yes _____   No _____

Name of exercise 9: _____
Weight: _____   Reps: _____
Set 1: _____
Set 2: _____
Muscles worked: _____
Set 3: _____
Set 4: _____
Stretched?   Yes _____   No _____

Cardiovascular Training

Warmed up   Yes _____   No _____

Time of day: _____   For how long?   Heart Rate
Type 1: _____
Type 2: _____
Type 3: _____
Type 4: _____
Stretched?   Yes _____   No _____

Name of exercise 2: _____
Weight: _____   Reps: _____
Set 1: _____
Set 2: _____
Muscles worked: _____
Set 3: _____
Set 4: _____
Stretched?   Yes _____   No _____

Name of exercise 4: _____
Weight: _____   Reps: _____
Set 1: _____
Set 2: _____
Muscles worked: _____
Set 3: _____
Set 4: _____
Stretched?   Yes _____   No _____

Name of exercise 6: _____
Weight: _____   Reps: _____
Set 1: _____
Set 2: _____
Muscles worked: _____
Set 3: _____
Set 4: _____
Stretched?   Yes _____   No _____

Name of exercise 8: _____
Weight: _____   Reps: _____
Set 1: _____
Set 2: _____
Muscles worked: _____
Set 3: _____
Set 4: _____
Stretched?   Yes _____   No _____

Name of exercise 10: _____
Weight: _____   Reps: _____
Set 1: _____
Set 2: _____
Muscles worked: _____
Set 3: _____
Set 4: _____
Stretched?   Yes _____   No _____

Evening Reflection

Did I put my faith in Action today?   Yes _____   No _____
I prayed for somone today   Yes _____   No _____
I read my Bible today   Yes _____   No _____
I helped someone in need today   Yes _____   No _____
I got 6 1/2 to 8 hours of sleep last night   Yes _____   No _____
I know I ate right today   Yes _____   No _____
I ate breakfast today   Yes _____   No _____
I ate starches after 4:00 p.m. today   Yes _____   No _____
I ate at least 4 meals today   Yes _____   No _____
I drank at least a gallon of water today   Yes _____   No _____
I had Courage to Change today   Yes _____   No _____
Tonight I forgive… _____

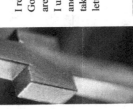

Captain's Log Statement of Faith

I realize that my actions don't earn my way into God's love or earn my way to heaven but that they are a reflection of my love affair with Jesus! I understand that by taking care of myself I honor and glorify God. I matter to God and the actions I take toward good health are daily written love letters telling God, "Thank you for my life"!

_____
Signature

"I press on toward the goal to win the prize for which God has called me heavenward in Christ Jesus."
Philippians 3:14

Captain's Log

"Each one should test his own actions. Then he can take pride in himself without comparing himself to somebody else, for each one should carry his own load." (Galatians 6:40)

Day: _____ Date: _____ / _____ / _____

Nutrition Log

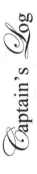

BREAKFAST Time: _____

	Type	Amt:		Type	Amt:
Protein	1. _____	_____		2. _____	_____
Complex Carbs	1. _____	_____		2. _____	_____
Fruit	1. _____	_____		2. _____	_____
Vegetables	1. _____	_____		2. _____	_____
Fat	1. _____	_____		2. _____	_____
Liquid/drink	1. _____	_____		2. _____	_____
Meal Replace.	1. _____	_____		2. _____	_____
Condiments	1. _____	_____		2. _____	_____
Other	1. _____	_____		2. _____	_____

SNACK 1 Time: _____

	Type	Amt:		Type	Amt:
Protein	1. _____	_____		2. _____	_____
Complex Carbs	1. _____	_____		2. _____	_____
Fruit	1. _____	_____		2. _____	_____
Vegetables	1. _____	_____		2. _____	_____
Fat	1. _____	_____		2. _____	_____
Liquid/drink	1. _____	_____		2. _____	_____
Meal Replace.	1. _____	_____		2. _____	_____
Condiments	1. _____	_____		2. _____	_____
Other	1. _____	_____		2. _____	_____

LUNCH Time: _____

	Type	Amt:		Type	Amt:
Protein	1. _____	_____		2. _____	_____
Complex Carbs	1. _____	_____		2. _____	_____
Fruit	1. _____	_____		2. _____	_____
Vegetables	1. _____	_____		2. _____	_____
Fat	1. _____	_____		2. _____	_____
Liquid/drink	1. _____	_____		2. _____	_____
Meal Replace.	1. _____	_____		2. _____	_____
Condiments	1. _____	_____		2. _____	_____
Other	1. _____	_____		2. _____	_____

SNACK 2 Time: _____

	Type	Amt:		Type	Amt:
Protein	1. _____	_____		2. _____	_____
Complex Carbs	1. _____	_____		2. _____	_____
Fruit	1. _____	_____		2. _____	_____
Vegetables	1. _____	_____		2. _____	_____
Fat	1. _____	_____		2. _____	_____
Liquid/drink	1. _____	_____		2. _____	_____
Meal Replace.	1. _____	_____		2. _____	_____
Condiments	1. _____	_____		2. _____	_____
Other	1. _____	_____		2. _____	_____

SNACK 3 Time: _____

	Type	Amt:		Type	Amt:
Protein	1. _____	_____		2. _____	_____
Complex Carbs	1. _____	_____		2. _____	_____
Fruit	1. _____	_____		2. _____	_____
Vegetables	1. _____	_____		2. _____	_____
Fat	1. _____	_____		2. _____	_____
Liquid/drink	1. _____	_____		2. _____	_____
Meal Replace.	1. _____	_____		2. _____	_____
Condiments	1. _____	_____		2. _____	_____
Other	1. _____	_____		2. _____	_____

DINNER Time: _____

	Type	Amt:		Type	Amt:
Protein	1. _____	_____		2. _____	_____
Complex Carbs	1. _____	_____		2. _____	_____
Fruit	1. _____	_____		2. _____	_____
Vegetables	1. _____	_____		2. _____	_____
Fat	1. _____	_____		2. _____	_____
Liquid/drink	1. _____	_____		2. _____	_____
Meal Replace.	1. _____	_____		2. _____	_____
Condiments	1. _____	_____		2. _____	_____
Other	1. _____	_____		2. _____	_____

Cardiovascular Training

Warmed up   Yes _____   No _____

Time of day: _____   For how long?   Heart Rate

Type 1: _____   _____   _____
Type 2: _____   _____   _____
Type 3: _____   _____   _____
Type 4: _____   _____   _____

Stretched?   Yes _____   No _____

Evening Reflection

Did I put my faith in Action today?   Yes _____   No _____
I prayed for somone today   Yes _____   No _____
I read my Bible today   Yes _____   No _____
I helped someone in need today   Yes _____   No _____
I got 6 1/2 to 8 hours of sleep last night Yes _____   No _____
I know I ate right today   Yes _____   No _____
I ate breakfast today   Yes _____   No _____
I ate starches after 4:00 p.m. today   Yes _____   No _____
I ate at least 4 meals today   Yes _____   No _____
I drank at least a gallon of water today   Yes _____   No _____
I had Courage to Change today   Yes _____   No _____
Tonight I forgive…

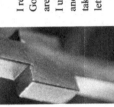

Captain's Log Statement of Faith

I realize that my actions don't earn my way into God's love or earn my way to heaven but that they are a reflection of my love affair with Jesus! I understand that by taking care of myself I honor and glorify God. I matter to God and the actions I take toward good health are daily written love letters telling God, "Thank you for my life"!

_____
Signature

Resistance Training

Time of day: _____

Warmed up   Yes _____   No _____

Name of exercise 1:   Weight: Reps:
_____
Set 1:   _____   _____
Set 2:   _____   _____
Muscles worked:
_____   Set 3:   _____   _____
Set 4:   _____   _____

Stretched?   Yes _____   No _____

Name of exercise 2:   Weight: Reps:
_____
Set 1:   _____   _____
Set 2:   _____   _____
Muscles worked:
_____   Set 3:   _____   _____
Set 4:   _____   _____

Stretched?   Yes _____   No _____

Name of exercise 3:   Weight: Reps:
_____
Set 1:   _____   _____
Set 2:   _____   _____
Muscles worked:
_____   Set 3:   _____   _____
Set 4:   _____   _____

Stretched?   Yes _____   No _____

Name of exercise 4:   Weight: Reps:
_____
Set 1:   _____   _____
Set 2:   _____   _____
Muscles worked:
_____   Set 3:   _____   _____
Set 4:   _____   _____

Stretched?   Yes _____   No _____

Name of exercise 5:   Weight: Reps:
_____
Set 1:   _____   _____
Set 2:   _____   _____
Muscles worked:
_____   Set 3:   _____   _____
Set 4:   _____   _____

Stretched?   Yes _____   No _____

Name of exercise 6:   Weight: Reps:
_____
Set 1:   _____   _____
Set 2:   _____   _____
Muscles worked:
_____   Set 3:   _____   _____
Set 4:   _____   _____

Stretched?   Yes _____   No _____

Name of exercise 7:   Weight: Reps:
_____
Set 1:   _____   _____
Set 2:   _____   _____
Muscles worked:
_____   Set 3:   _____   _____
Set 4:   _____   _____

Stretched?   Yes _____   No _____

Name of exercise 8:   Weight: Reps:
_____
Set 1:   _____   _____
Set 2:   _____   _____
Muscles worked:
_____   Set 3:   _____   _____
Set 4:   _____   _____

Stretched?   Yes _____   No _____

Name of exercise 9:   Weight: Reps:
_____
Set 1:   _____   _____
Set 2:   _____   _____
Muscles worked:
_____   Set 3:   _____   _____
Set 4:   _____   _____

Stretched?   Yes _____   No _____

Name of exercise 10:   Weight: Reps:
_____
Set 1:   _____   _____
Set 2:   _____   _____
Muscles worked:
_____   Set 3:   _____   _____
Set 4:   _____   _____

Stretched?   Yes _____   No _____

"I press on toward the goal to win the prize for which God has called me heavenward in Christ Jesus."
Philippians 3:14

STRESS!

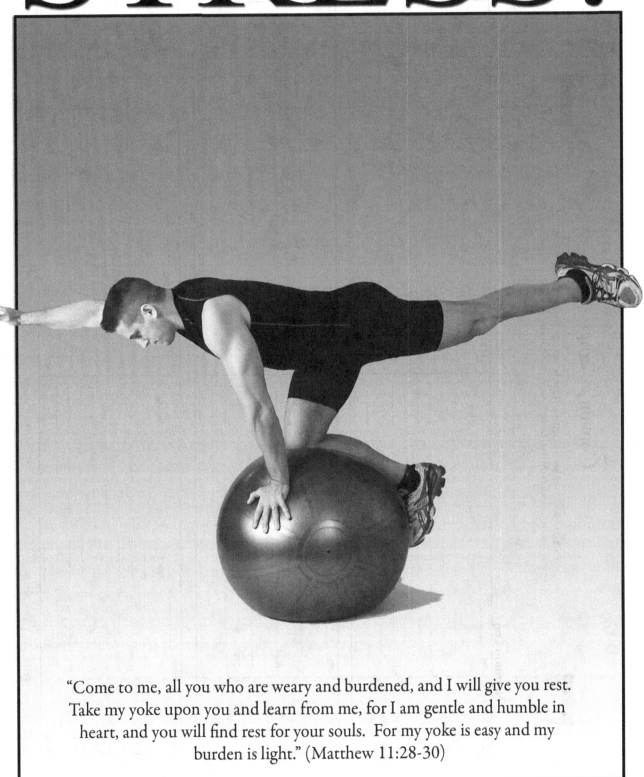

"Come to me, all you who are weary and burdened, and I will give you rest. Take my yoke upon you and learn from me, for I am gentle and humble in heart, and you will find rest for your souls. For my yoke is easy and my burden is light." (Matthew 11:28-30)

WEEK FIVE

Captain's Log

Day: _____   Date: _____ / _____ / _____

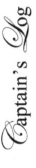
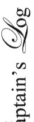

Nutrition Log

BREAKFAST	Time: _____						
	Type	Amt:	Type	Amt:			
Protein	1.		2.				
Complex Carbs	1.		2.				
Fruit	1.		2.				
Vegetables	1.		2.				
Fat	1.		2.				
Liquid/drink	1.		2.				
Meal Replace.	1.		2.				
Condiments	1.		2.				
Other	1.		2.				

LUNCH	Time: _____			
	Type	Amt:	Type	Amt:
Protein	1.		2.	
Complex Carbs	1.		2.	
Fruit	1.		2.	
Vegetables	1.		2.	
Fat	1.		2.	
Liquid/drink	1.		2.	
Meal Replace.	1.		2.	
Condiments	1.		2.	
Other	1.		2.	

SNACK 3	Time: _____			
	Type	Amt:	Type	Amt:
Protein	1.		2.	
Complex Carbs	1.		2.	
Fruit	1.		2.	
Vegetables	1.		2.	
Fat	1.		2.	
Liquid/drink	1.		2.	
Meal Replace.	1.		2.	
Condiments	1.		2.	
Other	1.		2.	

SNACK 1	Time: _____			
	Type	Amt:	Type	Amt:
Protein	1.		2.	
Complex Carbs	1.		2.	
Fruit	1.		2.	
Vegetables	1.		2.	
Fat	1.		2.	
Liquid/drink	1.		2.	
Meal Replace.	1.		2.	
Condiments	1.		2.	
Other	1.		2.	

SNACK 2	Time: _____			
	Type	Amt:	Type	Amt:
Protein	1.		2.	
Complex Carbs	1.		2.	
Fruit	1.		2.	
Vegetables	1.		2.	
Fat	1.		2.	
Liquid/drink	1.		2.	
Meal Replace.	1.		2.	
Condiments	1.		2.	
Other	1.		2.	

DINNER	Time: _____			
	Type	Amt:	Type	Amt:
Protein	1.		2.	
Complex Carbs	1.		2.	
Fruit	1.		2.	
Vegetables	1.		2.	
Fat	1.		2.	
Liquid/drink	1.		2.	
Meal Replace.	1.		2.	
Condiments	1.		2.	
Other	1.		2.	

Cardiovascular Training

Warmed up   Yes _____   No _____

Time of day: _____	For how long?	Heart Rate
Type 1:	_____	_____
Type 2:	_____	_____
Type 3:	_____	_____
Type 4:	_____	_____
Stretched? Yes _____ No _____		

Evening Reflection

Did I put my faith in Action today?	Yes _____	No _____
I prayed for somone today	Yes _____	No _____
I read my Bible today	Yes _____	No _____
I helped someone in need today	Yes _____	No _____
I got 6 1/2 to 8 hours of sleep last night	Yes _____	No _____
I know I ate right today	Yes _____	No _____
I ate breakfast today	Yes _____	No _____
I ate starches after 4:00 p.m. today	Yes _____	No _____
I ate at least 4 meals today	Yes _____	No _____
I drank at least a gallon of water today	Yes _____	No _____
I had Courage to Change today	Yes _____	No _____
Tonight I forgive….		

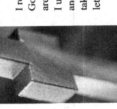

Captain's Log Statement of Faith

I realize that my actions don't earn my way into God's love or earn my way to heaven but that they are a reflection of my love affair with Jesus! I understand that by taking care of myself I honor and glorify God. I matter to God and the actions I take toward good health are daily written love letters telling God, "Thank you for my life"!

_____
Signature

Resistance Training

Time of day: _____

Warmed up   Yes _____   No _____

Name of exercise 1:	Weight:	Reps:
	Set 1: _____	
	Set 2: _____	
Muscles worked:	Set 3: _____	
	Set 4: _____	
Stretched? Yes _____ No _____		

Name of exercise 2:	Weight:	Reps:
	Set 1: _____	
	Set 2: _____	
Muscles worked:	Set 3: _____	
	Set 4: _____	
Stretched? Yes _____ No _____		

Name of exercise 3:	Weight:	Reps:
	Set 1: _____	
	Set 2: _____	
Muscles worked:	Set 3: _____	
	Set 4: _____	
Stretched? Yes _____ No _____		

Name of exercise 4:	Weight:	Reps:
	Set 1: _____	
	Set 2: _____	
Muscles worked:	Set 3: _____	
	Set 4: _____	
Stretched? Yes _____ No _____		

Name of exercise 5:	Weight:	Reps:
	Set 1: _____	
	Set 2: _____	
Muscles worked:	Set 3: _____	
	Set 4: _____	
Stretched? Yes _____ No _____		

Name of exercise 6:	Weight:	Reps:
	Set 1: _____	
	Set 2: _____	
Muscles worked:	Set 3: _____	
	Set 4: _____	
Stretched? Yes _____ No _____		

Name of exercise 7:	Weight:	Reps:
	Set 1: _____	
	Set 2: _____	
Muscles worked:	Set 3: _____	
	Set 4: _____	
Stretched? Yes _____ No _____		

Name of exercise 8:	Weight:	Reps:
	Set 1: _____	
	Set 2: _____	
Muscles worked:	Set 3: _____	
	Set 4: _____	
Stretched? Yes _____ No _____		

Name of exercise 9:	Weight:	Reps:
	Set 1: _____	
	Set 2: _____	
Muscles worked:	Set 3: _____	
	Set 4: _____	
Stretched? Yes _____ No _____		

Name of exercise 10:	Weight:	Reps:
	Set 1: _____	
	Set 2: _____	
Muscles worked:	Set 3: _____	
	Set 4: _____	
Stretched? Yes _____ No _____		

"I press on toward the goal to win the prize for which God has called me heavenward in Christ Jesus."

Philippians 3:14

Captain's Log

"Each one should test his own actions. Then he can take pride in himself without comparing himself to somebody else, for each one should carry his own load." (Galatians 6:40)

Day: _____   Date: _____ / _____ / _____

Nutrition Log

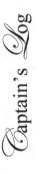

BREAKFAST   Time: _____

	Type	Amt:
	1.	
Protein	2.	
Complex Carbs	1.	
	2.	
Fruit	1.	
	2.	
Vegetables	1.	
	2.	
Fat	1.	
	2.	
Liquid/drink	1.	
	2.	
Meal Replace.	1.	
	2.	
Condiments	1.	
	2.	
Other	1.	
	2.	

LUNCH   Time: _____

	Type	Amt:
	1.	
Protein	2.	
Complex Carbs	1.	
	2.	
Fruit	1.	
	2.	
Vegetables	1.	
	2.	
Fat	1.	
	2.	
Liquid/drink	1.	
	2.	
Meal Replace.	1.	
	2.	
Condiments	1.	
	2.	
Other	1.	
	2.	

SNACK 3   Time: _____

	Type	Amt:
	1.	
Protein	2.	
Complex Carbs	1.	
	2.	
Fruit	1.	
	2.	
Vegetables	1.	
	2.	
Fat	1.	
	2.	
Liquid/drink	1.	
	2.	
Meal Replace.	1.	
	2.	
Condiments	1.	
	2.	
Other	1.	
	2.	

SNACK 1   Time: _____

	Type	Amt:
	1.	
Protein	2.	
Complex Carbs	1.	
	2.	
Fruit	1.	
	2.	
Vegetables	1.	
	2.	
Fat	1.	
	2.	
Liquid/drink	1.	
	2.	
Meal Replace.	1.	
	2.	
Condiments	1.	
	2.	
Other	1.	
	2.	

SNACK 2   Time: _____

	Type	Amt:
	1.	
Protein	2.	
Complex Carbs	1.	
	2.	
Fruit	1.	
	2.	
Vegetables	1.	
	2.	
Fat	1.	
	2.	
Liquid/drink	1.	
	2.	
Meal Replace.	1.	
	2.	
Condiments	1.	
	2.	
Other	1.	
	2.	

DINNER   Time: _____

	Type	Amt:
	1.	
Protein	2.	
Complex Carbs	1.	
	2.	
Fruit	1.	
	2.	
Vegetables	1.	
	2.	
Fat	1.	
	2.	
Liquid/drink	1.	
	2.	
Meal Replace.	1.	
	2.	
Condiments	1.	
	2.	
Other	1.	
	2.	

Time of day:______________

Resistance Training

Warmed up Yes______ No_____

Name of exercise 1:	Weight:	Reps:	Name of exercise 2:	Weight:	Reps:
______________	Set 1:_____	________	______________	Set 1:_____	________
______________	Set 2:_____	________	______________	Set 2:_____	________
Muscles worked:	Set 3:_____	________	Muscles worked:	Set 3:_____	________
______________	Set 4:_____	________	______________	Set 4:_____	________
Stretched? Yes______	No______		Stretched? Yes______	No______	

Name of exercise 3:	Weight:	Reps:	Name of exercise 4:	Weight:	Reps:
______________	Set 1:_____	________	______________	Set 1:_____	________
______________	Set 2:_____	________	______________	Set 2:_____	________
Muscles worked:	Set 3:_____	________	Muscles worked:	Set 3:_____	________
______________	Set 4:_____	________	______________	Set 4:_____	________
Stretched? Yes______	No______		Stretched? Yes______	No______	

Name of exercise 5:	Weight:	Reps:	Name of exercise 6:	Weight:	Reps:
______________	Set 1:_____	________	______________	Set 1:_____	________
______________	Set 2:_____	________	______________	Set 2:_____	________
Muscles worked:	Set 3:_____	________	Muscles worked:	Set 3:_____	________
______________	Set 4:_____	________	______________	Set 4:_____	________
Stretched? Yes______	No______		Stretched? Yes______	No______	

Name of exercise 7:	Weight:	Reps:	Name of exercise 8:	Weight:	Reps:
______________	Set 1:_____	________	______________	Set 1:_____	________
______________	Set 2:_____	________	______________	Set 2:_____	________
Muscles worked:	Set 3:_____	________	Muscles worked:	Set 3:_____	________
______________	Set 4:_____	________	______________	Set 4:_____	________
Stretched? Yes______	No______		Stretched? Yes______	No______	

Name of exercise 9:	Weight:	Reps:	Name of exercise 10:	Weight:	Reps:
______________	Set 1:_____	________	______________	Set 1:_____	________
______________	Set 2:_____	________	______________	Set 2:_____	________
Muscles worked:	Set 3:_____	________	Muscles worked:	Set 3:_____	________
______________	Set 4:_____	________	______________	Set 4:_____	________
Stretched? Yes______	No______		Stretched? Yes______	No______	

Cardiovascular Training

Warmed up Yes______ No______

Time of day:______________	For how long?	Heart Rate
Type 1:______________	________	________
Type 2:______________	________	________
Type 3:______________	________	________
Type 4:______________	________	________
Stretched? Yes______ No______		

Evening Reflection

Did I put my faith in Action today?	Yes______	No______
I prayed for somone today	Yes______	No______
I read my Bible today	Yes______	No______
I helped someone in need today	Yes______	No______
I got 6 1/2 to 8 hours of sleep last night	Yes______	No______
I know I ate right today	Yes______	No______
I ate breakfast today	Yes______	No______
I ate starches after 4:00 p.m. today	Yes______	No______
I ate at least 4 meals today	Yes______	No______
I drank at least a gallon of water today	Yes______	No______
I had Courage to Change today	Yes______	No______

Tonight I forgive...______________ ______________

______________ ______________

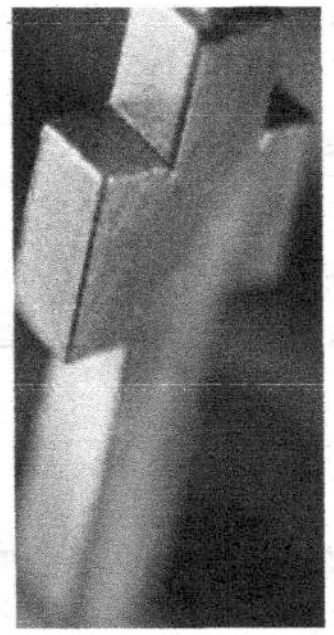

Captain's Log Statement of Faith

I realize that my actions don't earn my way into God's love or earn my way to heaven but that they are a reflection of my love affair with Jesus!
I understand that by taking care of myself I honor and glorify God. I matter to God and the actions I take toward good health are daily written love letters telling God, "Thank you for my life"!

____

Signature

"I press on toward the goal to win the prize for which God has called me heavenward in Christ Jesus."
Philippians 3:14

Captain's Log

Day: _____   Date: _____ / _____ / _____

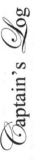

Nutrition Log

BREAKFAST Time: _____

	Type	Amt:		Type	Amt:
Protein	1.			2.	
Complex Carbs	1.			2.	
Fruit	1.			2.	
Vegetables	1.			2.	
Fat	1.			2.	
Liquid/drink	1.			2.	
Meal Replace.	1.			2.	
Condiments	1.			2.	
Other	1.			2.	

LUNCH Time: _____

	Type	Amt:		Type	Amt:
Protein	1.			2.	
Complex Carbs	1.			2.	
Fruit	1.			2.	
Vegetables	1.			2.	
Fat	1.			2.	
Liquid/drink	1.			2.	
Meal Replace.	1.			2.	
Condiments	1.			2.	
Other	1.			2.	

SNACK 3 Time: _____

	Type	Amt:		Type	Amt:
Protein	1.			2.	
Complex Carbs	1.			2.	
Fruit	1.			2.	
Vegetables	1.			2.	
Fat	1.			2.	
Liquid/drink	1.			2.	
Meal Replace.	1.			2.	
Condiments	1.			2.	
Other	1.			2.	

SNACK 1 Time: _____

	Type	Amt:		Type	Amt:
Protein	1.			2.	
Complex Carbs	1.			2.	
Fruit	1.			2.	
Vegetables	1.			2.	
Fat	1.			2.	
Liquid/drink	1.			2.	
Meal Replace.	1.			2.	
Condiments	1.			2.	
Other	1.			2.	

SNACK 2 Time: _____

	Type	Amt:		Type	Amt:
Protein	1.			2.	
Complex Carbs	1.			2.	
Fruit	1.			2.	
Vegetables	1.			2.	
Fat	1.			2.	
Liquid/drink	1.			2.	
Meal Replace.	1.			2.	
Condiments	1.			2.	
Other	1.			2.	

DINNER Time: _____

	Type	Amt:		Type	Amt:
Protein	1.			2.	
Complex Carbs	1.			2.	
Fruit	1.			2.	
Vegetables	1.			2.	
Fat	1.			2.	
Liquid/drink	1.			2.	
Meal Replace.	1.			2.	
Condiments	1.			2.	
Other	1.			2.	

Cardiovascular Training

Warmed up   Yes _____   No _____

Time of day: _____	For how long?	Heart Rate
Type 1: _____	_____	_____
Type 2: _____	_____	_____
Type 3: _____	_____	_____
Type 4: _____	_____	_____

Stretched?   Yes _____   No _____

Resistance Training

Time of day: _____

Warmed up   Yes _____   No _____

Name of exercise 1: _____
_____

	Weight:	Reps:
Set 1:	_____	_____
Set 2:	_____	_____
Set 3:	_____	_____
Set 4:	_____	_____

Muscles worked: _____

Stretched?   Yes _____   No _____

Name of exercise 2: _____
_____

	Weight:	Reps:
Set 1:	_____	_____
Set 2:	_____	_____
Set 3:	_____	_____
Set 4:	_____	_____

Muscles worked: _____

Stretched?   Yes _____   No _____

Name of exercise 3: _____
_____

	Weight:	Reps:
Set 1:	_____	_____
Set 2:	_____	_____
Set 3:	_____	_____
Set 4:	_____	_____

Muscles worked: _____

Stretched?   Yes _____   No _____

Name of exercise 4: _____
_____

	Weight:	Reps:
Set 1:	_____	_____
Set 2:	_____	_____
Set 3:	_____	_____
Set 4:	_____	_____

Muscles worked: _____

Stretched?   Yes _____   No _____

Name of exercise 5: _____
_____

	Weight:	Reps:
Set 1:	_____	_____
Set 2:	_____	_____
Set 3:	_____	_____
Set 4:	_____	_____

Muscles worked: _____

Stretched?   Yes _____   No _____

Name of exercise 6: _____
_____

	Weight:	Reps:
Set 1:	_____	_____
Set 2:	_____	_____
Set 3:	_____	_____
Set 4:	_____	_____

Muscles worked: _____

Stretched?   Yes _____   No _____

Name of exercise 7: _____
_____

	Weight:	Reps:
Set 1:	_____	_____
Set 2:	_____	_____
Set 3:	_____	_____
Set 4:	_____	_____

Muscles worked: _____

Stretched?   Yes _____   No _____

Name of exercise 8: _____
_____

	Weight:	Reps:
Set 1:	_____	_____
Set 2:	_____	_____
Set 3:	_____	_____
Set 4:	_____	_____

Muscles worked: _____

Stretched?   Yes _____   No _____

Name of exercise 9: _____
_____

	Weight:	Reps:
Set 1:	_____	_____
Set 2:	_____	_____
Set 3:	_____	_____
Set 4:	_____	_____

Muscles worked: _____

Stretched?   Yes _____   No _____

Name of exercise 10: _____
_____

	Weight:	Reps:
Set 1:	_____	_____
Set 2:	_____	_____
Set 3:	_____	_____
Set 4:	_____	_____

Muscles worked: _____

Stretched?   Yes _____   No _____

Evening Reflection

Did I put my faith in Action today?	Yes _____	No _____
I prayed for somone today	Yes _____	No _____
I read my Bible today	Yes _____	No _____
I helped someone in need today	Yes _____	No _____
I got 6 1/2 to 8 hours of sleep last night	Yes _____	No _____
I know I ate right today	Yes _____	No _____
I ate breakfast today	Yes _____	No _____
I ate starches after 4:00 p.m. today	Yes _____	No _____
I ate at least 4 meals today	Yes _____	No _____
I drank at least a gallon of water today	Yes _____	No _____
I had Courage to Change today	Yes _____	No _____
Tonight I forgive…		_____

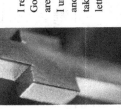

Captain's Log Statement of Faith

I realize that my actions don't earn my way into God's love or earn my way to heaven but that they are a reflection of my love affair with Jesus! I understand that by taking care of myself I honor and glorify God. I matter to God and the actions I take toward good health are daily written love letters telling God, "Thank you for my life"!

_____
Signature

"I press on toward the goal to win the prize for which God has called me heavenward in Christ Jesus."
Philippians 3:14

Captain's Log

"Each one should test his own actions. Then he can take pride in himself without comparing himself to somebody else, for each one should carry his own load." (Galatians 6:40)

Day: _____   Date: _____ / _____ / _____

Nutrition Log

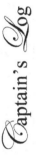
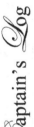

BREAKFAST — Time: _____

	Type	Amt:	Type	Amt:
Protein	1.		2.	
Complex Carbs	1.		2.	
Fruit	1.		2.	
Vegetables	1.		2.	
Fat	1.		2.	
Liquid/drink	1.		2.	
Meal Replace.	1.		2.	
Condiments	1.		2.	
Other	1.		2.	

LUNCH — Time: _____

	Type	Amt:	Type	Amt:
Protein	1.		2.	
Complex Carbs	1.		2.	
Fruit	1.		2.	
Vegetables	1.		2.	
Fat	1.		2.	
Liquid/drink	1.		2.	
Meal Replace.	1.		2.	
Condiments	1.		2.	
Other	1.		2.	

SNACK 3 — Time: _____

	Type	Amt:	Type	Amt:
Protein	1.		2.	
Complex Carbs	1.		2.	
Fruit	1.		2.	
Vegetables	1.		2.	
Fat	1.		2.	
Liquid/drink	1.		2.	
Meal Replace.	1.		2.	
Condiments	1.		2.	
Other	1.		2.	

SNACK 1 — Time: _____

	Type	Amt:	Type	Amt:
Protein	1.		2.	
Complex Carbs	1.		2.	
Fruit	1.		2.	
Vegetables	1.		2.	
Fat	1.		2.	
Liquid/drink	1.		2.	
Meal Replace.	1.		2.	
Condiments	1.		2.	
Other	1.		2.	

SNACK 2 — Time: _____

	Type	Amt:	Type	Amt:
Protein	1.		2.	
Complex Carbs	1.		2.	
Fruit	1.		2.	
Vegetables	1.		2.	
Fat	1.		2.	
Liquid/drink	1.		2.	
Meal Replace.	1.		2.	
Condiments	1.		2.	
Other	1.		2.	

DINNER — Time: _____

	Type	Amt:	Type	Amt:
Protein	1.		2.	
Complex Carbs	1.		2.	
Fruit	1.		2.	
Vegetables	1.		2.	
Fat	1.		2.	
Liquid/drink	1.		2.	
Meal Replace.	1.		2.	
Condiments	1.		2.	
Other	1.		2.	

Cardiovascular Training

Warmed up Yes _____ No _____

Time of day: _____	For how long?	Heart Rate
Type 1: _____	_____	_____
Type 2: _____	_____	_____
Type 3: _____	_____	_____
Type 4: _____	_____	_____

Stretched? Yes _____ No _____

Evening Reflection

Did I put my faith in Action today?	Yes _____	No _____
I prayed for somone today	Yes _____	No _____
I read my Bible today	Yes _____	No _____
I helped someone in need today	Yes _____	No _____
I got 6 1/2 to 8 hours of sleep last night	Yes _____	No _____
I know I ate right today	Yes _____	No _____
I ate breakfast today	Yes _____	No _____
I ate starches after 4:00 p.m. today	Yes _____	No _____
I ate at least 4 meals today	Yes _____	No _____
I drank at least a gallon of water today	Yes _____	No _____
I had Courage to Change today	Yes _____	No _____
Tonight I forgive…		

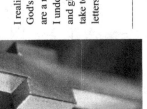

Captain's Log Statement of Faith

I realize that my actions don't earn my way into God's love or earn my way to heaven but that they are a reflection of my love affair with Jesus! I understand that by taking care of myself I honor and glorify God. I matter to God and the actions I take toward good health are daily written love letters telling God, "Thank you for my life"!

_____   **Signature**

"I press on toward the goal to win the prize for which God has called me heavenward in Christ Jesus."
Philippians 3:14

Resistance Training

Time of day: _____

Warmed up Yes _____ No _____

Name of exercise 1:	Weight:	Reps:
	Set 1: _____	_____
	Set 2: _____	_____
Muscles worked:	Set 3: _____	_____
	Set 4: _____	_____
Stretched? Yes _____	No _____	

Name of exercise 2:	Weight:	Reps:
	Set 1: _____	_____
	Set 2: _____	_____
Muscles worked:	Set 3: _____	_____
	Set 4: _____	_____
Stretched? Yes _____	No _____	

Name of exercise 3:	Weight:	Reps:
	Set 1: _____	_____
	Set 2: _____	_____
Muscles worked:	Set 3: _____	_____
	Set 4: _____	_____
Stretched? Yes _____	No _____	

Name of exercise 4:	Weight:	Reps:
	Set 1: _____	_____
	Set 2: _____	_____
Muscles worked:	Set 3: _____	_____
	Set 4: _____	_____
Stretched? Yes _____	No _____	

Name of exercise 5:	Weight:	Reps:
	Set 1: _____	_____
	Set 2: _____	_____
Muscles worked:	Set 3: _____	_____
	Set 4: _____	_____
Stretched? Yes _____	No _____	

Name of exercise 6:	Weight:	Reps:
	Set 1: _____	_____
	Set 2: _____	_____
Muscles worked:	Set 3: _____	_____
	Set 4: _____	_____
Stretched? Yes _____	No _____	

Name of exercise 7:	Weight:	Reps:
	Set 1: _____	_____
	Set 2: _____	_____
Muscles worked:	Set 3: _____	_____
	Set 4: _____	_____
Stretched? Yes _____	No _____	

Name of exercise 8:	Weight:	Reps:
	Set 1: _____	_____
	Set 2: _____	_____
Muscles worked:	Set 3: _____	_____
	Set 4: _____	_____
Stretched? Yes _____	No _____	

Name of exercise 9:	Weight:	Reps:
	Set 1: _____	_____
	Set 2: _____	_____
Muscles worked:	Set 3: _____	_____
	Set 4: _____	_____
Stretched? Yes _____	No _____	

Name of exercise 10:	Weight:	Reps:
	Set 1: _____	_____
	Set 2: _____	_____
Muscles worked:	Set 3: _____	_____
	Set 4: _____	_____
Stretched? Yes _____	No _____	

Captain's Log

"Each one should test his own actions. Then he can take pride in himself without comparing himself to somebody else, for each one should carry his own load." (Galatians 6:40)

Day: _____ Date: _____ / _____ / _____

Nutrition Log

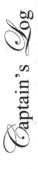

BREAKFAST   Time: _____

	Type	Amt:		Type	Amt:
Protein	1.			2.	
Complex Carbs	1.			2.	
Fruit	1.			2.	
Vegetables	1.			2.	
Fat	1.			2.	
Liquid/drink	1.			2.	
Meal Replace.	1.			2.	
Condiments	1.			2.	
Other	1.			2.	

SNACK 1   Time: _____

	Type	Amt:		Type	Amt:
Protein	1.			2.	
Complex Carbs	1.			2.	
Fruit	1.			2.	
Vegetables	1.			2.	
Fat	1.			2.	
Liquid/drink	1.			2.	
Meal Replace.	1.			2.	
Condiments	1.			2.	
Other	1.			2.	

LUNCH   Time: _____

	Type	Amt:		Type	Amt:
Protein	1.			2.	
Complex Carbs	1.			2.	
Fruit	1.			2.	
Vegetables	1.			2.	
Fat	1.			2.	
Liquid/drink	1.			2.	
Meal Replace.	1.			2.	
Condiments	1.			2.	
Other	1.			2.	

SNACK 2   Time: _____

	Type	Amt:		Type	Amt:
Protein	1.			2.	
Complex Carbs	1.			2.	
Fruit	1.			2.	
Vegetables	1.			2.	
Fat	1.			2.	
Liquid/drink	1.			2.	
Meal Replace.	1.			2.	
Condiments	1.			2.	
Other	1.			2.	

SNACK 3   Time: _____

	Type	Amt:		Type	Amt:
Protein	1.			2.	
Complex Carbs	1.			2.	
Fruit	1.			2.	
Vegetables	1.			2.	
Fat	1.			2.	
Liquid/drink	1.			2.	
Meal Replace.	1.			2.	
Condiments	1.			2.	
Other	1.			2.	

DINNER   Time: _____

	Type	Amt:		Type	Amt:
Protein	1.			2.	
Complex Carbs	1.			2.	
Fruit	1.			2.	
Vegetables	1.			2.	
Fat	1.			2.	
Liquid/drink	1.			2.	
Meal Replace.	1.			2.	
Condiments	1.			2.	
Other	1.			2.	

Cardiovascular Training

Warmed up   Yes_____   No_____

	For how long?	Heart Rate
Type 1:	_____	_____
Type 2:	_____	_____
Type 3:	_____	_____
Type 4:	_____	_____

Time of day: _____

Stretched?   Yes_____   No_____

Evening Reflection

	Yes	No
Did I put my faith in Action today?	Yes_____	No_____
I prayed for somone today	Yes_____	No_____
I read my Bible today	Yes_____	No_____
I helped someone in need today	Yes_____	No_____
I got 6 1/2 to 8 hours of sleep last night	Yes_____	No_____
I know I ate right today	Yes_____	No_____
I ate breakfast today	Yes_____	No_____
I ate starches after 4:00 p.m. today	Yes_____	No_____
I ate at least 4 meals today	Yes_____	No_____
I drank at least a gallon of water today	Yes_____	No_____
I had Courage to Change today	Yes_____	No_____
Tonight I forgive….		

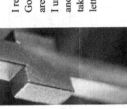

Captain's Log Statement of Faith

I realize that my actions don't earn my way into God's love or earn my way to heaven but that they are a reflection of my love affair with Jesus! I understand that by taking care of myself I honor and glorify God. I matter to God and the actions I take toward good health are daily written love letters telling God, "Thank you for my life"!

_____
Signature

Resistance Training

Time of day: _____

Warmed up   Yes_____   No_____

Name of exercise 1:

	Weight:	Reps:
Set 1:	_____	_____
Set 2:	_____	_____
Set 3:	_____	_____
Set 4:	_____	_____

Muscles worked: _____

Stretched?   Yes_____   No_____

Name of exercise 2:

	Weight:	Reps:
Set 1:	_____	_____
Set 2:	_____	_____
Set 3:	_____	_____
Set 4:	_____	_____

Muscles worked: _____

Stretched?   Yes_____   No_____

Name of exercise 3:

	Weight:	Reps:
Set 1:	_____	_____
Set 2:	_____	_____
Set 3:	_____	_____
Set 4:	_____	_____

Muscles worked: _____

Stretched?   Yes_____   No_____

Name of exercise 4:

	Weight:	Reps:
Set 1:	_____	_____
Set 2:	_____	_____
Set 3:	_____	_____
Set 4:	_____	_____

Muscles worked: _____

Stretched?   Yes_____   No_____

Name of exercise 5:

	Weight:	Reps:
Set 1:	_____	_____
Set 2:	_____	_____
Set 3:	_____	_____
Set 4:	_____	_____

Muscles worked: _____

Stretched?   Yes_____   No_____

Name of exercise 6:

	Weight:	Reps:
Set 1:	_____	_____
Set 2:	_____	_____
Set 3:	_____	_____
Set 4:	_____	_____

Muscles worked: _____

Stretched?   Yes_____   No_____

Name of exercise 7:

	Weight:	Reps:
Set 1:	_____	_____
Set 2:	_____	_____
Set 3:	_____	_____
Set 4:	_____	_____

Muscles worked: _____

Stretched?   Yes_____   No_____

Name of exercise 8:

	Weight:	Reps:
Set 1:	_____	_____
Set 2:	_____	_____
Set 3:	_____	_____
Set 4:	_____	_____

Muscles worked: _____

Stretched?   Yes_____   No_____

Name of exercise 9:

	Weight:	Reps:
Set 1:	_____	_____
Set 2:	_____	_____
Set 3:	_____	_____
Set 4:	_____	_____

Muscles worked: _____

Stretched?   Yes_____   No_____

Name of exercise 10:

	Weight:	Reps:
Set 1:	_____	_____
Set 2:	_____	_____
Set 3:	_____	_____
Set 4:	_____	_____

Muscles worked: _____

Stretched?   Yes_____   No_____

"I press on toward the goal to win the prize for which God has called me heavenward in Christ Jesus."
Philippians 3:14

Captain's Log

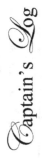

"Each one should test his own actions. Then he can take pride in himself without comparing himself to somebody else, for each one should carry his own load." (Galatians 6:40)

Day: _____   Date: _____ / _____ / _____

Nutrition Log

BREAKFAST   Time: _____

	Type	Amt:	Type	Amt:
Protein	1. _____	_____	2. _____	_____
Complex Carbs	1. _____	_____	2. _____	_____
Fruit	1. _____	_____	2. _____	_____
Vegetables	1. _____	_____	2. _____	_____
Fat	1. _____	_____	2. _____	_____
Liquid/drink	1. _____	_____	2. _____	_____
Meal Replace.	1. _____	_____	2. _____	_____
Condiments	1. _____	_____	2. _____	_____
Other	1. _____	_____	2. _____	_____

LUNCH   Time: _____

	Type	Amt:	Type	Amt:
Protein	1. _____	_____	2. _____	_____
Complex Carbs	1. _____	_____	2. _____	_____
Fruit	1. _____	_____	2. _____	_____
Vegetables	1. _____	_____	2. _____	_____
Fat	1. _____	_____	2. _____	_____
Liquid/drink	1. _____	_____	2. _____	_____
Meal Replace.	1. _____	_____	2. _____	_____
Condiments	1. _____	_____	2. _____	_____
Other	1. _____	_____	2. _____	_____

SNACK 3   Time: _____

	Type	Amt:	Type	Amt:
Protein	1. _____	_____	2. _____	_____
Complex Carbs	1. _____	_____	2. _____	_____
Fruit	1. _____	_____	2. _____	_____
Vegetables	1. _____	_____	2. _____	_____
Fat	1. _____	_____	2. _____	_____
Liquid/drink	1. _____	_____	2. _____	_____
Meal Replace.	1. _____	_____	2. _____	_____
Condiments	1. _____	_____	2. _____	_____
Other	1. _____	_____	2. _____	_____

SNACK 1   Time: _____

	Type	Amt:	Type	Amt:
Protein	1. _____	_____	2. _____	_____
Complex Carbs	1. _____	_____	2. _____	_____
Fruit	1. _____	_____	2. _____	_____
Vegetables	1. _____	_____	2. _____	_____
Fat	1. _____	_____	2. _____	_____
Liquid/drink	1. _____	_____	2. _____	_____
Meal Replace.	1. _____	_____	2. _____	_____
Condiments	1. _____	_____	2. _____	_____
Other	1. _____	_____	2. _____	_____

SNACK 2   Time: _____

	Type	Amt:	Type	Amt:
Protein	1. _____	_____	2. _____	_____
Complex Carbs	1. _____	_____	2. _____	_____
Fruit	1. _____	_____	2. _____	_____
Vegetables	1. _____	_____	2. _____	_____
Fat	1. _____	_____	2. _____	_____
Liquid/drink	1. _____	_____	2. _____	_____
Meal Replace.	1. _____	_____	2. _____	_____
Condiments	1. _____	_____	2. _____	_____
Other	1. _____	_____	2. _____	_____

DINNER   Time: _____

	Type	Amt:	Type	Amt:
Protein	1. _____	_____	2. _____	_____
Complex Carbs	1. _____	_____	2. _____	_____
Fruit	1. _____	_____	2. _____	_____
Vegetables	1. _____	_____	2. _____	_____
Fat	1. _____	_____	2. _____	_____
Liquid/drink	1. _____	_____	2. _____	_____
Meal Replace.	1. _____	_____	2. _____	_____
Condiments	1. _____	_____	2. _____	_____
Other	1. _____	_____	2. _____	_____

Cardiovascular Training

Warmed up   Yes _____   No _____

Time of day: _____	For how long?	Heart Rate
Type 1:	_____	_____
Type 2:	_____	_____
Type 3:	_____	_____
Type 4:	_____	_____
Stretched? Yes _____ No _____		

Evening Reflection

Did I put my faith in Action today?	Yes _____	No _____
I prayed for somone today	Yes _____	No _____
I read my Bible today	Yes _____	No _____
I helped someone in need today	Yes _____	No _____
I got 6 1/2 to 8 hours of sleep last night	Yes _____	No _____
I know I ate right today	Yes _____	No _____
I ate breakfast today	Yes _____	No _____
I ate starches after 4:00 p.m. today	Yes _____	No _____
I ate at least 4 meals today	Yes _____	No _____
I drank at least a gallon of water today	Yes _____	No _____
I had Courage to Change today	Yes _____	No _____
Tonight I forgive…		

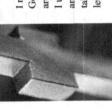

Captain's Log Statement of Faith

I realize that my actions don't earn my way into God's love or earn my way to heaven but that they are a reflection of my love affair with Jesus! I understand that by taking care of myself I honor and glorify God. I matter to God and the actions I take toward good health are daily written love letters telling God, "Thank you for my life"!

_____
Signature

Resistance Training

Time of day: _____

Warmed up   Yes _____   No _____

Name of exercise 1:

	Weight:	Reps:
Set 1:	_____	_____
Set 2:	_____	_____
Set 3:	_____	_____
Set 4:	_____	_____

Muscles worked: _____

Stretched?   Yes _____   No _____

Name of exercise 2:

	Weight:	Reps:
Set 1:	_____	_____
Set 2:	_____	_____
Set 3:	_____	_____
Set 4:	_____	_____

Muscles worked: _____

Stretched?   Yes _____   No _____

Name of exercise 3:

	Weight:	Reps:
Set 1:	_____	_____
Set 2:	_____	_____
Set 3:	_____	_____
Set 4:	_____	_____

Muscles worked: _____

Stretched?   Yes _____   No _____

Name of exercise 4:

	Weight:	Reps:
Set 1:	_____	_____
Set 2:	_____	_____
Set 3:	_____	_____
Set 4:	_____	_____

Muscles worked: _____

Stretched?   Yes _____   No _____

Name of exercise 5:

	Weight:	Reps:
Set 1:	_____	_____
Set 2:	_____	_____
Set 3:	_____	_____
Set 4:	_____	_____

Muscles worked: _____

Stretched?   Yes _____   No _____

Name of exercise 6:

	Weight:	Reps:
Set 1:	_____	_____
Set 2:	_____	_____
Set 3:	_____	_____
Set 4:	_____	_____

Muscles worked: _____

Stretched?   Yes _____   No _____

Name of exercise 7:

	Weight:	Reps:
Set 1:	_____	_____
Set 2:	_____	_____
Set 3:	_____	_____
Set 4:	_____	_____

Muscles worked: _____

Stretched?   Yes _____   No _____

Name of exercise 8:

	Weight:	Reps:
Set 1:	_____	_____
Set 2:	_____	_____
Set 3:	_____	_____
Set 4:	_____	_____

Muscles worked: _____

Stretched?   Yes _____   No _____

Name of exercise 9:

	Weight:	Reps:
Set 1:	_____	_____
Set 2:	_____	_____
Set 3:	_____	_____
Set 4:	_____	_____

Muscles worked: _____

Stretched?   Yes _____   No _____

Name of exercise 10:

	Weight:	Reps:
Set 1:	_____	_____
Set 2:	_____	_____
Set 3:	_____	_____
Set 4:	_____	_____

Muscles worked: _____

Stretched?   Yes _____   No _____

"I press on toward the goal to win the prize for which God has called me heavenward in Christ Jesus."
Philippians 3:14

Captain's Log

"Each one should test his own actions. Then he can take pride in himself without comparing himself to somebody else, for each one should carry his own load." (Galatians 6:40)

Day: _____   Date: _____ / _____ / _____

Nutrition Log

BREAKFAST	Time: _____				SNACK 1	Time: _____			
	Type	Amt:	Type	Amt:		Type	Amt:	Type	Amt:
Protein	1.		2.		Protein	1.		2.	
Complex Carbs	1.		2.		Complex Carbs	1.		2.	
Fruit	1.		2.		Fruit	1.		2.	
Vegetables	1.		2.		Vegetables	1.		2.	
Fat	1.		2.		Fat	1.		2.	
Liquid/drink	1.		2.		Liquid/drink	1.		2.	
Meal Replace.	1.		2.		Meal Replace.	1.		2.	
Condiments	1.		2.		Condiments	1.		2.	
Other	1.		2.		Other	1.		2.	

LUNCH	Time: _____				SNACK 2	Time: _____			
	Type	Amt:	Type	Amt:		Type	Amt:	Type	Amt:
Protein	1.		2.		Protein	1.		2.	
Complex Carbs	1.		2.		Complex Carbs	1.		2.	
Fruit	1.		2.		Fruit	1.		2.	
Vegetables	1.		2.		Vegetables	1.		2.	
Fat	1.		2.		Fat	1.		2.	
Liquid/drink	1.		2.		Liquid/drink	1.		2.	
Meal Replace.	1.		2.		Meal Replace.	1.		2.	
Condiments	1.		2.		Condiments	1.		2.	
Other	1.		2.		Other	1.		2.	

SNACK 3	Time: _____				DINNER	Time: _____			
	Type	Amt:	Type	Amt:		Type	Amt:	Type	Amt:
Protein	1.		2.		Protein	1.		2.	
Complex Carbs	1.		2.		Complex Carbs	1.		2.	
Fruit	1.		2.		Fruit	1.		2.	
Vegetables	1.		2.		Vegetables	1.		2.	
Fat	1.		2.		Fat	1.		2.	
Liquid/drink	1.		2.		Liquid/drink	1.		2.	
Meal Replace.	1.		2.		Meal Replace.	1.		2.	
Condiments	1.		2.		Condiments	1.		2.	
Other	1.		2.		Other	1.		2.	

Cardiovascular Training

Warmed up   Yes _____   No _____

Time of day: _____	For how long?	Heart Rate
Type 1:	_____	_____
Type 2:	_____	_____
Type 3:	_____	_____
Type 4:	_____	_____
Stretched? Yes _____ No _____		

Evening Reflection

Did I put my faith in Action today?	Yes _____	No _____
I prayed for somone today	Yes _____	No _____
I read my Bible today	Yes _____	No _____
I helped someone in need today	Yes _____	No _____
I got 6 1/2 to 8 hours of sleep last night	Yes _____	No _____
I know I ate right today	Yes _____	No _____
I ate breakfast today	Yes _____	No _____
I ate starches after 4:00 p.m. today	Yes _____	No _____
I ate at least 4 meals today	Yes _____	No _____
I drank at least a gallon of water today	Yes _____	No _____
I had Courage to Change today	Yes _____	No _____
Tonight I forgive…		

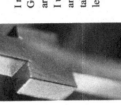

Captain's Log Statement of Faith

I realize that my actions don't earn my way into God's love or earn my way to heaven but that they are a reflection of my love affair with Jesus! I understand that by taking care of myself I honor and glorify God. I matter to God and the actions I take toward good health are daily written love letters telling God, "Thank you for my life"!

_____
Signature

Resistance Training

Time of day: _____

Warmed up   Yes _____   No _____

Name of exercise 1:

	Weight:	Reps:
Set 1:	_____	_____
Set 2:	_____	_____
Muscles worked:		
Set 3:	_____	_____
Set 4:	_____	_____
Stretched? Yes _____ No _____		

Name of exercise 2:

	Weight:	Reps:
Set 1:	_____	_____
Set 2:	_____	_____
Muscles worked:		
Set 3:	_____	_____
Set 4:	_____	_____
Stretched? Yes _____ No _____		

Name of exercise 3:

	Weight:	Reps:
Set 1:	_____	_____
Set 2:	_____	_____
Muscles worked:		
Set 3:	_____	_____
Set 4:	_____	_____
Stretched? Yes _____ No _____		

Name of exercise 4:

	Weight:	Reps:
Set 1:	_____	_____
Set 2:	_____	_____
Muscles worked:		
Set 3:	_____	_____
Set 4:	_____	_____
Stretched? Yes _____ No _____		

Name of exercise 5:

	Weight:	Reps:
Set 1:	_____	_____
Set 2:	_____	_____
Muscles worked:		
Set 3:	_____	_____
Set 4:	_____	_____
Stretched? Yes _____ No _____		

Name of exercise 6:

	Weight:	Reps:
Set 1:	_____	_____
Set 2:	_____	_____
Muscles worked:		
Set 3:	_____	_____
Set 4:	_____	_____
Stretched? Yes _____ No _____		

Name of exercise 7:

	Weight:	Reps:
Set 1:	_____	_____
Set 2:	_____	_____
Muscles worked:		
Set 3:	_____	_____
Set 4:	_____	_____
Stretched? Yes _____ No _____		

Name of exercise 8:

	Weight:	Reps:
Set 1:	_____	_____
Set 2:	_____	_____
Muscles worked:		
Set 3:	_____	_____
Set 4:	_____	_____
Stretched? Yes _____ No _____		

Name of exercise 9:

	Weight:	Reps:
Set 1:	_____	_____
Set 2:	_____	_____
Muscles worked:		
Set 3:	_____	_____
Set 4:	_____	_____
Stretched? Yes _____ No _____		

Name of exercise 10:

	Weight:	Reps:
Set 1:	_____	_____
Set 2:	_____	_____
Muscles worked:		
Set 3:	_____	_____
Set 4:	_____	_____
Stretched? Yes _____ No _____		

"I press on toward the goal to win the prize for which God has called me heavenward in Christ Jesus."
Philippians 3:14

THE PROCESS OF CHANGE

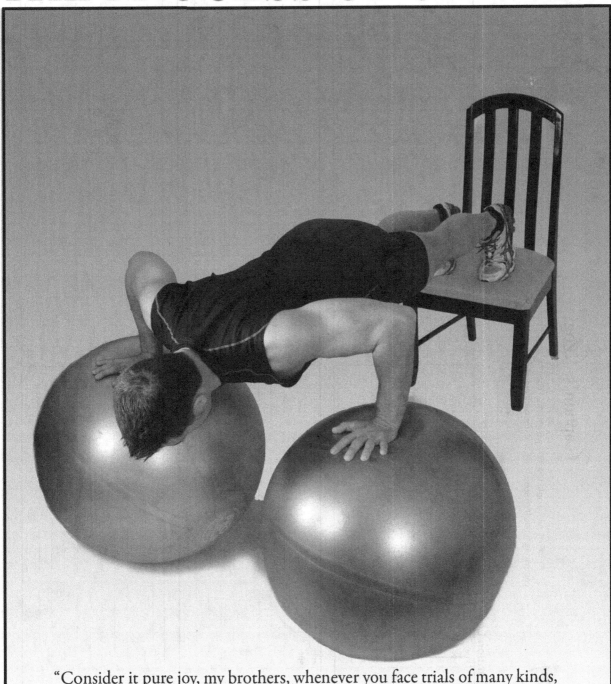

"Consider it pure joy, my brothers, whenever you face trials of many kinds, because you know that the testing of your faith develops perseverance. Perseverance must finish its work so that you may be mature and complete, not lacking anything." (James 1:2)

WEEK SIX

Captain's Log

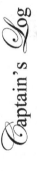

"Each one should test his own actions. Then he can take pride in himself without comparing himself to somebody else, for each one should carry his own load." (Galatians 6:40)

Day: _____ Date: _____ / _____ / _____

Nutrition Log

BREAKFAST Time: _____

	Type	Amt:		Type	Amt:
Protein	1.			2.	
Complex Carbs	1.			2.	
Fruit	1.			2.	
Vegetables	1.			2.	
Fat	1.			2.	
Liquid/drink	1.			2.	
Meal Replace.	1.			2.	
Condiments	1.			2.	
Other	1.			2.	

LUNCH Time: _____

	Type	Amt:		Type	Amt:
Protein	1.			2.	
Complex Carbs	1.			2.	
Fruit	1.			2.	
Vegetables	1.			2.	
Fat	1.			2.	
Liquid/drink	1.			2.	
Meal Replace.	1.			2.	
Condiments	1.			2.	
Other	1.			2.	

SNACK 3 Time: _____

	Type	Amt:		Type	Amt:
Protein	1.			2.	
Complex Carbs	1.			2.	
Fruit	1.			2.	
Vegetables	1.			2.	
Fat	1.			2.	
Liquid/drink	1.			2.	
Meal Replace.	1.			2.	
Condiments	1.			2.	
Other	1.			2.	

SNACK 1 Time: _____

	Type	Amt:		Type	Amt:
Protein	1.			2.	
Complex Carbs	1.			2.	
Fruit	1.			2.	
Vegetables	1.			2.	
Fat	1.			2.	
Liquid/drink	1.			2.	
Meal Replace.	1.			2.	
Condiments	1.			2.	
Other	1.			2.	

SNACK 2 Time: _____

	Type	Amt:		Type	Amt:
Protein	1.			2.	
Complex Carbs	1.			2.	
Fruit	1.			2.	
Vegetables	1.			2.	
Fat	1.			2.	
Liquid/drink	1.			2.	
Meal Replace.	1.			2.	
Condiments	1.			2.	
Other	1.			2.	

DINNER Time: _____

	Type	Amt:		Type	Amt:
Protein	1.			2.	
Complex Carbs	1.			2.	
Fruit	1.			2.	
Vegetables	1.			2.	
Fat	1.			2.	
Liquid/drink	1.			2.	
Meal Replace.	1.			2.	
Condiments	1.			2.	
Other	1.			2.	

Resistance Training

Time of day: _____

Warmed up   Yes _____   No _____

Name of exercise 1:
_____
Weight: _____   Reps: _____
Set 1: _____
Set 2: _____
Muscles worked: _____
Set 3: _____
Set 4: _____
Stretched?   Yes _____   No _____

Name of exercise 2:
_____
Weight: _____   Reps: _____
Set 1: _____
Set 2: _____
Muscles worked: _____
Set 3: _____
Set 4: _____
Stretched?   Yes _____   No _____

Name of exercise 3:
_____
Weight: _____   Reps: _____
Set 1: _____
Set 2: _____
Muscles worked: _____
Set 3: _____
Set 4: _____
Stretched?   Yes _____   No _____

Name of exercise 4:
_____
Weight: _____   Reps: _____
Set 1: _____
Set 2: _____
Muscles worked: _____
Set 3: _____
Set 4: _____
Stretched?   Yes _____   No _____

Name of exercise 5:
_____
Weight: _____   Reps: _____
Set 1: _____
Set 2: _____
Muscles worked: _____
Set 3: _____
Set 4: _____
Stretched?   Yes _____   No _____

Name of exercise 6:
_____
Weight: _____   Reps: _____
Set 1: _____
Set 2: _____
Muscles worked: _____
Set 3: _____
Set 4: _____
Stretched?   Yes _____   No _____

Name of exercise 7:
_____
Weight: _____   Reps: _____
Set 1: _____
Set 2: _____
Muscles worked: _____
Set 3: _____
Set 4: _____
Stretched?   Yes _____   No _____

Name of exercise 8:
_____
Weight: _____   Reps: _____
Set 1: _____
Set 2: _____
Muscles worked: _____
Set 3: _____
Set 4: _____
Stretched?   Yes _____   No _____

Name of exercise 9:
_____
Weight: _____   Reps: _____
Set 1: _____
Set 2: _____
Muscles worked: _____
Set 3: _____
Set 4: _____
Stretched?   Yes _____   No _____

Name of exercise 10:
_____
Weight: _____   Reps: _____
Set 1: _____
Set 2: _____
Muscles worked: _____
Set 3: _____
Set 4: _____
Stretched?   Yes _____   No _____

Cardiovascular Training

Warmed up   Yes _____   No _____

Time of day: _____

For how long?   Heart Rate

Type 1: _____
Type 2: _____
Type 3: _____
Type 4: _____

Stretched?   Yes _____   No _____

Evening Reflection

Did I put my faith in Action today?   Yes _____   No _____
I prayed for somone today   Yes _____   No _____
I read my Bible today   Yes _____   No _____
I helped someone in need today   Yes _____   No _____
I got 6 1/2 to 8 hours of sleep last night   Yes _____   No _____
I know I ate right today   Yes _____   No _____
I ate breakfast today   Yes _____   No _____
I ate starches after 4:00 p.m. today   Yes _____   No _____
I ate at least 4 meals today   Yes _____   No _____
I drank at least a gallon of water today   Yes _____   No _____
I had Courage to Change today   Yes _____   No _____
Tonight I forgive… _____

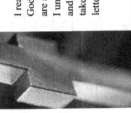

Captain's Log Statement of Faith

I realize that my actions don't earn my way into God's love or earn my way to heaven but that they are a reflection of my love affair with Jesus! I understand that by taking care of myself I honor and glorify God. I matter to God and the actions I take toward good health are daily written love letters telling God, "Thank you for my life"!

_____
Signature

"I press on toward the goal to win the prize for which God has called me heavenward in Christ Jesus."
Philippians 3:14

Captain's Log

Day: _____   Date: _____ / _____ / _____

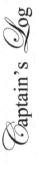

Nutrition Log

BREAKFAST Time: _____

	Amt:		Type	Amt:
Protein	1. _____		2. _____	_____
Complex Carbs	1. _____		2. _____	_____
Fruit	1. _____		2. _____	_____
Vegetables	1. _____		2. _____	_____
Fat	1. _____		2. _____	_____
Liquid/drink	1. _____		2. _____	_____
Meal Replace.	1. _____		2. _____	_____
Condiments	1. _____		2. _____	_____
Other	1. _____		2. _____	_____

LUNCH Time: _____

	Amt:		Type	Amt:
Protein	1. _____		2. _____	_____
Complex Carbs	1. _____		2. _____	_____
Fruit	1. _____		2. _____	_____
Vegetables	1. _____		2. _____	_____
Fat	1. _____		2. _____	_____
Liquid/drink	1. _____		2. _____	_____
Meal Replace.	1. _____		2. _____	_____
Condiments	1. _____		2. _____	_____
Other	1. _____		2. _____	_____

SNACK 3 Time: _____

	Amt:		Type	Amt:
Protein	1. _____		2. _____	_____
Complex Carbs	1. _____		2. _____	_____
Fruit	1. _____		2. _____	_____
Vegetables	1. _____		2. _____	_____
Fat	1. _____		2. _____	_____
Liquid/drink	1. _____		2. _____	_____
Meal Replace.	1. _____		2. _____	_____
Condiments	1. _____		2. _____	_____
Other	1. _____		2. _____	_____

SNACK 1 Time: _____

	Type	Amt:	Type	Amt:
Protein	1. _____		2. _____	_____
Complex Carbs	1. _____		2. _____	_____
Fruit	1. _____		2. _____	_____
Vegetables	1. _____		2. _____	_____
Fat	1. _____		2. _____	_____
Liquid/drink	1. _____		2. _____	_____
Meal Replace.	1. _____		2. _____	_____
Condiments	1. _____		2. _____	_____
Other	1. _____		2. _____	_____

SNACK 2 Time: _____

	Type	Amt:	Type	Amt:
Protein	1. _____		2. _____	_____
Complex Carbs	1. _____		2. _____	_____
Fruit	1. _____		2. _____	_____
Vegetables	1. _____		2. _____	_____
Fat	1. _____		2. _____	_____
Liquid/drink	1. _____		2. _____	_____
Meal Replace.	1. _____		2. _____	_____
Condiments	1. _____		2. _____	_____
Other	1. _____		2. _____	_____

DINNER Time: _____

	Type	Amt:	Type	Amt:
Protein	1. _____		2. _____	_____
Complex Carbs	1. _____		2. _____	_____
Fruit	1. _____		2. _____	_____
Vegetables	1. _____		2. _____	_____
Fat	1. _____		2. _____	_____
Liquid/drink	1. _____		2. _____	_____
Meal Replace.	1. _____		2. _____	_____
Condiments	1. _____		2. _____	_____
Other	1. _____		2. _____	_____

Cardiovascular Training

Warmed up   Yes _____   No _____

Time of day: _____	For how long?	Heart Rate
Type 1:	_____	_____
Type 2:	_____	_____
Type 3:	_____	_____
Type 4:	_____	_____

Stretched?   Yes _____   No _____

Evening Reflection

Did I put my faith in Action today?	Yes _____	No _____
I prayed for somone today	Yes _____	No _____
I read my Bible today	Yes _____	No _____
I helped someone in need today	Yes _____	No _____
I got 6 1/2 to 8 hours of sleep last night	Yes _____	No _____
I know I ate right today	Yes _____	No _____
I ate breakfast today	Yes _____	No _____
I ate starches after 4:00 p.m. today	Yes _____	No _____
I ate at least 4 meals today	Yes _____	No _____
I drank at least a gallon of water today	Yes _____	No _____
I had Courage to Change today	Yes _____	No _____
Tonight I forgive...		

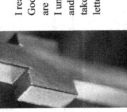

Captain's Log Statement of Faith

I realize that my actions don't earn my way into God's love or earn my way to heaven but that they are a reflection of my love affair with Jesus! I understand that by taking care of myself I honor and glorify God. I matter to God and the actions I take toward good health are daily written love letters telling God, "Thank you for my life"!

_____
Signature

Resistance Training

Time of day: _____

Warmed up   Yes _____   No _____

Name of exercise 1: _____

	Weight:	Reps:
Set 1:	_____	_____
Set 2:	_____	_____
Set 3:	_____	_____
Set 4:	_____	_____

Muscles worked: _____

Stretched?   Yes _____   No _____

Name of exercise 2: _____

	Weight:	Reps:
Set 1:	_____	_____
Set 2:	_____	_____
Set 3:	_____	_____
Set 4:	_____	_____

Muscles worked: _____

Stretched?   Yes _____   No _____

Name of exercise 3: _____

	Weight:	Reps:
Set 1:	_____	_____
Set 2:	_____	_____
Set 3:	_____	_____
Set 4:	_____	_____

Muscles worked: _____

Stretched?   Yes _____   No _____

Name of exercise 4: _____

	Weight:	Reps:
Set 1:	_____	_____
Set 2:	_____	_____
Set 3:	_____	_____
Set 4:	_____	_____

Muscles worked: _____

Stretched?   Yes _____   No _____

Name of exercise 5: _____

	Weight:	Reps:
Set 1:	_____	_____
Set 2:	_____	_____
Set 3:	_____	_____
Set 4:	_____	_____

Muscles worked: _____

Stretched?   Yes _____   No _____

Name of exercise 6: _____

	Weight:	Reps:
Set 1:	_____	_____
Set 2:	_____	_____
Set 3:	_____	_____
Set 4:	_____	_____

Muscles worked: _____

Stretched?   Yes _____   No _____

Name of exercise 7: _____

	Weight:	Reps:
Set 1:	_____	_____
Set 2:	_____	_____
Set 3:	_____	_____
Set 4:	_____	_____

Muscles worked: _____

Stretched?   Yes _____   No _____

Name of exercise 8: _____

	Weight:	Reps:
Set 1:	_____	_____
Set 2:	_____	_____
Set 3:	_____	_____
Set 4:	_____	_____

Muscles worked: _____

Stretched?   Yes _____   No _____

Name of exercise 9: _____

	Weight:	Reps:
Set 1:	_____	_____
Set 2:	_____	_____
Set 3:	_____	_____
Set 4:	_____	_____

Muscles worked: _____

Stretched?   Yes _____   No _____

Name of exercise 10: _____

	Weight:	Reps:
Set 1:	_____	_____
Set 2:	_____	_____
Set 3:	_____	_____
Set 4:	_____	_____

Muscles worked: _____

Stretched?   Yes _____   No _____

"I press on toward the goal to win the prize for which God has called me heavenward in Christ Jesus."
Philippians 3:14

Captain's Log

Day: _____ Date: _____ / _____ / _____

Nutrition Log

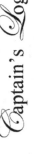

BREAKFAST Time: _____

	Type	Amt:
Protein	1. _____	_____
Complex Carbs	1. _____	_____
Fruit	1. _____	_____
Vegetables	1. _____	_____
Fat	1. _____	_____
Liquid/drink	1. _____	_____
Meal Replace.	1. _____	_____
Condiments	1. _____	_____
Other	1. _____	_____

Type	Amt:
2. _____	_____
2. _____	_____
2. _____	_____
2. _____	_____
2. _____	_____
2. _____	_____
2. _____	_____
2. _____	_____
2. _____	_____

SNACK 1 Time: _____

	Type	Amt:
Protein	1. _____	_____
Complex Carbs	1. _____	_____
Fruit	1. _____	_____
Vegetables	1. _____	_____
Fat	1. _____	_____
Liquid/drink	1. _____	_____
Meal Replace.	1. _____	_____
Condiments	1. _____	_____
Other	1. _____	_____

Type	Amt:
2. _____	_____
2. _____	_____
2. _____	_____
2. _____	_____
2. _____	_____
2. _____	_____
2. _____	_____
2. _____	_____
2. _____	_____

LUNCH Time: _____

	Type	Amt:
Protein	1. _____	_____
Complex Carbs	1. _____	_____
Fruit	1. _____	_____
Vegetables	1. _____	_____
Fat	1. _____	_____
Liquid/drink	1. _____	_____
Meal Replace.	1. _____	_____
Condiments	1. _____	_____
Other	1. _____	_____

Type	Amt:
2. _____	_____
2. _____	_____
2. _____	_____
2. _____	_____
2. _____	_____
2. _____	_____
2. _____	_____
2. _____	_____
2. _____	_____

SNACK 2 Time: _____

	Type	Amt:
Protein	1. _____	_____
Complex Carbs	1. _____	_____
Fruit	1. _____	_____
Vegetables	1. _____	_____
Fat	1. _____	_____
Liquid/drink	1. _____	_____
Meal Replace.	1. _____	_____
Condiments	1. _____	_____
Other	1. _____	_____

Type	Amt:
2. _____	_____
2. _____	_____
2. _____	_____
2. _____	_____
2. _____	_____
2. _____	_____
2. _____	_____
2. _____	_____
2. _____	_____

SNACK 3 Time: _____

	Type	Amt:
Protein	1. _____	_____
Complex Carbs	1. _____	_____
Fruit	1. _____	_____
Vegetables	1. _____	_____
Fat	1. _____	_____
Liquid/drink	1. _____	_____
Meal Replace.	1. _____	_____
Condiments	1. _____	_____
Other	1. _____	_____

Type	Amt:
2. _____	_____
2. _____	_____
2. _____	_____
2. _____	_____
2. _____	_____
2. _____	_____
2. _____	_____
2. _____	_____
2. _____	_____

DINNER Time: _____

	Type	Amt:
Protein	1. _____	_____
Complex Carbs	1. _____	_____
Fruit	1. _____	_____
Vegetables	1. _____	_____
Fat	1. _____	_____
Liquid/drink	1. _____	_____
Meal Replace.	1. _____	_____
Condiments	1. _____	_____
Other	1. _____	_____

Type	Amt:
2. _____	_____
2. _____	_____
2. _____	_____
2. _____	_____
2. _____	_____
2. _____	_____
2. _____	_____
2. _____	_____
2. _____	_____

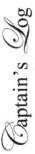

Cardiovascular Training

Warmed up   Yes _____   No _____

Time of day: _____	For how long?	Heart Rate
Type 1: _____	_____	_____
Type 2: _____	_____	_____
Type 3: _____	_____	_____
Type 4: _____	_____	_____

Stretched?   Yes _____   No _____

Evening Reflection

Did I put my faith in Action today?	Yes _____	No _____
I prayed for somone today	Yes _____	No _____
I read my Bible today	Yes _____	No _____
I helped someone in need today	Yes _____	No _____
I got 6 1/2 to 8 hours of sleep last night	Yes _____	No _____
I know I ate right today	Yes _____	No _____
I ate breakfast today	Yes _____	No _____
I ate starches after 4:00 p.m. today	Yes _____	No _____
I ate at least 4 meals today	Yes _____	No _____
I drank at least a gallon of water today	Yes _____	No _____
I had Courage to Change today	Yes _____	No _____
Tonight I forgive….		

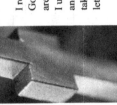

Captain's Log Statement of Faith

I realize that my actions don't earn my way into God's love or earn my way to heaven but that they are a reflection of my love affair with Jesus! I understand that by taking care of myself I honor and glorify God. I matter to God and the actions I take toward good health are daily written love letters telling God, "Thank you for my life"!

_____
Signature

Resistance Training

Time of day: _____

Warmed up   Yes _____   No _____

Name of exercise 1: _____

	Weight:	Reps:
Set 1:	_____	_____
Set 2:	_____	_____
Set 3:	_____	_____
Set 4:	_____	_____

Muscles worked: _____

Stretched?   Yes _____   No _____

Name of exercise 2: _____

	Weight:	Reps:
Set 1:	_____	_____
Set 2:	_____	_____
Set 3:	_____	_____
Set 4:	_____	_____

Muscles worked: _____

Stretched?   Yes _____   No _____

Name of exercise 3: _____

	Weight:	Reps:
Set 1:	_____	_____
Set 2:	_____	_____
Set 3:	_____	_____
Set 4:	_____	_____

Muscles worked: _____

Stretched?   Yes _____   No _____

Name of exercise 4: _____

	Weight:	Reps:
Set 1:	_____	_____
Set 2:	_____	_____
Set 3:	_____	_____
Set 4:	_____	_____

Muscles worked: _____

Stretched?   Yes _____   No _____

Name of exercise 5: _____

	Weight:	Reps:
Set 1:	_____	_____
Set 2:	_____	_____
Set 3:	_____	_____
Set 4:	_____	_____

Muscles worked: _____

Stretched?   Yes _____   No _____

Name of exercise 6: _____

	Weight:	Reps:
Set 1:	_____	_____
Set 2:	_____	_____
Set 3:	_____	_____
Set 4:	_____	_____

Muscles worked: _____

Stretched?   Yes _____   No _____

Name of exercise 7: _____

	Weight:	Reps:
Set 1:	_____	_____
Set 2:	_____	_____
Set 3:	_____	_____
Set 4:	_____	_____

Muscles worked: _____

Stretched?   Yes _____   No _____

Name of exercise 8: _____

	Weight:	Reps:
Set 1:	_____	_____
Set 2:	_____	_____
Set 3:	_____	_____
Set 4:	_____	_____

Muscles worked: _____

Stretched?   Yes _____   No _____

Name of exercise 9: _____

	Weight:	Reps:
Set 1:	_____	_____
Set 2:	_____	_____
Set 3:	_____	_____
Set 4:	_____	_____

Muscles worked: _____

Stretched?   Yes _____   No _____

Name of exercise 10: _____

	Weight:	Reps:
Set 1:	_____	_____
Set 2:	_____	_____
Set 3:	_____	_____
Set 4:	_____	_____

Muscles worked: _____

Stretched?   Yes _____   No _____

"I press on toward the goal to win the prize for which God has called me heavenward in Christ Jesus."
Philippians 3:14

Captain's Log

"Each one should test his own actions. Then he can take pride in himself without comparing himself to somebody else, for each one should carry his own load." (Galatians 6:40)

Day: _____   Date: _____ / _____ / _____

Nutrition Log

BREAKFAST   Time: _____

	Type	Amt:		Type	Amt:
Protein	1. _____	_____	2. _____	_____
Complex Carbs	1. _____	_____	2. _____	_____
Fruit	1. _____	_____	2. _____	_____
Vegetables	1. _____	_____	2. _____	_____
Fat	1. _____	_____	2. _____	_____
Liquid/drink	1. _____	_____	2. _____	_____
Meal Replace.	1. _____	_____	2. _____	_____
Condiments	1. _____	_____	2. _____	_____
Other	1. _____	_____	2. _____	_____

LUNCH   Time: _____

	Type	Amt:		Type	Amt:
Protein	1. _____	_____	2. _____	_____
Complex Carbs	1. _____	_____	2. _____	_____
Fruit	1. _____	_____	2. _____	_____
Vegetables	1. _____	_____	2. _____	_____
Fat	1. _____	_____	2. _____	_____
Liquid/drink	1. _____	_____	2. _____	_____
Meal Replace.	1. _____	_____	2. _____	_____
Condiments	1. _____	_____	2. _____	_____
Other	1. _____	_____	2. _____	_____

SNACK 3   Time: _____

	Type	Amt:		Type	Amt:
Protein	1. _____	_____	2. _____	_____
Complex Carbs	1. _____	_____	2. _____	_____
Fruit	1. _____	_____	2. _____	_____
Vegetables	1. _____	_____	2. _____	_____
Fat	1. _____	_____	2. _____	_____
Liquid/drink	1. _____	_____	2. _____	_____
Meal Replace.	1. _____	_____	2. _____	_____
Condiments	1. _____	_____	2. _____	_____
Other	1. _____	_____	2. _____	_____

SNACK 1   Time: _____

	Type	Amt:		Type	Amt:
Protein	1. _____	_____	2. _____	_____
Complex Carbs	1. _____	_____	2. _____	_____
Fruit	1. _____	_____	2. _____	_____
Vegetables	1. _____	_____	2. _____	_____
Fat	1. _____	_____	2. _____	_____
Liquid/drink	1. _____	_____	2. _____	_____
Meal Replace.	1. _____	_____	2. _____	_____
Condiments	1. _____	_____	2. _____	_____
Other	1. _____	_____	2. _____	_____

SNACK 2   Time: _____

	Type	Amt:		Type	Amt:
Protein	1. _____	_____	2. _____	_____
Complex Carbs	1. _____	_____	2. _____	_____
Fruit	1. _____	_____	2. _____	_____
Vegetables	1. _____	_____	2. _____	_____
Fat	1. _____	_____	2. _____	_____
Liquid/drink	1. _____	_____	2. _____	_____
Meal Replace.	1. _____	_____	2. _____	_____
Condiments	1. _____	_____	2. _____	_____
Other	1. _____	_____	2. _____	_____

DINNER   Time: _____

	Type	Amt:		Type	Amt:
Protein	1. _____	_____	2. _____	_____
Complex Carbs	1. _____	_____	2. _____	_____
Fruit	1. _____	_____	2. _____	_____
Vegetables	1. _____	_____	2. _____	_____
Fat	1. _____	_____	2. _____	_____
Liquid/drink	1. _____	_____	2. _____	_____
Meal Replace.	1. _____	_____	2. _____	_____
Condiments	1. _____	_____	2. _____	_____
Other	1. _____	_____	2. _____	_____

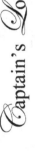
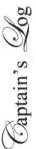

Cardiovascular Training

Warmed up   Yes _____   No _____

Time of day: _____	For how long?	Heart Rate
Type 1:	_____	_____
Type 2:	_____	_____
Type 3:	_____	_____
Type 4:	_____	_____
Stretched? Yes _____ No _____		

Evening Reflection

Did I put my faith in Action today?	Yes _____	No _____
I prayed for somone today	Yes _____	No _____
I read my Bible today	Yes _____	No _____
I helped someone in need today	Yes _____	No _____
I got 6 1/2 to 8 hours of sleep last night	Yes _____	No _____
I know I ate right today	Yes _____	No _____
I ate breakfast today	Yes _____	No _____
I ate starches after 4:00 p.m. today	Yes _____	No _____
I ate at least 4 meals today	Yes _____	No _____
I drank at least a gallon of water today	Yes _____	No _____
I had Courage to Change today	Yes _____	No _____
Tonight I forgive… _____		

Captain's Log Statement of Faith

I realize that my actions don't earn my way into God's love or earn my way to heaven but that they are a reflection of my love affair with Jesus! I understand that by taking care of myself I honor and glorify God. I matter to God and the actions I take toward good health are daily written love letters telling God, "Thank you for my life"!

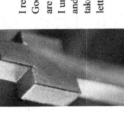

_____
Signature

Resistance Training

Time of day: _____

Warmed up   Yes _____   No _____

Name of exercise 1:
_____   Weight: _____   Reps: _____
Set 1: _____
Set 2: _____
Muscles worked: _____   Set 3: _____
Set 4: _____
Stretched?   Yes _____   No _____

Name of exercise 2:
_____   Weight: _____   Reps: _____
Set 1: _____
Set 2: _____
Muscles worked: _____   Set 3: _____
Set 4: _____
Stretched?   Yes _____   No _____

Name of exercise 3:
_____   Weight: _____   Reps: _____
Set 1: _____
Set 2: _____
Muscles worked: _____   Set 3: _____
Set 4: _____
Stretched?   Yes _____   No _____

Name of exercise 4:
_____   Weight: _____   Reps: _____
Set 1: _____
Set 2: _____
Muscles worked: _____   Set 3: _____
Set 4: _____
Stretched?   Yes _____   No _____

Name of exercise 5:
_____   Weight: _____   Reps: _____
Set 1: _____
Set 2: _____
Muscles worked: _____   Set 3: _____
Set 4: _____
Stretched?   Yes _____   No _____

Name of exercise 6:
_____   Weight: _____   Reps: _____
Set 1: _____
Set 2: _____
Muscles worked: _____   Set 3: _____
Set 4: _____
Stretched?   Yes _____   No _____

Name of exercise 7:
_____   Weight: _____   Reps: _____
Set 1: _____
Set 2: _____
Muscles worked: _____   Set 3: _____
Set 4: _____
Stretched?   Yes _____   No _____

Name of exercise 8:
_____   Weight: _____   Reps: _____
Set 1: _____
Set 2: _____
Muscles worked: _____   Set 3: _____
Set 4: _____
Stretched?   Yes _____   No _____

Name of exercise 9:
_____   Weight: _____   Reps: _____
Set 1: _____
Set 2: _____
Muscles worked: _____   Set 3: _____
Set 4: _____
Stretched?   Yes _____   No _____

Name of exercise 10:
_____   Weight: _____   Reps: _____
Set 1: _____
Set 2: _____
Muscles worked: _____   Set 3: _____
Set 4: _____
Stretched?   Yes _____   No _____

"I press on toward the goal to win the prize for which God has called me heavenward in Christ Jesus."

Philippians 3:14

Captain's Log

"Each one should test his own actions. Then he can take pride in himself without comparing himself to somebody else, for each one should carry his own load." (Galatians 6:40)

Day: _____ Date: _____ / _____ / _____

Nutrition Log

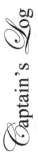

BREAKFAST Time: _____

	Type	Amt:		Type	Amt:
Protein	1.			2.	
Complex Carbs	1.			2.	
Fruit	1.			2.	
Vegetables	1.			2.	
Fat	1.			2.	
Liquid/drink	1.			2.	
Meal Replace.	1.			2.	
Condiments	1.			2.	
Other	1.			2.	

LUNCH Time: _____

	Type	Amt:		Type	Amt:
Protein	1.			2.	
Complex Carbs	1.			2.	
Fruit	1.			2.	
Vegetables	1.			2.	
Fat	1.			2.	
Liquid/drink	1.			2.	
Meal Replace.	1.			2.	
Condiments	1.			2.	
Other	1.			2.	

SNACK 3 Time: _____

	Type	Amt:		Type	Amt:
Protein	1.			2.	
Complex Carbs	1.			2.	
Fruit	1.			2.	
Vegetables	1.			2.	
Fat	1.			2.	
Liquid/drink	1.			2.	
Meal Replace.	1.			2.	
Condiments	1.			2.	
Other	1.			2.	

SNACK 1 Time: _____

	Type	Amt:		Type	Amt:
Protein	1.			2.	
Complex Carbs	1.			2.	
Fruit	1.			2.	
Vegetables	1.			2.	
Fat	1.			2.	
Liquid/drink	1.			2.	
Meal Replace.	1.			2.	
Condiments	1.			2.	
Other	1.			2.	

SNACK 2 Time: _____

	Type	Amt:		Type	Amt:
Protein	1.			2.	
Complex Carbs	1.			2.	
Fruit	1.			2.	
Vegetables	1.			2.	
Fat	1.			2.	
Liquid/drink	1.			2.	
Meal Replace.	1.			2.	
Condiments	1.			2.	
Other	1.			2.	

DINNER Time: _____

	Type	Amt:		Type	Amt:
Protein	1.			2.	
Complex Carbs	1.			2.	
Fruit	1.			2.	
Vegetables	1.			2.	
Fat	1.			2.	
Liquid/drink	1.			2.	
Meal Replace.	1.			2.	
Condiments	1.			2.	
Other	1.			2.	

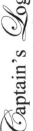

Resistance Training

Time of day: _____

Warmed up   Yes _____   No _____

Name of exercise 1: _____   Weight: _____   Reps: _____

_____

Set 1: _____
Set 2: _____
Set 3: _____
Set 4: _____

Muscles worked: _____

Stretched?   Yes _____   No _____

Name of exercise 3: _____   Weight: _____   Reps: _____

_____

Set 1: _____
Set 2: _____
Set 3: _____
Set 4: _____

Muscles worked: _____

Stretched?   Yes _____   No _____

Name of exercise 5: _____   Weight: _____   Reps: _____

_____

Set 1: _____
Set 2: _____
Set 3: _____
Set 4: _____

Muscles worked: _____

Stretched?   Yes _____   No _____

Name of exercise 7: _____   Weight: _____   Reps: _____

_____

Set 1: _____
Set 2: _____
Set 3: _____
Set 4: _____

Muscles worked: _____

Stretched?   Yes _____   No _____

Name of exercise 9: _____   Weight: _____   Reps: _____

_____

Set 1: _____
Set 2: _____
Set 3: _____
Set 4: _____

Muscles worked: _____

Stretched?   Yes _____   No _____

Cardiovascular Training

Warmed up   Yes _____   No _____

Time of day: _____   For how long?   Heart Rate

Type 1: _____
Type 2: _____
Type 3: _____
Type 4: _____

Stretched?   Yes _____   No _____

Name of exercise 2: _____   Weight: _____   Reps: _____

_____

Set 1: _____
Set 2: _____
Set 3: _____
Set 4: _____

Muscles worked: _____

Stretched?   Yes _____   No _____

Name of exercise 4: _____   Weight: _____   Reps: _____

_____

Set 1: _____
Set 2: _____
Set 3: _____
Set 4: _____

Muscles worked: _____

Stretched?   Yes _____   No _____

Name of exercise 6: _____   Weight: _____   Reps: _____

_____

Set 1: _____
Set 2: _____
Set 3: _____
Set 4: _____

Muscles worked: _____

Stretched?   Yes _____   No _____

Name of exercise 8: _____   Weight: _____   Reps: _____

_____

Set 1: _____
Set 2: _____
Set 3: _____
Set 4: _____

Muscles worked: _____

Stretched?   Yes _____   No _____

Name of exercise 10: _____   Weight: _____   Reps: _____

_____

Set 1: _____
Set 2: _____
Set 3: _____
Set 4: _____

Muscles worked: _____

Stretched?   Yes _____   No _____

Evening Reflection

Did I put my faith in Action today?	Yes _____	No _____
I prayed for somone today	Yes _____	No _____
I read my Bible today	Yes _____	No _____
I helped someone in need today	Yes _____	No _____
I got 6 1/2 to 8 hours of sleep last night	Yes _____	No _____
I know I ate right today	Yes _____	No _____
I ate breakfast today	Yes _____	No _____
I ate starches after 4:00 p.m. today	Yes _____	No _____
I ate at least 4 meals today	Yes _____	No _____
I drank at least a gallon of water today	Yes _____	No _____
I had Courage to Change today	Yes _____	No _____
Tonight I forgive… _____		

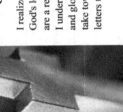

Captain's Log Statement of Faith

I realize that my actions don't earn my way into God's love or earn my way to heaven but that they are a reflection of my love affair with Jesus! I understand that by taking care of myself I honor and glorify God. I matter to God and the actions I take toward good health are daily written love letters telling God, "Thank you for my life"!

_____

Signature

"I press on toward the goal to win the prize for which God has called me heavenward in Christ Jesus."
Philippians 3:14

Captain's Log

Day: _____ Date: _____ / _____ / _____

Nutrition Log

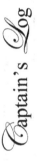
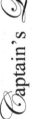

BREAKFAST Time: _____

	Type	Amt:	Type	Amt:
Protein	1.		2.	
Complex Carbs	1.		2.	
Fruit	1.		2.	
Vegetables	1.		2.	
Fat	1.		2.	
Liquid/drink	1.		2.	
Meal Replace.	1.		2.	
Condiments	1.		2.	
Other	1.		2.	

SNACK 1 Time: _____

	Type	Amt:	Type	Amt:
Protein	1.		2.	
Complex Carbs	1.		2.	
Fruit	1.		2.	
Vegetables	1.		2.	
Fat	1.		2.	
Liquid/drink	1.		2.	
Meal Replace.	1.		2.	
Condiments	1.		2.	
Other	1.		2.	

LUNCH Time: _____

	Type	Amt:	Type	Amt:
Protein	1.		2.	
Complex Carbs	1.		2.	
Fruit	1.		2.	
Vegetables	1.		2.	
Fat	1.		2.	
Liquid/drink	1.		2.	
Meal Replace.	1.		2.	
Condiments	1.		2.	
Other	1.		2.	

SNACK 2 Time: _____

	Type	Amt:	Type	Amt:
Protein	1.		2.	
Complex Carbs	1.		2.	
Fruit	1.		2.	
Vegetables	1.		2.	
Fat	1.		2.	
Liquid/drink	1.		2.	
Meal Replace.	1.		2.	
Condiments	1.		2.	
Other	1.		2.	

SNACK 3 Time: _____

	Type	Amt:	Type	Amt:
Protein	1.		2.	
Complex Carbs	1.		2.	
Fruit	1.		2.	
Vegetables	1.		2.	
Fat	1.		2.	
Liquid/drink	1.		2.	
Meal Replace.	1.		2.	
Condiments	1.		2.	
Other	1.		2.	

DINNER Time: _____

	Type	Amt:	Type	Amt:
Protein	1.		2.	
Complex Carbs	1.		2.	
Fruit	1.		2.	
Vegetables	1.		2.	
Fat	1.		2.	
Liquid/drink	1.		2.	
Meal Replace.	1.		2.	
Condiments	1.		2.	
Other	1.		2.	

Resistance Training

Time of day: _____

Warmed up   Yes _____   No _____

Name of exercise 1:
_____
Weight: _____   Reps: _____
Set 1: _____
Set 2: _____
Muscles worked: _____
Set 3: _____
Set 4: _____
Stretched?   Yes _____   No _____

Name of exercise 3:
_____
Weight: _____   Reps: _____
Set 1: _____
Set 2: _____
Muscles worked: _____
Set 3: _____
Set 4: _____
Stretched?   Yes _____   No _____

Name of exercise 5:
_____
Weight: _____   Reps: _____
Set 1: _____
Set 2: _____
Muscles worked: _____
Set 3: _____
Set 4: _____
Stretched?   Yes _____   No _____

Name of exercise 7:
_____
Weight: _____   Reps: _____
Set 1: _____
Set 2: _____
Muscles worked: _____
Set 3: _____
Set 4: _____
Stretched?   Yes _____   No _____

Name of exercise 9:
_____
Weight: _____   Reps: _____
Set 1: _____
Set 2: _____
Muscles worked: _____
Set 3: _____
Set 4: _____
Stretched?   Yes _____   No _____

Cardiovascular Training

Warmed up   Yes _____   No _____

Time of day: _____   For how long?   Heart Rate
Type 1: _____
Type 2: _____
Type 3: _____
Type 4: _____
Stretched?   Yes _____   No _____

Evening Reflection

Did I put my faith in Action today?   Yes _____   No _____
I prayed for somone today   Yes _____   No _____
I read my Bible today   Yes _____   No _____
I helped someone in need today   Yes _____   No _____
I got 6 1/2 to 8 hours of sleep last night   Yes _____   No _____
I know I ate right today   Yes _____   No _____
I ate breakfast today   Yes _____   No _____
I ate starches after 4:00 p.m. today   Yes _____   No _____
I ate at least 4 meals today   Yes _____   No _____
I drank at least a gallon of water today   Yes _____   No _____
I had Courage to Change today   Yes _____   No _____
Tonight I forgive… _____

Name of exercise 2:
_____
Weight: _____   Reps: _____
Set 1: _____
Set 2: _____
Muscles worked: _____
Set 3: _____
Set 4: _____
Stretched?   Yes _____   No _____

Name of exercise 4:
_____
Weight: _____   Reps: _____
Set 1: _____
Set 2: _____
Muscles worked: _____
Set 3: _____
Set 4: _____
Stretched?   Yes _____   No _____

Name of exercise 6:
_____
Weight: _____   Reps: _____
Set 1: _____
Set 2: _____
Muscles worked: _____
Set 3: _____
Set 4: _____
Stretched?   Yes _____   No _____

Name of exercise 8:
_____
Weight: _____   Reps: _____
Set 1: _____
Set 2: _____
Muscles worked: _____
Set 3: _____
Set 4: _____
Stretched?   Yes _____   No _____

Name of exercise 10:
_____
Weight: _____   Reps: _____
Set 1: _____
Set 2: _____
Muscles worked: _____
Set 3: _____
Set 4: _____
Stretched?   Yes _____   No _____

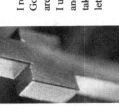

Captain's Log Statement of Faith

I realize that my actions don't earn my way into God's love or earn my way to heaven but that they are a reflection of my love affair with Jesus! I understand that by taking care of myself I honor and glorify God. I matter to God and the actions I take toward good health are daily written love letters telling God, "Thank you for my life"!

_____
Signature

"I press on toward the goal to win the prize for which God has called me heavenward in Christ Jesus."
Philippians 3:14

Captain's Log

"Each one should test his own actions. Then he can take pride in himself without comparing himself to somebody else, for each one should carry his own load." (Galatians 6:40)

Day: _____ Date: _____ / _____ / _____

Nutrition Log

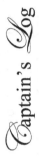

BREAKFAST
Time: _____

	Type 1.	Amt:	Type 2.	Amt:
Protein				
Complex Carbs				
Fruit				
Vegetables				
Fat				
Liquid/drink				
Meal Replace.				
Condiments				
Other				

LUNCH
Time: _____

	Type 1.	Amt:	Type 2.	Amt:
Protein				
Complex Carbs				
Fruit				
Vegetables				
Fat				
Liquid/drink				
Meal Replace.				
Condiments				
Other				

SNACK 3
Time: _____

	Type 1.	Amt:	Type 2.	Amt:
Protein				
Complex Carbs				
Fruit				
Vegetables				
Fat				
Liquid/drink				
Meal Replace.				
Condiments				
Other				

SNACK 1
Time: _____

	Type 1.	Amt:	Type 2.	Amt:
Protein				
Complex Carbs				
Fruit				
Vegetables				
Fat				
Liquid/drink				
Meal Replace.				
Condiments				
Other				

SNACK 2
Time: _____

	Type 1.	Amt:	Type 2.	Amt:
Protein				
Complex Carbs				
Fruit				
Vegetables				
Fat				
Liquid/drink				
Meal Replace.				
Condiments				
Other				

DINNER
Time: _____

	Type 1.	Amt:	Type 2.	Amt:
Protein				
Complex Carbs				
Fruit				
Vegetables				
Fat				
Liquid/drink				
Meal Replace.				
Condiments				
Other				

Cardiovascular Training

Warmed up   Yes _____   No _____

Time of day: _____	For how long?	Heart Rate
Type 1:	_____	_____
Type 2:	_____	_____
Type 3:	_____	_____
Type 4:	_____	_____
Stretched? Yes _____ No _____		

Evening Reflection

Did I put my faith in Action today?	Yes _____	No _____
I prayed for somone today	Yes _____	No _____
I read my Bible today	Yes _____	No _____
I helped someone in need today	Yes _____	No _____
I got 6 1/2 to 8 hours of sleep last night	Yes _____	No _____
I know I ate right today	Yes _____	No _____
I ate breakfast today	Yes _____	No _____
I ate starches after 4:00 p.m. today	Yes _____	No _____
I ate at least 4 meals today	Yes _____	No _____
I drank at least a gallon of water today	Yes _____	No _____
I had Courage to Change today	Yes _____	No _____
Tonight I forgive……		

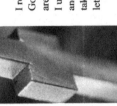

Captain's Log Statement of Faith

I realize that my actions don't earn my way into God's love or earn my way to heaven but that they are a reflection of my love affair with Jesus! I understand that by taking care of myself I honor and glorify God. I matter to God and the actions I take toward good health are daily written love letters telling God, "Thank you for my life"!

_____
Signature

"I press on toward the goal to win the prize for which God has called me heavenward in Christ Jesus."
Philippians 3:14

Resistance Training

Time of day: _____

Warmed up   Yes _____   No _____

Name of exercise 1: _____

	Weight:	Reps:
Set 1:	_____	_____
Set 2:	_____	_____
Set 3:	_____	_____
Set 4:	_____	_____

Muscles worked: _____

Stretched?   Yes _____   No _____

Name of exercise 2: _____

	Weight:	Reps:
Set 1:	_____	_____
Set 2:	_____	_____
Set 3:	_____	_____
Set 4:	_____	_____

Muscles worked: _____

Stretched?   Yes _____   No _____

Name of exercise 3: _____

	Weight:	Reps:
Set 1:	_____	_____
Set 2:	_____	_____
Set 3:	_____	_____
Set 4:	_____	_____

Muscles worked: _____

Stretched?   Yes _____   No _____

Name of exercise 4: _____

	Weight:	Reps:
Set 1:	_____	_____
Set 2:	_____	_____
Set 3:	_____	_____
Set 4:	_____	_____

Muscles worked: _____

Stretched?   Yes _____   No _____

Name of exercise 5: _____

	Weight:	Reps:
Set 1:	_____	_____
Set 2:	_____	_____
Set 3:	_____	_____
Set 4:	_____	_____

Muscles worked: _____

Stretched?   Yes _____   No _____

Name of exercise 6: _____

	Weight:	Reps:
Set 1:	_____	_____
Set 2:	_____	_____
Set 3:	_____	_____
Set 4:	_____	_____

Muscles worked: _____

Stretched?   Yes _____   No _____

Name of exercise 7: _____

	Weight:	Reps:
Set 1:	_____	_____
Set 2:	_____	_____
Set 3:	_____	_____
Set 4:	_____	_____

Muscles worked: _____

Stretched?   Yes _____   No _____

Name of exercise 8: _____

	Weight:	Reps:
Set 1:	_____	_____
Set 2:	_____	_____
Set 3:	_____	_____
Set 4:	_____	_____

Muscles worked: _____

Stretched?   Yes _____   No _____

Name of exercise 9: _____

	Weight:	Reps:
Set 1:	_____	_____
Set 2:	_____	_____
Set 3:	_____	_____
Set 4:	_____	_____

Muscles worked: _____

Stretched?   Yes _____   No _____

Name of exercise 10: _____

	Weight:	Reps:
Set 1:	_____	_____
Set 2:	_____	_____
Set 3:	_____	_____
Set 4:	_____	_____

Muscles worked: _____

Stretched?   Yes _____   No _____

THE CHILD IN YOU

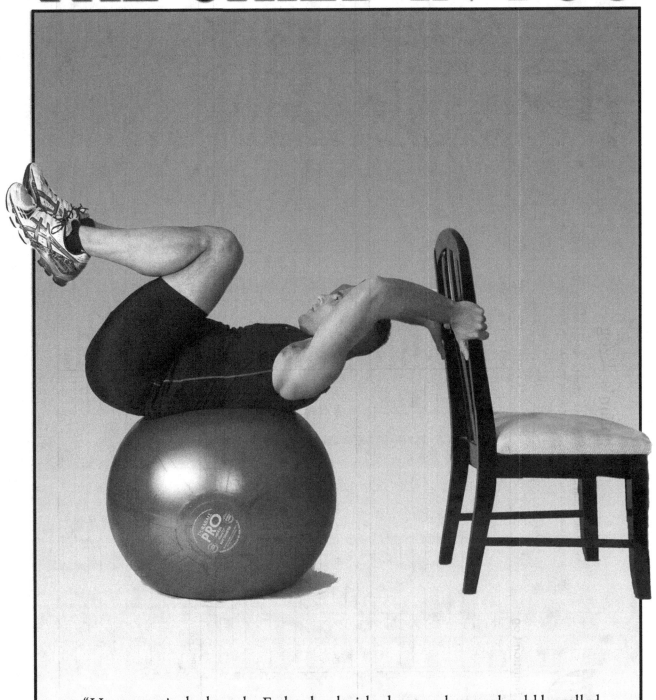

"How great is the love the Father has lavished on us, that we should be called children of God! And that is what we are!" (1 John 3:1),

WEEK SEVEN

Captain's Log

"Each one should test his own actions. Then he can take pride in himself without comparing himself to somebody else, for each one should carry his own load." (Galatians 6:40)

Day: _____ Date: _____ / _____ / _____

Nutrition Log

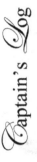

BREAKFAST	Time: _____			SNACK 1	Time: _____		
	Type	Amt:	Type	Amt:		Type	Amt:	Type	Amt:
Protein	1.		2.		Protein	1.		2.
Complex Carbs	1.		2.		Complex Carbs	1.		2.
Fruit	1.		2.		Fruit	1.		2.
Vegetables	1.		2.		Vegetables	1.		2.
Fat	1.		2.		Fat	1.		2.
Liquid/drink	1.		2.		Liquid/drink	1.		2.
Meal Replace.	1.		2.		Meal Replace.	1.		2.
Condiments	1.		2.		Condiments	1.		2.
Other	1.		2.		Other	1.		2.

LUNCH	Time: _____			SNACK 2	Time: _____		
	Type	Amt:	Type	Amt:		Type	Amt:	Type	Amt:
Protein	1.		2.		Protein	1.		2.
Complex Carbs	1.		2.		Complex Carbs	1.		2.
Fruit	1.		2.		Fruit	1.		2.
Vegetables	1.		2.		Vegetables	1.		2.
Fat	1.		2.		Fat	1.		2.
Liquid/drink	1.		2.		Liquid/drink	1.		2.
Meal Replace.	1.		2.		Meal Replace.	1.		2.
Condiments	1.		2.		Condiments	1.		2.
Other	1.		2.		Other	1.		2.

SNACK 3	Time: _____			DINNER	Time: _____		
	Type	Amt:	Type	Amt:		Type	Amt:	Type	Amt:
Protein	1.		2.		Protein	1.		2.
Complex Carbs	1.		2.		Complex Carbs	1.		2.
Fruit	1.		2.		Fruit	1.		2.
Vegetables	1.		2.		Vegetables	1.		2.
Fat	1.		2.		Fat	1.		2.
Liquid/drink	1.		2.		Liquid/drink	1.		2.
Meal Replace.	1.		2.		Meal Replace.	1.		2.
Condiments	1.		2.		Condiments	1.		2.
Other	1.		2.		Other	1.		2.

Cardiovascular Training

Warmed up Yes _____ No _____

| Time of day: _____ | For how long? _____ | Heart Rate _____ |

Type 1: _____
Type 2: _____
Type 3: _____
Type 4: _____

Stretched? Yes _____ No _____

Evening Reflection

Did I put my faith in Action today?	Yes _____	No _____
I prayed for somone today	Yes _____	No _____
I read my Bible today	Yes _____	No _____
I helped someone in need today	Yes _____	No _____
I got 6 1/2 to 8 hours of sleep last night	Yes _____	No _____
I know I ate right today	Yes _____	No _____
I ate breakfast today	Yes _____	No _____
I ate starches after 4:00 p.m. today	Yes _____	No _____
I ate at least 4 meals today	Yes _____	No _____
I drank at least a gallon of water today	Yes _____	No _____
I had Courage to Change today	Yes _____	No _____
Tonight I forgive…. _____		

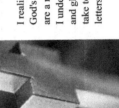

Captain's Log Statement of Faith

I realize that my actions don't earn my way into God's love or earn my way to heaven but that they are a reflection of my love affair with Jesus! I understand that by taking care of myself I honor and glorify God. I matter to God and the actions I take toward good health are daily written love letters telling God, "Thank you for my life"!

_____
Signature

Resistance Training

Time of day: _____

Warmed up Yes _____ No _____

Name of exercise 1: | Weight: | Reps:
Set 1: _____
Set 2: _____
Set 3: _____
Set 4: _____
Muscles worked:
Stretched? Yes _____ No _____

Name of exercise 2: | Weight: | Reps:
Set 1: _____
Set 2: _____
Set 3: _____
Set 4: _____
Muscles worked:
Stretched? Yes _____ No _____

Name of exercise 3: | Weight: | Reps:
Set 1: _____
Set 2: _____
Set 3: _____
Set 4: _____
Muscles worked:
Stretched? Yes _____ No _____

Name of exercise 4: | Weight: | Reps:
Set 1: _____
Set 2: _____
Set 3: _____
Set 4: _____
Muscles worked:
Stretched? Yes _____ No _____

Name of exercise 5: | Weight: | Reps:
Set 1: _____
Set 2: _____
Set 3: _____
Set 4: _____
Muscles worked:
Stretched? Yes _____ No _____

Name of exercise 6: | Weight: | Reps:
Set 1: _____
Set 2: _____
Set 3: _____
Set 4: _____
Muscles worked:
Stretched? Yes _____ No _____

Name of exercise 7: | Weight: | Reps:
Set 1: _____
Set 2: _____
Set 3: _____
Set 4: _____
Muscles worked:
Stretched? Yes _____ No _____

Name of exercise 8: | Weight: | Reps:
Set 1: _____
Set 2: _____
Set 3: _____
Set 4: _____
Muscles worked:
Stretched? Yes _____ No _____

Name of exercise 9: | Weight: | Reps:
Set 1: _____
Set 2: _____
Set 3: _____
Set 4: _____
Muscles worked:
Stretched? Yes _____ No _____

Name of exercise 10: | Weight: | Reps:
Set 1: _____
Set 2: _____
Set 3: _____
Set 4: _____
Muscles worked:
Stretched? Yes _____ No _____

"I press on toward the goal to win the prize for which God has called me heavenward in Christ Jesus."
Philippians 3:14

Captain's Log

"Each one should test his own actions. Then he can take pride in himself without comparing himself to somebody else, for each one should carry his own load." (Galatians 6:40)

Day: _____   Date: ____ / ____ / ____

Nutrition Log

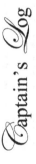
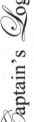

BREAKFAST Time: _____

	Type	Amt:	Type	Amt:
Protein	1.		2.	
Complex Carbs	1.		2.	
Fruit	1.		2.	
Vegetables	1.		2.	
Fat	1.		2.	
Liquid/drink	1.		2.	
Meal Replace.	1.		2.	
Condiments	1.		2.	
Other	1.		2.	

LUNCH Time: _____

	Type	Amt:	Type	Amt:
Protein	1.		2.	
Complex Carbs	1.		2.	
Fruit	1.		2.	
Vegetables	1.		2.	
Fat	1.		2.	
Liquid/drink	1.		2.	
Meal Replace.	1.		2.	
Condiments	1.		2.	
Other	1.		2.	

SNACK 3 Time: _____

	Type	Amt:	Type	Amt:
Protein	1.		2.	
Complex Carbs	1.		2.	
Fruit	1.		2.	
Vegetables	1.		2.	
Fat	1.		2.	
Liquid/drink	1.		2.	
Meal Replace.	1.		2.	
Condiments	1.		2.	
Other	1.		2.	

SNACK 1 Time: _____

	Type	Amt:	Type	Amt:
Protein	1.		2.	
Complex Carbs	1.		2.	
Fruit	1.		2.	
Vegetables	1.		2.	
Fat	1.		2.	
Liquid/drink	1.		2.	
Meal Replace.	1.		2.	
Condiments	1.		2.	
Other	1.		2.	

SNACK 2 Time: _____

	Type	Amt:	Type	Amt:
Protein	1.		2.	
Complex Carbs	1.		2.	
Fruit	1.		2.	
Vegetables	1.		2.	
Fat	1.		2.	
Liquid/drink	1.		2.	
Meal Replace.	1.		2.	
Condiments	1.		2.	
Other	1.		2.	

DINNER Time: _____

	Type	Amt:	Type	Amt:
Protein	1.		2.	
Complex Carbs	1.		2.	
Fruit	1.		2.	
Vegetables	1.		2.	
Fat	1.		2.	
Liquid/drink	1.		2.	
Meal Replace.	1.		2.	
Condiments	1.		2.	
Other	1.		2.	

Cardiovascular Training

Warmed up   Yes _____   No _____

Time of day: _____	For how long?	Heart Rate
Type 1:	_____	_____
Type 2:	_____	_____
Type 3:	_____	_____
Type 4:	_____	_____
Stretched? Yes _____ No _____		

Evening Reflection

Did I put my faith in Action today?	Yes _____	No _____
I prayed for somone today	Yes _____	No _____
I read my Bible today	Yes _____	No _____
I helped someone in need today	Yes _____	No _____
I got 6 1/2 to 8 hours of sleep last night	Yes _____	No _____
I know I ate right today	Yes _____	No _____
I ate breakfast today	Yes _____	No _____
I ate starches after 4:00 p.m. today	Yes _____	No _____
I ate at least 4 meals today	Yes _____	No _____
I drank at least a gallon of water today	Yes _____	No _____
I had Courage to Change today	Yes _____	No _____
Tonight I forgive… _____		

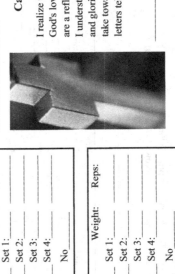

Captain's Log Statement of Faith

I realize that my actions don't earn my way into God's love or earn my way to heaven but that they are a reflection of my love affair with Jesus! I understand that by taking care of myself I honor and glorify God. I matter to God and the actions I take toward good health are daily written love letters telling God, "Thank you for my life"!

Signature _____

Resistance Training

Time of day: _____

Warmed up   Yes _____   No _____

Name of exercise 1:	Weight:	Reps:
_____	Set 1: _____	
_____	Set 2: _____	
Muscles worked:	Set 3: _____	
_____	Set 4: _____	
Stretched? Yes _____ No _____		

Name of exercise 2:	Weight:	Reps:
_____	Set 1: _____	
_____	Set 2: _____	
Muscles worked:	Set 3: _____	
_____	Set 4: _____	
Stretched? Yes _____ No _____		

Name of exercise 3:	Weight:	Reps:
_____	Set 1: _____	
_____	Set 2: _____	
Muscles worked:	Set 3: _____	
_____	Set 4: _____	
Stretched? Yes _____ No _____		

Name of exercise 4:	Weight:	Reps:
_____	Set 1: _____	
_____	Set 2: _____	
Muscles worked:	Set 3: _____	
_____	Set 4: _____	
Stretched? Yes _____ No _____		

Name of exercise 5:	Weight:	Reps:
_____	Set 1: _____	
_____	Set 2: _____	
Muscles worked:	Set 3: _____	
_____	Set 4: _____	
Stretched? Yes _____ No _____		

Name of exercise 6:	Weight:	Reps:
_____	Set 1: _____	
_____	Set 2: _____	
Muscles worked:	Set 3: _____	
_____	Set 4: _____	
Stretched? Yes _____ No _____		

Name of exercise 7:	Weight:	Reps:
_____	Set 1: _____	
_____	Set 2: _____	
Muscles worked:	Set 3: _____	
_____	Set 4: _____	
Stretched? Yes _____ No _____		

Name of exercise 8:	Weight:	Reps:
_____	Set 1: _____	
_____	Set 2: _____	
Muscles worked:	Set 3: _____	
_____	Set 4: _____	
Stretched? Yes _____ No _____		

Name of exercise 9:	Weight:	Reps:
_____	Set 1: _____	
_____	Set 2: _____	
Muscles worked:	Set 3: _____	
_____	Set 4: _____	
Stretched? Yes _____ No _____		

Name of exercise 10:	Weight:	Reps:
_____	Set 1: _____	
_____	Set 2: _____	
Muscles worked:	Set 3: _____	
_____	Set 4: _____	
Stretched? Yes _____ No _____		

"I press on toward the goal to win the prize for which God has called me heavenward in Christ Jesus."
Philippians 3:14

Captain's Log

Nutrition Log

"Each one should test his own actions. Then he can take pride in himself without comparing himself to somebody else, for each one should carry his own load." (Galatians 6:40)

Day: _____   Date: _____ / _____ / _____

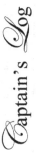
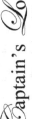

BREAKFAST
Time: _____

	Type	Amt:	Type	Amt:
Protein	1.	___	2.	___
Complex Carbs	1.	___	2.	___
Fruit	1.	___	2.	___
Vegetables	1.	___	2.	___
Fat	1.	___	2.	___
Liquid/drink	1.	___	2.	___
Meal Replace.	1.	___	2.	___
Condiments	1.	___	2.	___
Other	1.	___	2.	___

SNACK 1
Time: _____

	Type	Amt:	Type	Amt:
Protein	1.	___	2.	___
Complex Carbs	1.	___	2.	___
Fruit	1.	___	2.	___
Vegetables	1.	___	2.	___
Fat	1.	___	2.	___
Liquid/drink	1.	___	2.	___
Meal Replace.	1.	___	2.	___
Condiments	1.	___	2.	___
Other	1.	___	2.	___

LUNCH
Time: _____

	Type	Amt:	Type	Amt:
Protein	1.	___	2.	___
Complex Carbs	1.	___	2.	___
Fruit	1.	___	2.	___
Vegetables	1.	___	2.	___
Fat	1.	___	2.	___
Liquid/drink	1.	___	2.	___
Meal Replace.	1.	___	2.	___
Condiments	1.	___	2.	___
Other	1.	___	2.	___

SNACK 2
Time: _____

	Type	Amt:	Type	Amt:
Protein	1.	___	2.	___
Complex Carbs	1.	___	2.	___
Fruit	1.	___	2.	___
Vegetables	1.	___	2.	___
Fat	1.	___	2.	___
Liquid/drink	1.	___	2.	___
Meal Replace.	1.	___	2.	___
Condiments	1.	___	2.	___
Other	1.	___	2.	___

SNACK 3
Time: _____

	Type	Amt:	Type	Amt:
Protein	1.	___	2.	___
Complex Carbs	1.	___	2.	___
Fruit	1.	___	2.	___
Vegetables	1.	___	2.	___
Fat	1.	___	2.	___
Liquid/drink	1.	___	2.	___
Meal Replace.	1.	___	2.	___
Condiments	1.	___	2.	___
Other	1.	___	2.	___

DINNER
Time: _____

	Type	Amt:	Type	Amt:
Protein	1.	___	2.	___
Complex Carbs	1.	___	2.	___
Fruit	1.	___	2.	___
Vegetables	1.	___	2.	___
Fat	1.	___	2.	___
Liquid/drink	1.	___	2.	___
Meal Replace.	1.	___	2.	___
Condiments	1.	___	2.	___
Other	1.	___	2.	___

Cardiovascular Training

Warmed up Yes_____ No_____

Time of day: _____	For how long?	Heart Rate
Type 1: _____	_____	_____
Type 2: _____	_____	_____
Type 3: _____	_____	_____
Type 4: _____	_____	_____
Stretched? Yes_____ No_____		

Evening Reflection

Did I put my faith in Action today?	Yes_____	No_____
I prayed for somone today	Yes_____	No_____
I read my Bible today	Yes_____	No_____
I helped someone in need today	Yes_____	No_____
I got 6 1/2 to 8 hours of sleep last night	Yes_____	No_____
I know I ate right today	Yes_____	No_____
I ate breakfast today	Yes_____	No_____
I ate starches after 4:00 p.m. today	Yes_____	No_____
I ate at least 4 meals today	Yes_____	No_____
I drank at least a gallon of water today	Yes_____	No_____
I had Courage to Change today	Yes_____	No_____
Tonight I forgive…_____		

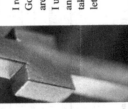

Captain's Log Statement of Faith

I realize that my actions don't earn my way into God's love or earn my way to heaven but that they are a reflection of my love affair with Jesus! I understand that by taking care of myself I honor and glorify God. I matter to God and the actions I take toward good health are daily written love letters telling God, "Thank you for my life"!

_____ **Signature**

Resistance Training

Time of day: _____

Warmed up Yes_____ No_____

Name of exercise 1:

	Weight:	Reps:
	Set 1: _____	_____
	Set 2: _____	_____
Muscles worked:	Set 3: _____	_____
_____	Set 4: _____	_____
Stretched? Yes_____ No_____		

Name of exercise 2:

	Weight:	Reps:
	Set 1: _____	_____
	Set 2: _____	_____
Muscles worked:	Set 3: _____	_____
_____	Set 4: _____	_____
Stretched? Yes_____ No_____		

Name of exercise 3:

	Weight:	Reps:
	Set 1: _____	_____
	Set 2: _____	_____
Muscles worked:	Set 3: _____	_____
_____	Set 4: _____	_____
Stretched? Yes_____ No_____		

Name of exercise 4:

	Weight:	Reps:
	Set 1: _____	_____
	Set 2: _____	_____
Muscles worked:	Set 3: _____	_____
_____	Set 4: _____	_____
Stretched? Yes_____ No_____		

Name of exercise 5:

	Weight:	Reps:
	Set 1: _____	_____
	Set 2: _____	_____
Muscles worked:	Set 3: _____	_____
_____	Set 4: _____	_____
Stretched? Yes_____ No_____		

Name of exercise 6:

	Weight:	Reps:
	Set 1: _____	_____
	Set 2: _____	_____
Muscles worked:	Set 3: _____	_____
_____	Set 4: _____	_____
Stretched? Yes_____ No_____		

Name of exercise 7:

	Weight:	Reps:
	Set 1: _____	_____
	Set 2: _____	_____
Muscles worked:	Set 3: _____	_____
_____	Set 4: _____	_____
Stretched? Yes_____ No_____		

Name of exercise 8:

	Weight:	Reps:
	Set 1: _____	_____
	Set 2: _____	_____
Muscles worked:	Set 3: _____	_____
_____	Set 4: _____	_____
Stretched? Yes_____ No_____		

Name of exercise 9:

	Weight:	Reps:
	Set 1: _____	_____
	Set 2: _____	_____
Muscles worked:	Set 3: _____	_____
_____	Set 4: _____	_____
Stretched? Yes_____ No_____		

Name of exercise 10:

	Weight:	Reps:
	Set 1: _____	_____
	Set 2: _____	_____
Muscles worked:	Set 3: _____	_____
_____	Set 4: _____	_____
Stretched? Yes_____ No_____		

"I press on toward the goal to win the prize for which God has called me heavenward in Christ Jesus."
Philippians 3:14

Captain's Log

"Each one should test his own actions. Then he can take pride in himself without comparing himself to somebody else, for each one should carry his own load." (Galatians 6:40)

Day: _____ Date: _____ / _____ / _____

Nutrition Log

BREAKFAST — Time: _____

	Type	Amt:	Type	Amt:
Protein	1.		2.	
Complex Carbs	1.		2.	
Fruit	1.		2.	
Vegetables	1.		2.	
Fat	1.		2.	
Liquid/drink	1.		2.	
Meal Replace.	1.		2.	
Condiments	1.		2.	
Other	1.		2.	

LUNCH — Time: _____

	Type	Amt:	Type	Amt:
Protein	1.		2.	
Complex Carbs	1.		2.	
Fruit	1.		2.	
Vegetables	1.		2.	
Fat	1.		2.	
Liquid/drink	1.		2.	
Meal Replace.	1.		2.	
Condiments	1.		2.	
Other	1.		2.	

SNACK 3 — Time: _____

	Type	Amt:	Type	Amt:
Protein	1.		2.	
Complex Carbs	1.		2.	
Fruit	1.		2.	
Vegetables	1.		2.	
Fat	1.		2.	
Liquid/drink	1.		2.	
Meal Replace.	1.		2.	
Condiments	1.		2.	
Other	1.		2.	

SNACK 1 — Time: _____

	Type	Amt:	Type	Amt:
Protein	1.		2.	
Complex Carbs	1.		2.	
Fruit	1.		2.	
Vegetables	1.		2.	
Fat	1.		2.	
Liquid/drink	1.		2.	
Meal Replace.	1.		2.	
Condiments	1.		2.	
Other	1.		2.	

SNACK 2 — Time: _____

	Type	Amt:	Type	Amt:
Protein	1.		2.	
Complex Carbs	1.		2.	
Fruit	1.		2.	
Vegetables	1.		2.	
Fat	1.		2.	
Liquid/drink	1.		2.	
Meal Replace.	1.		2.	
Condiments	1.		2.	
Other	1.		2.	

DINNER — Time: _____

	Type	Amt:	Type	Amt:
Protein	1.		2.	
Complex Carbs	1.		2.	
Fruit	1.		2.	
Vegetables	1.		2.	
Fat	1.		2.	
Liquid/drink	1.		2.	
Meal Replace.	1.		2.	
Condiments	1.		2.	
Other	1.		2.	

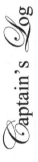
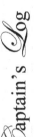

Resistance Training

Time of day: _____
Warmed up   Yes _____   No _____

Name of exercise 1: _____
Weight: | Reps:
Set 1: _____
Set 2: _____
Muscles worked: _____
Set 3: _____
Set 4: _____
Stretched?   Yes _____   No _____

Name of exercise 3: _____
Weight: | Reps:
Set 1: _____
Set 2: _____
Muscles worked: _____
Set 3: _____
Set 4: _____
Stretched?   Yes _____   No _____

Name of exercise 5: _____
Weight: | Reps:
Set 1: _____
Set 2: _____
Muscles worked: _____
Set 3: _____
Set 4: _____
Stretched?   Yes _____   No _____

Name of exercise 7: _____
Weight: | Reps:
Set 1: _____
Set 2: _____
Muscles worked: _____
Set 3: _____
Set 4: _____
Stretched?   Yes _____   No _____

Name of exercise 9: _____
Weight: | Reps:
Set 1: _____
Set 2: _____
Muscles worked: _____
Set 3: _____
Set 4: _____
Stretched?   Yes _____   No _____

Cardiovascular Training

Warmed up   Yes _____   No _____

Time of day: _____

	For how long?	Heart Rate
Type 1:		
Type 2:		
Type 3:		
Type 4:		

Stretched?   Yes _____   No _____

Name of exercise 2: _____
Weight: | Reps:
Set 1: _____
Set 2: _____
Muscles worked: _____
Set 3: _____
Set 4: _____
Stretched?   Yes _____   No _____

Name of exercise 4: _____
Weight: | Reps:
Set 1: _____
Set 2: _____
Muscles worked: _____
Set 3: _____
Set 4: _____
Stretched?   Yes _____   No _____

Name of exercise 6: _____
Weight: | Reps:
Set 1: _____
Set 2: _____
Muscles worked: _____
Set 3: _____
Set 4: _____
Stretched?   Yes _____   No _____

Name of exercise 8: _____
Weight: | Reps:
Set 1: _____
Set 2: _____
Muscles worked: _____
Set 3: _____
Set 4: _____
Stretched?   Yes _____   No _____

Name of exercise 10: _____
Weight: | Reps:
Set 1: _____
Set 2: _____
Muscles worked: _____
Set 3: _____
Set 4: _____
Stretched?   Yes _____   No _____

Evening Reflection

Did I put my faith in Action today?	Yes _____	No _____
I prayed for somone today	Yes _____	No _____
I read my Bible today	Yes _____	No _____
I helped someone in need today	Yes _____	No _____
I got 6 1/2 to 8 hours of sleep last night	Yes _____	No _____
I know I ate right today	Yes _____	No _____
I ate breakfast today	Yes _____	No _____
I ate starches after 4:00 p.m. today	Yes _____	No _____
I ate at least 4 meals today	Yes _____	No _____
I drank at least a gallon of water today	Yes _____	No _____
I had Courage to Change today	Yes _____	No _____
Tonight I forgive…		

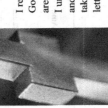

Captain's Log Statement of Faith

I realize that my actions don't earn my way into
God's love or earn my way to heaven but that they
are a reflection of my love affair with Jesus!
I understand that by taking care of myself I honor
and glorify God. I matter to God and the actions I
take toward good health are daily written love
letters telling God, "Thank you for my life"!

_____
Signature

"I press on toward the goal to win the prize for which God has called me heavenward in Christ Jesus."
Philippians 3:14

Captain's Log

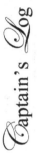

"Each one should test his own actions. Then he can take pride in himself without comparing himself to somebody else, for each one should carry his own load." (Galatians 6:40)

Day: _____ Date: _____ / _____ / _____

Nutrition Log

BREAKFAST Time: _____

	Type	Amt:	Type	Amt:
Protein	1.	_____	2.	_____
Complex Carbs	1.	_____	2.	_____
Fruit	1.	_____	2.	_____
Vegetables	1.	_____	2.	_____
Fat	1.	_____	2.	_____
Liquid/drink	1.	_____	2.	_____
Meal Replace.	1.	_____	2.	_____
Condiments	1.	_____	2.	_____
Other	1.	_____	2.	_____

SNACK 1 Time: _____

	Type	Amt:	Type	Amt:
Protein	1.	_____	2.	_____
Complex Carbs	1.	_____	2.	_____
Fruit	1.	_____	2.	_____
Vegetables	1.	_____	2.	_____
Fat	1.	_____	2.	_____
Liquid/drink	1.	_____	2.	_____
Meal Replace.	1.	_____	2.	_____
Condiments	1.	_____	2.	_____
Other	1.	_____	2.	_____

LUNCH Time: _____

	Type	Amt:	Type	Amt:
Protein	1.	_____	2.	_____
Complex Carbs	1.	_____	2.	_____
Fruit	1.	_____	2.	_____
Vegetables	1.	_____	2.	_____
Fat	1.	_____	2.	_____
Liquid/drink	1.	_____	2.	_____
Meal Replace.	1.	_____	2.	_____
Condiments	1.	_____	2.	_____
Other	1.	_____	2.	_____

SNACK 2 Time: _____

	Type	Amt:	Type	Amt:
Protein	1.	_____	2.	_____
Complex Carbs	1.	_____	2.	_____
Fruit	1.	_____	2.	_____
Vegetables	1.	_____	2.	_____
Fat	1.	_____	2.	_____
Liquid/drink	1.	_____	2.	_____
Meal Replace.	1.	_____	2.	_____
Condiments	1.	_____	2.	_____
Other	1.	_____	2.	_____

SNACK 3 Time: _____

	Type	Amt:	Type	Amt:
Protein	1.	_____	2.	_____
Complex Carbs	1.	_____	2.	_____
Fruit	1.	_____	2.	_____
Vegetables	1.	_____	2.	_____
Fat	1.	_____	2.	_____
Liquid/drink	1.	_____	2.	_____
Meal Replace.	1.	_____	2.	_____
Condiments	1.	_____	2.	_____
Other	1.	_____	2.	_____

DINNER Time: _____

	Type	Amt:	Type	Amt:
Protein	1.	_____	2.	_____
Complex Carbs	1.	_____	2.	_____
Fruit	1.	_____	2.	_____
Vegetables	1.	_____	2.	_____
Fat	1.	_____	2.	_____
Liquid/drink	1.	_____	2.	_____
Meal Replace.	1.	_____	2.	_____
Condiments	1.	_____	2.	_____
Other	1.	_____	2.	_____

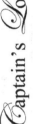

Cardiovascular Training

Warmed up   Yes _____   No _____

Time of day: _____	For how long?	Heart Rate
Type 1:	_____	_____
Type 2:	_____	_____
Type 3:	_____	_____
Type 4:	_____	_____
Stretched? Yes _____ No _____		

Evening Reflection

Did I put my faith in Action today?	Yes _____	No _____
I prayed for somone today	Yes _____	No _____
I read my Bible today	Yes _____	No _____
I helped someone in need today	Yes _____	No _____
I got 6 1/2 to 8 hours of sleep last night	Yes _____	No _____
I know I ate right today	Yes _____	No _____
I ate breakfast today	Yes _____	No _____
I ate starches after 4:00 p.m. today	Yes _____	No _____
I ate at least 4 meals today	Yes _____	No _____
I drank at least a gallon of water today	Yes _____	No _____
I had Courage to Change today	Yes _____	No _____
Tonight I forgive…		

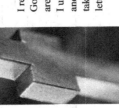

Captain's Log Statement of Faith

I realize that my actions don't earn my way into God's love or earn my way to heaven but that they are a reflection of my love affair with Jesus! I understand that by taking care of myself I honor and glorify God. I matter to God and the actions I take toward good health are daily written love letters telling God, "Thank you for my life"!

_____   **Signature**

"I press on toward the goal to win the prize for which God has called me heavenward in Christ Jesus."

Philippians 3:14

Resistance Training

Time of day: _____

Warmed up   Yes _____   No _____

Name of exercise 1: _____

	Weight:	Reps:
Set 1:	_____	_____
Set 2:	_____	_____
Set 3:	_____	_____
Set 4:	_____	_____

Muscles worked: _____

Stretched?   Yes _____   No _____

Name of exercise 2: _____

	Weight:	Reps:
Set 1:	_____	_____
Set 2:	_____	_____
Set 3:	_____	_____
Set 4:	_____	_____

Muscles worked: _____

Stretched?   Yes _____   No _____

Name of exercise 3: _____

	Weight:	Reps:
Set 1:	_____	_____
Set 2:	_____	_____
Set 3:	_____	_____
Set 4:	_____	_____

Muscles worked: _____

Stretched?   Yes _____   No _____

Name of exercise 4: _____

	Weight:	Reps:
Set 1:	_____	_____
Set 2:	_____	_____
Set 3:	_____	_____
Set 4:	_____	_____

Muscles worked: _____

Stretched?   Yes _____   No _____

Name of exercise 5: _____

	Weight:	Reps:
Set 1:	_____	_____
Set 2:	_____	_____
Set 3:	_____	_____
Set 4:	_____	_____

Muscles worked: _____

Stretched?   Yes _____   No _____

Name of exercise 6: _____

	Weight:	Reps:
Set 1:	_____	_____
Set 2:	_____	_____
Set 3:	_____	_____
Set 4:	_____	_____

Muscles worked: _____

Stretched?   Yes _____   No _____

Name of exercise 7: _____

	Weight:	Reps:
Set 1:	_____	_____
Set 2:	_____	_____
Set 3:	_____	_____
Set 4:	_____	_____

Muscles worked: _____

Stretched?   Yes _____   No _____

Name of exercise 8: _____

	Weight:	Reps:
Set 1:	_____	_____
Set 2:	_____	_____
Set 3:	_____	_____
Set 4:	_____	_____

Muscles worked: _____

Stretched?   Yes _____   No _____

Name of exercise 9: _____

	Weight:	Reps:
Set 1:	_____	_____
Set 2:	_____	_____
Set 3:	_____	_____
Set 4:	_____	_____

Muscles worked: _____

Stretched?   Yes _____   No _____

Name of exercise 10: _____

	Weight:	Reps:
Set 1:	_____	_____
Set 2:	_____	_____
Set 3:	_____	_____
Set 4:	_____	_____

Muscles worked: _____

Stretched?   Yes _____   No _____

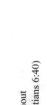

Captain's Log

"Each one should test his own actions. Then he can take pride in himself without comparing himself to somebody else, for each one should carry his own load." (Galatians 6:40)

Day: _____   Date: _____ / _____ / _____

Nutrition Log

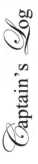
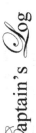

BREAKFAST   Time: _____

	Type	Amt:		Type	Amt:
Protein	1.			2.	
Complex Carbs	1.			2.	
Fruit	1.			2.	
Vegetables	1.			2.	
Fat	1.			2.	
Liquid/drink	1.			2.	
Meal Replace.	1.			2.	
Condiments	1.			2.	
Other	1.			2.	

SNACK 1   Time: _____

	Type	Amt:		Type	Amt:
Protein	1.			2.	
Complex Carbs	1.			2.	
Fruit	1.			2.	
Vegetables	1.			2.	
Fat	1.			2.	
Liquid/drink	1.			2.	
Meal Replace.	1.			2.	
Condiments	1.			2.	
Other	1.			2.	

LUNCH   Time: _____

	Type	Amt:		Type	Amt:
Protein	1.			2.	
Complex Carbs	1.			2.	
Fruit	1.			2.	
Vegetables	1.			2.	
Fat	1.			2.	
Liquid/drink	1.			2.	
Meal Replace.	1.			2.	
Condiments	1.			2.	
Other	1.			2.	

SNACK 2   Time: _____

	Type	Amt:		Type	Amt:
Protein	1.			2.	
Complex Carbs	1.			2.	
Fruit	1.			2.	
Vegetables	1.			2.	
Fat	1.			2.	
Liquid/drink	1.			2.	
Meal Replace.	1.			2.	
Condiments	1.			2.	
Other	1.			2.	

SNACK 3   Time: _____

	Type	Amt:		Type	Amt:
Protein	1.			2.	
Complex Carbs	1.			2.	
Fruit	1.			2.	
Vegetables	1.			2.	
Fat	1.			2.	
Liquid/drink	1.			2.	
Meal Replace.	1.			2.	
Condiments	1.			2.	
Other	1.			2.	

DINNER   Time: _____

	Type	Amt:		Type	Amt:
Protein	1.			2.	
Complex Carbs	1.			2.	
Fruit	1.			2.	
Vegetables	1.			2.	
Fat	1.			2.	
Liquid/drink	1.			2.	
Meal Replace.	1.			2.	
Condiments	1.			2.	
Other	1.			2.	

Cardiovascular Training

Warmed up Yes _____ No _____

Time of day: _____	For how long?	Heart Rate
Type 1:	_____	_____
Type 2:	_____	_____
Type 3:	_____	_____
Type 4:	_____	_____
Stretched? Yes _____ No _____		

Resistance Training

Time of day: _____

Warmed up Yes _____ No _____

Name of exercise 1: _____
	Weight:	Reps:
Set 1:	_____	_____
Set 2:	_____	_____
Set 3:	_____	_____
Set 4:	_____	_____

Muscles worked: _____

Stretched? Yes _____ No _____

Name of exercise 2: _____
	Weight:	Reps:
Set 1:	_____	_____
Set 2:	_____	_____
Set 3:	_____	_____
Set 4:	_____	_____

Muscles worked: _____

Stretched? Yes _____ No _____

Name of exercise 3: _____
	Weight:	Reps:
Set 1:	_____	_____
Set 2:	_____	_____
Set 3:	_____	_____
Set 4:	_____	_____

Muscles worked: _____

Stretched? Yes _____ No _____

Name of exercise 4: _____
	Weight:	Reps:
Set 1:	_____	_____
Set 2:	_____	_____
Set 3:	_____	_____
Set 4:	_____	_____

Muscles worked: _____

Stretched? Yes _____ No _____

Name of exercise 5: _____
	Weight:	Reps:
Set 1:	_____	_____
Set 2:	_____	_____
Set 3:	_____	_____
Set 4:	_____	_____

Muscles worked: _____

Stretched? Yes _____ No _____

Name of exercise 6: _____
	Weight:	Reps:
Set 1:	_____	_____
Set 2:	_____	_____
Set 3:	_____	_____
Set 4:	_____	_____

Muscles worked: _____

Stretched? Yes _____ No _____

Name of exercise 7: _____
	Weight:	Reps:
Set 1:	_____	_____
Set 2:	_____	_____
Set 3:	_____	_____
Set 4:	_____	_____

Muscles worked: _____

Stretched? Yes _____ No _____

Name of exercise 8: _____
	Weight:	Reps:
Set 1:	_____	_____
Set 2:	_____	_____
Set 3:	_____	_____
Set 4:	_____	_____

Muscles worked: _____

Stretched? Yes _____ No _____

Name of exercise 9: _____
	Weight:	Reps:
Set 1:	_____	_____
Set 2:	_____	_____
Set 3:	_____	_____
Set 4:	_____	_____

Muscles worked: _____

Stretched? Yes _____ No _____

Name of exercise 10: _____
	Weight:	Reps:
Set 1:	_____	_____
Set 2:	_____	_____
Set 3:	_____	_____
Set 4:	_____	_____

Muscles worked: _____

Stretched? Yes _____ No _____

Evening Reflection

Did I put my faith in Action today?	Yes _____	No _____
I prayed for somone today	Yes _____	No _____
I read my Bible today	Yes _____	No _____
I helped someone in need today	Yes _____	No _____
I got 6 1/2 to 8 hours of sleep last night	Yes _____	No _____
I know I ate right today	Yes _____	No _____
I ate breakfast today	Yes _____	No _____
I ate starches after 4:00 p.m. today	Yes _____	No _____
I ate at least 4 meals today	Yes _____	No _____
I drank at least a gallon of water today	Yes _____	No _____
I had Courage to Change today	Yes _____	No _____
Tonight I forgive…		

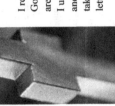

Captain's Log Statement of Faith

I realize that my actions don't earn my way into God's love or earn my way to heaven but that they are a reflection of my love affair with Jesus! I understand that by taking care of myself I honor and glorify God. I matter to God and the actions I take toward good health are daily written love letters telling God, "Thank you for my life"!

_____
Signature

"I press on toward the goal to win the prize for which God has called me heavenward in Christ Jesus."
Philippians 3:14

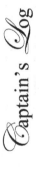

Captain's Log

"Each one should test his own actions. Then he can take pride in himself without comparing himself to somebody else, for each one should carry his own load." (Galatians 6:40)

Day: _____ Date: _____ / _____ / _____

Nutrition Log

BREAKFAST Time: _____

	Amt:	Type	Amt:	Type
Protein		1. _____		2. _____
Complex Carbs		1. _____		2. _____
Fruit		1. _____		2. _____
Vegetables		1. _____		2. _____
Fat		1. _____		2. _____
Liquid/drink		1. _____		2. _____
Meal Replace.		1. _____		2. _____
Condiments		1. _____		2. _____
Other		1. _____		2. _____

SNACK 1 Time: _____

	Amt:	Type	Amt:	Type
Protein		1. _____		2. _____
Complex Carbs		1. _____		2. _____
Fruit		1. _____		2. _____
Vegetables		1. _____		2. _____
Fat		1. _____		2. _____
Liquid/drink		1. _____		2. _____
Meal Replace.		1. _____		2. _____
Condiments		1. _____		2. _____
Other		1. _____		2. _____

LUNCH Time: _____

	Amt:	Type	Amt:	Type
Protein		1. _____		2. _____
Complex Carbs		1. _____		2. _____
Fruit		1. _____		2. _____
Vegetables		1. _____		2. _____
Fat		1. _____		2. _____
Liquid/drink		1. _____		2. _____
Meal Replace.		1. _____		2. _____
Condiments		1. _____		2. _____
Other		1. _____		2. _____

SNACK 2 Time: _____

	Amt:	Type	Amt:	Type
Protein		1. _____		2. _____
Complex Carbs		1. _____		2. _____
Fruit		1. _____		2. _____
Vegetables		1. _____		2. _____
Fat		1. _____		2. _____
Liquid/drink		1. _____		2. _____
Meal Replace.		1. _____		2. _____
Condiments		1. _____		2. _____
Other		1. _____		2. _____

SNACK 3 Time: _____

	Amt:	Type	Amt:	Type
Protein		1. _____		2. _____
Complex Carbs		1. _____		2. _____
Fruit		1. _____		2. _____
Vegetables		1. _____		2. _____
Fat		1. _____		2. _____
Liquid/drink		1. _____		2. _____
Meal Replace.		1. _____		2. _____
Condiments		1. _____		2. _____
Other		1. _____		2. _____

DINNER Time: _____

	Amt:	Type	Amt:	Type
Protein		1. _____		2. _____
Complex Carbs		1. _____		2. _____
Fruit		1. _____		2. _____
Vegetables		1. _____		2. _____
Fat		1. _____		2. _____
Liquid/drink		1. _____		2. _____
Meal Replace.		1. _____		2. _____
Condiments		1. _____		2. _____
Other		1. _____		2. _____

Cardiovascular Training

Time of day: _____

Warmed up Yes _____ No _____

	For how long?	Heart Rate
Type 1:	_____	_____
Type 2:	_____	_____
Type 3:	_____	_____
Type 4:	_____	_____
Stretched? Yes _____ No _____		

Evening Reflection

Did I put my faith in Action today?	Yes _____	No _____
I prayed for somone today	Yes _____	No _____
I read my Bible today	Yes _____	No _____
I helped someone in need today	Yes _____	No _____
I got 6 1/2 to 8 hours of sleep last night	Yes _____	No _____
I know I ate right today	Yes _____	No _____
I ate breakfast today	Yes _____	No _____
I ate starches after 4:00 p.m. today	Yes _____	No _____
I ate at least 4 meals today	Yes _____	No _____
I drank at least a gallon of water today	Yes _____	No _____
I had Courage to Change today	Yes _____	No _____
Tonight I forgive… _____		

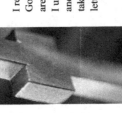

Captain's Log Statement of Faith

I realize that my actions don't earn my way into God's love or earn my way to heaven but that they are a reflection of my love affair with Jesus! I understand that by taking care of myself I honor and glorify God. I matter to God and the actions I take toward good health are daily written love letters telling God, "Thank you for my life"!

_____
Signature

Resistance Training

Time of day: _____

Warmed up Yes _____ No _____

Name of exercise 1: _____

	Weight:	Reps:
Set 1:	_____	_____
Set 2:	_____	_____
Set 3:	_____	_____
Set 4:	_____	_____

Muscles worked: _____

Stretched? Yes _____ No _____

Name of exercise 2: _____

	Weight:	Reps:
Set 1:	_____	_____
Set 2:	_____	_____
Set 3:	_____	_____
Set 4:	_____	_____

Muscles worked: _____

Stretched? Yes _____ No _____

Name of exercise 3: _____

	Weight:	Reps:
Set 1:	_____	_____
Set 2:	_____	_____
Set 3:	_____	_____
Set 4:	_____	_____

Muscles worked: _____

Stretched? Yes _____ No _____

Name of exercise 4: _____

	Weight:	Reps:
Set 1:	_____	_____
Set 2:	_____	_____
Set 3:	_____	_____
Set 4:	_____	_____

Muscles worked: _____

Stretched? Yes _____ No _____

Name of exercise 5: _____

	Weight:	Reps:
Set 1:	_____	_____
Set 2:	_____	_____
Set 3:	_____	_____
Set 4:	_____	_____

Muscles worked: _____

Stretched? Yes _____ No _____

Name of exercise 6: _____

	Weight:	Reps:
Set 1:	_____	_____
Set 2:	_____	_____
Set 3:	_____	_____
Set 4:	_____	_____

Muscles worked: _____

Stretched? Yes _____ No _____

Name of exercise 7: _____

	Weight:	Reps:
Set 1:	_____	_____
Set 2:	_____	_____
Set 3:	_____	_____
Set 4:	_____	_____

Muscles worked: _____

Stretched? Yes _____ No _____

Name of exercise 8: _____

	Weight:	Reps:
Set 1:	_____	_____
Set 2:	_____	_____
Set 3:	_____	_____
Set 4:	_____	_____

Muscles worked: _____

Stretched? Yes _____ No _____

Name of exercise 9: _____

	Weight:	Reps:
Set 1:	_____	_____
Set 2:	_____	_____
Set 3:	_____	_____
Set 4:	_____	_____

Muscles worked: _____

Stretched? Yes _____ No _____

Name of exercise 10: _____

	Weight:	Reps:
Set 1:	_____	_____
Set 2:	_____	_____
Set 3:	_____	_____
Set 4:	_____	_____

Muscles worked: _____

Stretched? Yes _____ No _____

"I press on toward the goal to win the prize for which God has called me heavenward in Christ Jesus."
Philippians 3:14

A LOVE LETTER

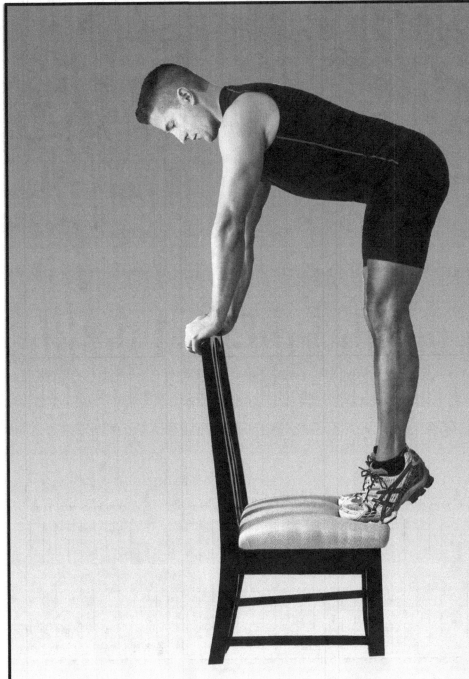

"I have no greater joy than to hear that my children are walking in the truth."
(3 John 1:4) "So there is hope for your future," declares the LORD.
"Your children (you) will return to their own land." (Jeremiah 31:17)

WEEK EIGHT

Captain's Log

"Each one should test his own actions. Then he can take pride in himself without comparing himself to somebody else, for each one should carry his own load." (Galatians 6:40)

Day: _____   Date: _____ / _____ / _____

Nutrition Log

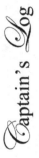
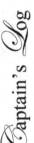

BREAKFAST Time: _____

	Type	Amt:		Type	Amt:
Protein	1.			2.	
Complex Carbs	1.			2.	
Fruit	1.			2.	
Vegetables	1.			2.	
Fat	1.			2.	
Liquid/drink	1.			2.	
Meal Replace.	1.			2.	
Condiments	1.			2.	
Other	1.			2.	

SNACK 1 Time: _____

	Type	Amt:		Type	Amt:
Protein	1.			2.	
Complex Carbs	1.			2.	
Fruit	1.			2.	
Vegetables	1.			2.	
Fat	1.			2.	
Liquid/drink	1.			2.	
Meal Replace.	1.			2.	
Condiments	1.			2.	
Other	1.			2.	

LUNCH Time: _____

	Type	Amt:		Type	Amt:
Protein	1.			2.	
Complex Carbs	1.			2.	
Fruit	1.			2.	
Vegetables	1.			2.	
Fat	1.			2.	
Liquid/drink	1.			2.	
Meal Replace.	1.			2.	
Condiments	1.			2.	
Other	1.			2.	

SNACK 2 Time: _____

	Type	Amt:		Type	Amt:
Protein	1.			2.	
Complex Carbs	1.			2.	
Fruit	1.			2.	
Vegetables	1.			2.	
Fat	1.			2.	
Liquid/drink	1.			2.	
Meal Replace.	1.			2.	
Condiments	1.			2.	
Other	1.			2.	

SNACK 3 Time: _____

	Type	Amt:		Type	Amt:
Protein	1.			2.	
Complex Carbs	1.			2.	
Fruit	1.			2.	
Vegetables	1.			2.	
Fat	1.			2.	
Liquid/drink	1.			2.	
Meal Replace.	1.			2.	
Condiments	1.			2.	
Other	1.			2.	

DINNER Time: _____

	Type	Amt:		Type	Amt:
Protein	1.			2.	
Complex Carbs	1.			2.	
Fruit	1.			2.	
Vegetables	1.			2.	
Fat	1.			2.	
Liquid/drink	1.			2.	
Meal Replace.	1.			2.	
Condiments	1.			2.	
Other	1.			2.	

Cardiovascular Training

Warmed up   Yes_____   No_____

Time of day: _____	For how long?	Heart Rate
Type 1: _____	_____	_____
Type 2: _____	_____	_____
Type 3: _____	_____	_____
Type 4: _____	_____	_____
Stretched? Yes_____ No_____		

Evening Reflection

Did I put my faith in Action today?	Yes_____	No_____
I prayed for somone today	Yes_____	No_____
I read my Bible today	Yes_____	No_____
I helped someone in need today	Yes_____	No_____
I got 6 1/2 to 8 hours of sleep last night	Yes_____	No_____
I know I ate right today	Yes_____	No_____
I ate breakfast today	Yes_____	No_____
I ate starches after 4:00 p.m. today	Yes_____	No_____
I ate at least 4 meals today	Yes_____	No_____
I drank at least a gallon of water today	Yes_____	No_____
I had Courage to Change today	Yes_____	No_____
Tonight I forgive…		

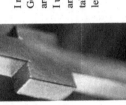

Captain's Log Statement of Faith

I realize that my actions don't earn my way into God's love or earn my way to heaven but that they are a reflection of my love affair with Jesus! I understand that by taking care of myself I honor and glorify God. I matter to God and the actions I take toward good health are daily written love letters telling God, "Thank you for my life"!

_____   **Signature**

Resistance Training

Time of day: _____

Warmed up   Yes_____   No_____

Name of exercise 1: _____

	Weight:	Reps:
Set 1:	_____	_____
Set 2:	_____	_____
Muscles worked:	Set 3: _____	_____
	Set 4: _____	_____
Stretched? Yes_____ No_____		

Name of exercise 2: _____

	Weight:	Reps:
Set 1:	_____	_____
Set 2:	_____	_____
Muscles worked:	Set 3: _____	_____
	Set 4: _____	_____
Stretched? Yes_____ No_____		

Name of exercise 3: _____

	Weight:	Reps:
Set 1:	_____	_____
Set 2:	_____	_____
Muscles worked:	Set 3: _____	_____
	Set 4: _____	_____
Stretched? Yes_____ No_____		

Name of exercise 4: _____

	Weight:	Reps:
Set 1:	_____	_____
Set 2:	_____	_____
Muscles worked:	Set 3: _____	_____
	Set 4: _____	_____
Stretched? Yes_____ No_____		

Name of exercise 5: _____

	Weight:	Reps:
Set 1:	_____	_____
Set 2:	_____	_____
Muscles worked:	Set 3: _____	_____
	Set 4: _____	_____
Stretched? Yes_____ No_____		

Name of exercise 6: _____

	Weight:	Reps:
Set 1:	_____	_____
Set 2:	_____	_____
Muscles worked:	Set 3: _____	_____
	Set 4: _____	_____
Stretched? Yes_____ No_____		

Name of exercise 7: _____

	Weight:	Reps:
Set 1:	_____	_____
Set 2:	_____	_____
Muscles worked:	Set 3: _____	_____
	Set 4: _____	_____
Stretched? Yes_____ No_____		

Name of exercise 8: _____

	Weight:	Reps:
Set 1:	_____	_____
Set 2:	_____	_____
Muscles worked:	Set 3: _____	_____
	Set 4: _____	_____
Stretched? Yes_____ No_____		

Name of exercise 9: _____

	Weight:	Reps:
Set 1:	_____	_____
Set 2:	_____	_____
Muscles worked:	Set 3: _____	_____
	Set 4: _____	_____
Stretched? Yes_____ No_____		

Name of exercise 10: _____

	Weight:	Reps:
Set 1:	_____	_____
Set 2:	_____	_____
Muscles worked:	Set 3: _____	_____
	Set 4: _____	_____
Stretched? Yes_____ No_____		

"I press on toward the goal to win the prize for which God has called me heavenward in Christ Jesus."

Philippians 3:14

Captain's Log

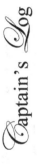

"Each one should test his own actions. Then he can take pride in himself without comparing himself to somebody else, for each one should carry his own load." (Galatians 6:40)

Day: _____   Date: ____ / ____ / ____

Nutrition Log

BREAKFAST   Time: _____

	Type	Amt:		Type	Amt:
Protein	1. _____	_____		2. _____	_____
Complex Carbs	1. _____	_____		2. _____	_____
Fruit	1. _____	_____		2. _____	_____
Vegetables	1. _____	_____		2. _____	_____
Fat	1. _____	_____		2. _____	_____
Liquid/drink	1. _____	_____		2. _____	_____
Meal Replace.	1. _____	_____		2. _____	_____
Condiments	1. _____	_____		2. _____	_____
Other	1. _____	_____		2. _____	_____

SNACK 1   Time: _____

	Type	Amt:		Type	Amt:
Protein	1. _____	_____		2. _____	_____
Complex Carbs	1. _____	_____		2. _____	_____
Fruit	1. _____	_____		2. _____	_____
Vegetables	1. _____	_____		2. _____	_____
Fat	1. _____	_____		2. _____	_____
Liquid/drink	1. _____	_____		2. _____	_____
Meal Replace.	1. _____	_____		2. _____	_____
Condiments	1. _____	_____		2. _____	_____
Other	1. _____	_____		2. _____	_____

LUNCH   Time: _____

	Type	Amt:		Type	Amt:
Protein	1. _____	_____		2. _____	_____
Complex Carbs	1. _____	_____		2. _____	_____
Fruit	1. _____	_____		2. _____	_____
Vegetables	1. _____	_____		2. _____	_____
Fat	1. _____	_____		2. _____	_____
Liquid/drink	1. _____	_____		2. _____	_____
Meal Replace.	1. _____	_____		2. _____	_____
Condiments	1. _____	_____		2. _____	_____
Other	1. _____	_____		2. _____	_____

SNACK 2   Time: _____

	Type	Amt:		Type	Amt:
Protein	1. _____	_____		2. _____	_____
Complex Carbs	1. _____	_____		2. _____	_____
Fruit	1. _____	_____		2. _____	_____
Vegetables	1. _____	_____		2. _____	_____
Fat	1. _____	_____		2. _____	_____
Liquid/drink	1. _____	_____		2. _____	_____
Meal Replace.	1. _____	_____		2. _____	_____
Condiments	1. _____	_____		2. _____	_____
Other	1. _____	_____		2. _____	_____

SNACK 3   Time: _____

	Type	Amt:		Type	Amt:
Protein	1. _____	_____		2. _____	_____
Complex Carbs	1. _____	_____		2. _____	_____
Fruit	1. _____	_____		2. _____	_____
Vegetables	1. _____	_____		2. _____	_____
Fat	1. _____	_____		2. _____	_____
Liquid/drink	1. _____	_____		2. _____	_____
Meal Replace.	1. _____	_____		2. _____	_____
Condiments	1. _____	_____		2. _____	_____
Other	1. _____	_____		2. _____	_____

DINNER   Time: _____

	Type	Amt:		Type	Amt:
Protein	1. _____	_____		2. _____	_____
Complex Carbs	1. _____	_____		2. _____	_____
Fruit	1. _____	_____		2. _____	_____
Vegetables	1. _____	_____		2. _____	_____
Fat	1. _____	_____		2. _____	_____
Liquid/drink	1. _____	_____		2. _____	_____
Meal Replace.	1. _____	_____		2. _____	_____
Condiments	1. _____	_____		2. _____	_____
Other	1. _____	_____		2. _____	_____

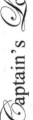

Cardiovascular Training

Warmed up   Yes _____   No _____

Time of day:	For how long?	Heart Rate
Type 1: _____	_____	_____
Type 2: _____	_____	_____
Type 3: _____	_____	_____
Type 4: _____	_____	_____
Stretched? Yes _____ No _____		

Evening Reflection

Did I put my faith in Action today?	Yes _____	No _____
I prayed for somone today	Yes _____	No _____
I read my Bible today	Yes _____	No _____
I helped someone in need today	Yes _____	No _____
I got 6 1/2 to 8 hours of sleep last night	Yes _____	No _____
I know I ate right today	Yes _____	No _____
I ate breakfast today	Yes _____	No _____
I ate starches after 4:00 p.m. today	Yes _____	No _____
I ate at least 4 meals today	Yes _____	No _____
I drank at least a gallon of water today	Yes _____	No _____
I had Courage to Change today	Yes _____	No _____
Tonight I forgive… _____		

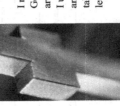

Captain's Log Statement of Faith

I realize that my actions don't earn my way into God's love or earn my way to heaven but that they are a reflection of my love affair with Jesus! I understand that by taking care of myself I honor and glorify God. I matter to God and the actions I take toward good health are daily written love letters telling God, "Thank you for my life"!

_____
Signature

Resistance Training

Time of day: _____

Warmed up   Yes _____   No _____

Name of exercise 1:	Weight:	Reps:
Set 1:	_____	_____
Set 2:	_____	_____
Muscles worked:	Set 3: _____	_____
	Set 4: _____	_____
Stretched? Yes _____ No _____		

Name of exercise 2:	Weight:	Reps:
Set 1:	_____	_____
Set 2:	_____	_____
Muscles worked:	Set 3: _____	_____
	Set 4: _____	_____
Stretched? Yes _____ No _____		

Name of exercise 3:	Weight:	Reps:
Set 1:	_____	_____
Set 2:	_____	_____
Muscles worked:	Set 3: _____	_____
	Set 4: _____	_____
Stretched? Yes _____ No _____		

Name of exercise 4:	Weight:	Reps:
Set 1:	_____	_____
Set 2:	_____	_____
Muscles worked:	Set 3: _____	_____
	Set 4: _____	_____
Stretched? Yes _____ No _____		

Name of exercise 5:	Weight:	Reps:
Set 1:	_____	_____
Set 2:	_____	_____
Muscles worked:	Set 3: _____	_____
	Set 4: _____	_____
Stretched? Yes _____ No _____		

Name of exercise 6:	Weight:	Reps:
Set 1:	_____	_____
Set 2:	_____	_____
Muscles worked:	Set 3: _____	_____
	Set 4: _____	_____
Stretched? Yes _____ No _____		

Name of exercise 7:	Weight:	Reps:
Set 1:	_____	_____
Set 2:	_____	_____
Muscles worked:	Set 3: _____	_____
	Set 4: _____	_____
Stretched? Yes _____ No _____		

Name of exercise 8:	Weight:	Reps:
Set 1:	_____	_____
Set 2:	_____	_____
Muscles worked:	Set 3: _____	_____
	Set 4: _____	_____
Stretched? Yes _____ No _____		

Name of exercise 9:	Weight:	Reps:
Set 1:	_____	_____
Set 2:	_____	_____
Muscles worked:	Set 3: _____	_____
	Set 4: _____	_____
Stretched? Yes _____ No _____		

Name of exercise 10:	Weight:	Reps:
Set 1:	_____	_____
Set 2:	_____	_____
Muscles worked:	Set 3: _____	_____
	Set 4: _____	_____
Stretched? Yes _____ No _____		

"I press on toward the goal to win the prize for which God has called me heavenward in Christ Jesus."

Philippians 3:14

Captain's Log

"Each one should test his own actions. Then he can take pride in himself without comparing himself to somebody else, for each one should carry his own load." (Galatians 6:40)

Day: _____   Date: ____ / ____ / ____

Nutrition Log

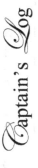

BREAKFAST	Time: _____			SNACK 1	Time: _____		
	Type	Amt:			Type	Amt:	
Protein	1. _____		2. _____	Protein	1. _____		2. _____
Complex Carbs	1. _____		2. _____	Complex Carbs	1. _____		2. _____
Fruit	1. _____		2. _____	Fruit	1. _____		2. _____
Vegetables	1. _____		2. _____	Vegetables	1. _____		2. _____
Fat	1. _____		2. _____	Fat	1. _____		2. _____
Liquid/drink	1. _____		2. _____	Liquid/drink	1. _____		2. _____
Meal Replace.	1. _____		2. _____	Meal Replace.	1. _____		2. _____
Condiments	1. _____		2. _____	Condiments	1. _____		2. _____
Other	1. _____		2. _____	Other	1. _____		2. _____

LUNCH	Time: _____			SNACK 2	Time: _____		
	Type	Amt:			Type	Amt:	
Protein	1. _____		2. _____	Protein	1. _____		2. _____
Complex Carbs	1. _____		2. _____	Complex Carbs	1. _____		2. _____
Fruit	1. _____		2. _____	Fruit	1. _____		2. _____
Vegetables	1. _____		2. _____	Vegetables	1. _____		2. _____
Fat	1. _____		2. _____	Fat	1. _____		2. _____
Liquid/drink	1. _____		2. _____	Liquid/drink	1. _____		2. _____
Meal Replace.	1. _____		2. _____	Meal Replace.	1. _____		2. _____
Condiments	1. _____		2. _____	Condiments	1. _____		2. _____
Other	1. _____		2. _____	Other	1. _____		2. _____

SNACK 3	Time: _____			DINNER	Time: _____		
	Type	Amt:			Type	Amt:	
Protein	1. _____		2. _____	Protein	1. _____		2. _____
Complex Carbs	1. _____		2. _____	Complex Carbs	1. _____		2. _____
Fruit	1. _____		2. _____	Fruit	1. _____		2. _____
Vegetables	1. _____		2. _____	Vegetables	1. _____		2. _____
Fat	1. _____		2. _____	Fat	1. _____		2. _____
Liquid/drink	1. _____		2. _____	Liquid/drink	1. _____		2. _____
Meal Replace.	1. _____		2. _____	Meal Replace.	1. _____		2. _____
Condiments	1. _____		2. _____	Condiments	1. _____		2. _____
Other	1. _____		2. _____	Other	1. _____		2. _____

Cardiovascular Training

Warmed up Yes _____ No _____

Time of day: _____

	For how long?	Heart Rate
Type 1:	_____	_____
Type 2:	_____	_____
Type 3:	_____	_____
Type 4:	_____	_____

Stretched? Yes _____ No _____

Evening Reflection

Did I put my faith in Action today?	Yes	No
I prayed for somone today	Yes	No
I read my Bible today	Yes	No
I helped someone in need today	Yes	No
I got 6 1/2 to 8 hours of sleep last night	Yes	No
I know I ate right today	Yes	No
I ate breakfast today	Yes	No
I ate starches after 4:00 p.m. today	Yes	No
I ate at least 4 meals today	Yes	No
I drank at least a gallon of water today	Yes	No
I had Courage to Change today	Yes	No
Tonight I forgive…		

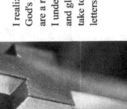

Captain's Log Statement of Faith

I realize that my actions don't earn my way into God's love or earn my way to heaven but that they are a reflection of my love affair with Jesus! I understand that by taking care of myself I honor and glorify God. I matter to God and the actions I take toward good health are daily written love letters telling God, "Thank you for my life"!

_____
Signature

Resistance Training

Time of day: _____ Warmed up Yes _____ No _____

Name of exercise 1: _____ Weight: _____ Reps: _____
Set 1: _____
Set 2: _____
Muscles worked: _____ Set 3: _____
Set 4: _____
Stretched? Yes _____ No _____

Name of exercise 2: _____ Weight: _____ Reps: _____
Set 1: _____
Set 2: _____
Muscles worked: _____ Set 3: _____
Set 4: _____
Stretched? Yes _____ No _____

Name of exercise 3: _____ Weight: _____ Reps: _____
Set 1: _____
Set 2: _____
Muscles worked: _____ Set 3: _____
Set 4: _____
Stretched? Yes _____ No _____

Name of exercise 4: _____ Weight: _____ Reps: _____
Set 1: _____
Set 2: _____
Muscles worked: _____ Set 3: _____
Set 4: _____
Stretched? Yes _____ No _____

Name of exercise 5: _____ Weight: _____ Reps: _____
Set 1: _____
Set 2: _____
Muscles worked: _____ Set 3: _____
Set 4: _____
Stretched? Yes _____ No _____

Name of exercise 6: _____ Weight: _____ Reps: _____
Set 1: _____
Set 2: _____
Muscles worked: _____ Set 3: _____
Set 4: _____
Stretched? Yes _____ No _____

Name of exercise 7: _____ Weight: _____ Reps: _____
Set 1: _____
Set 2: _____
Muscles worked: _____ Set 3: _____
Set 4: _____
Stretched? Yes _____ No _____

Name of exercise 8: _____ Weight: _____ Reps: _____
Set 1: _____
Set 2: _____
Muscles worked: _____ Set 3: _____
Set 4: _____
Stretched? Yes _____ No _____

Name of exercise 9: _____ Weight: _____ Reps: _____
Set 1: _____
Set 2: _____
Muscles worked: _____ Set 3: _____
Set 4: _____
Stretched? Yes _____ No _____

Name of exercise 10: _____ Weight: _____ Reps: _____
Set 1: _____
Set 2: _____
Muscles worked: _____ Set 3: _____
Set 4: _____
Stretched? Yes _____ No _____

"I press on toward the goal to win the prize for which God has called me heavenward in Christ Jesus."
Philippians 3:14

Captain's Log

"Each one should test his own actions. Then he can take pride in himself without comparing himself to somebody else, for each one should carry his own load." (Galatians 6:40)

Day: _____   Date: _____ / _____ / _____

Nutrition Log

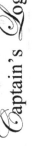
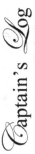

BREAKFAST Time: _____

	Type	Amt:	Type	Amt:
Protein	1.		2.	
Complex Carbs	1.		2.	
Fruit	1.		2.	
Vegetables	1.		2.	
Fat	1.		2.	
Liquid/drink	1.		2.	
Meal Replace.	1.		2.	
Condiments	1.		2.	
Other	1.		2.	

LUNCH Time: _____

	Type	Amt:	Type	Amt:
Protein	1.		2.	
Complex Carbs	1.		2.	
Fruit	1.		2.	
Vegetables	1.		2.	
Fat	1.		2.	
Liquid/drink	1.		2.	
Meal Replace.	1.		2.	
Condiments	1.		2.	
Other	1.		2.	

SNACK 3 Time: _____

	Type	Amt:	Type	Amt:
Protein	1.		2.	
Complex Carbs	1.		2.	
Fruit	1.		2.	
Vegetables	1.		2.	
Fat	1.		2.	
Liquid/drink	1.		2.	
Meal Replace.	1.		2.	
Condiments	1.		2.	
Other	1.		2.	

SNACK 1 Time: _____

	Type	Amt:	Type	Amt:
Protein	1.		2.	
Complex Carbs	1.		2.	
Fruit	1.		2.	
Vegetables	1.		2.	
Fat	1.		2.	
Liquid/drink	1.		2.	
Meal Replace.	1.		2.	
Condiments	1.		2.	
Other	1.		2.	

SNACK 2 Time: _____

	Type	Amt:	Type	Amt:
Protein	1.		2.	
Complex Carbs	1.		2.	
Fruit	1.		2.	
Vegetables	1.		2.	
Fat	1.		2.	
Liquid/drink	1.		2.	
Meal Replace.	1.		2.	
Condiments	1.		2.	
Other	1.		2.	

DINNER Time: _____

	Type	Amt:	Type	Amt:
Protein	1.		2.	
Complex Carbs	1.		2.	
Fruit	1.		2.	
Vegetables	1.		2.	
Fat	1.		2.	
Liquid/drink	1.		2.	
Meal Replace.	1.		2.	
Condiments	1.		2.	
Other	1.		2.	

Cardiovascular Training

Warmed up   Yes _____   No _____

Time of day: _____	For how long?	Heart Rate
Type 1:	_____	_____
Type 2:	_____	_____
Type 3:	_____	_____
Type 4:	_____	_____
Stretched?	Yes _____	No _____

Evening Reflection

Did I put my faith in Action today?	Yes _____	No _____
I prayed for somone today	Yes _____	No _____
I read my Bible today	Yes _____	No _____
I helped someone in need today	Yes _____	No _____
I got 6 1/2 to 8 hours of sleep last night	Yes _____	No _____
I know I ate right today	Yes _____	No _____
I ate breakfast today	Yes _____	No _____
I ate starches after 4:00 p.m. today	Yes _____	No _____
I ate at least 4 meals today	Yes _____	No _____
I drank at least a gallon of water today	Yes _____	No _____
I had Courage to Change today	Yes _____	No _____
Tonight I forgive…		

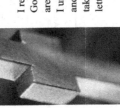

Captain's Log Statement of Faith

I realize that my actions don't earn my way into God's love or earn my way to heaven but that they are a reflection of my love affair with Jesus! I understand that by taking care of myself I honor and glorify God. I matter to God and the actions I take toward good health are daily written love letters telling God, "Thank you for my life"!

_____   **Signature**

Resistance Training

Time of day: _____

Warmed up   Yes _____   No _____

Name of exercise 1:

	Weight:	Reps:
Set 1:	_____	_____
Set 2:	_____	_____
Set 3:	_____	_____
Set 4:	_____	_____

Muscles worked: _____

Stretched?   Yes _____   No _____

Name of exercise 2:

	Weight:	Reps:
Set 1:	_____	_____
Set 2:	_____	_____
Set 3:	_____	_____
Set 4:	_____	_____

Muscles worked: _____

Stretched?   Yes _____   No _____

Name of exercise 3:

	Weight:	Reps:
Set 1:	_____	_____
Set 2:	_____	_____
Set 3:	_____	_____
Set 4:	_____	_____

Muscles worked: _____

Stretched?   Yes _____   No _____

Name of exercise 4:

	Weight:	Reps:
Set 1:	_____	_____
Set 2:	_____	_____
Set 3:	_____	_____
Set 4:	_____	_____

Muscles worked: _____

Stretched?   Yes _____   No _____

Name of exercise 5:

	Weight:	Reps:
Set 1:	_____	_____
Set 2:	_____	_____
Set 3:	_____	_____
Set 4:	_____	_____

Muscles worked: _____

Stretched?   Yes _____   No _____

Name of exercise 6:

	Weight:	Reps:
Set 1:	_____	_____
Set 2:	_____	_____
Set 3:	_____	_____
Set 4:	_____	_____

Muscles worked: _____

Stretched?   Yes _____   No _____

Name of exercise 7:

	Weight:	Reps:
Set 1:	_____	_____
Set 2:	_____	_____
Set 3:	_____	_____
Set 4:	_____	_____

Muscles worked: _____

Stretched?   Yes _____   No _____

Name of exercise 8:

	Weight:	Reps:
Set 1:	_____	_____
Set 2:	_____	_____
Set 3:	_____	_____
Set 4:	_____	_____

Muscles worked: _____

Stretched?   Yes _____   No _____

Name of exercise 9:

	Weight:	Reps:
Set 1:	_____	_____
Set 2:	_____	_____
Set 3:	_____	_____
Set 4:	_____	_____

Muscles worked: _____

Stretched?   Yes _____   No _____

Name of exercise 10:

	Weight:	Reps:
Set 1:	_____	_____
Set 2:	_____	_____
Set 3:	_____	_____
Set 4:	_____	_____

Muscles worked: _____

Stretched?   Yes _____   No _____

"I press on toward the goal to win the prize for which God has called me heavenward in Christ Jesus."
Philippians 3:14

Captain's Log

"Each one should test his own actions. Then he can take pride in himself without comparing himself to somebody else, for each one should carry his own load." (Galatians 6:40)

Day: _____   Date: _____ / _____ / _____

Nutrition Log

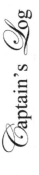

BREAKFAST   Time: _____

	Type	Amt:	Type	Amt:
Protein	1. _____	_____	2. _____	_____
Complex Carbs	1. _____	_____	2. _____	_____
Fruit	1. _____	_____	2. _____	_____
Vegetables	1. _____	_____	2. _____	_____
Fat	1. _____	_____	2. _____	_____
Liquid/drink	1. _____	_____	2. _____	_____
Meal Replace.	1. _____	_____	2. _____	_____
Condiments	1. _____	_____	2. _____	_____
Other	1. _____	_____	2. _____	_____

SNACK 1   Time: _____

	Type	Amt:	Type	Amt:
Protein	1. _____	_____	2. _____	_____
Complex Carbs	1. _____	_____	2. _____	_____
Fruit	1. _____	_____	2. _____	_____
Vegetables	1. _____	_____	2. _____	_____
Fat	1. _____	_____	2. _____	_____
Liquid/drink	1. _____	_____	2. _____	_____
Meal Replace.	1. _____	_____	2. _____	_____
Condiments	1. _____	_____	2. _____	_____
Other	1. _____	_____	2. _____	_____

LUNCH   Time: _____

	Type	Amt:	Type	Amt:
Protein	1. _____	_____	2. _____	_____
Complex Carbs	1. _____	_____	2. _____	_____
Fruit	1. _____	_____	2. _____	_____
Vegetables	1. _____	_____	2. _____	_____
Fat	1. _____	_____	2. _____	_____
Liquid/drink	1. _____	_____	2. _____	_____
Meal Replace.	1. _____	_____	2. _____	_____
Condiments	1. _____	_____	2. _____	_____
Other	1. _____	_____	2. _____	_____

SNACK 2   Time: _____

	Type	Amt:	Type	Amt:
Protein	1. _____	_____	2. _____	_____
Complex Carbs	1. _____	_____	2. _____	_____
Fruit	1. _____	_____	2. _____	_____
Vegetables	1. _____	_____	2. _____	_____
Fat	1. _____	_____	2. _____	_____
Liquid/drink	1. _____	_____	2. _____	_____
Meal Replace.	1. _____	_____	2. _____	_____
Condiments	1. _____	_____	2. _____	_____
Other	1. _____	_____	2. _____	_____

SNACK 3   Time: _____

	Type	Amt:	Type	Amt:
Protein	1. _____	_____	2. _____	_____
Complex Carbs	1. _____	_____	2. _____	_____
Fruit	1. _____	_____	2. _____	_____
Vegetables	1. _____	_____	2. _____	_____
Fat	1. _____	_____	2. _____	_____
Liquid/drink	1. _____	_____	2. _____	_____
Meal Replace.	1. _____	_____	2. _____	_____
Condiments	1. _____	_____	2. _____	_____
Other	1. _____	_____	2. _____	_____

DINNER   Time: _____

	Type	Amt:	Type	Amt:
Protein	1. _____	_____	2. _____	_____
Complex Carbs	1. _____	_____	2. _____	_____
Fruit	1. _____	_____	2. _____	_____
Vegetables	1. _____	_____	2. _____	_____
Fat	1. _____	_____	2. _____	_____
Liquid/drink	1. _____	_____	2. _____	_____
Meal Replace.	1. _____	_____	2. _____	_____
Condiments	1. _____	_____	2. _____	_____
Other	1. _____	_____	2. _____	_____

Resistance Training

Time of day: _____

Warmed up   Yes _____   No _____

Name of exercise 1: _____
Weight: _____   Reps: _____
Set 1: _____
Set 2: _____
Muscles worked: _____   Set 3: _____
Set 4: _____
Stretched?   Yes _____   No _____

Name of exercise 3: _____
Weight: _____   Reps: _____
Set 1: _____
Set 2: _____
Muscles worked: _____   Set 3: _____
Set 4: _____
Stretched?   Yes _____   No _____

Name of exercise 5: _____
Weight: _____   Reps: _____
Set 1: _____
Set 2: _____
Muscles worked: _____   Set 3: _____
Set 4: _____
Stretched?   Yes _____   No _____

Name of exercise 7: _____
Weight: _____   Reps: _____
Set 1: _____
Set 2: _____
Muscles worked: _____   Set 3: _____
Set 4: _____
Stretched?   Yes _____   No _____

Name of exercise 9: _____
Weight: _____   Reps: _____
Set 1: _____
Set 2: _____
Muscles worked: _____   Set 3: _____
Set 4: _____
Stretched?   Yes _____   No _____

Name of exercise 2: _____
Weight: _____   Reps: _____
Set 1: _____
Set 2: _____
Muscles worked: _____   Set 3: _____
Set 4: _____
Stretched?   Yes _____   No _____

Name of exercise 4: _____
Weight: _____   Reps: _____
Set 1: _____
Set 2: _____
Muscles worked: _____   Set 3: _____
Set 4: _____
Stretched?   Yes _____   No _____

Name of exercise 6: _____
Weight: _____   Reps: _____
Set 1: _____
Set 2: _____
Muscles worked: _____   Set 3: _____
Set 4: _____
Stretched?   Yes _____   No _____

Name of exercise 8: _____
Weight: _____   Reps: _____
Set 1: _____
Set 2: _____
Muscles worked: _____   Set 3: _____
Set 4: _____
Stretched?   Yes _____   No _____

Name of exercise 10: _____
Weight: _____   Reps: _____
Set 1: _____
Set 2: _____
Muscles worked: _____   Set 3: _____
Set 4: _____
Stretched?   Yes _____   No _____

Cardiovascular Training

Warmed up   Yes _____   No _____

Time of day: _____	For how long?	Heart Rate
Type 1:	_____	_____
Type 2:	_____	_____
Type 3:	_____	_____
Type 4:	_____	_____
Stretched? Yes _____ No _____		

Evening Reflection

Did I put my faith in Action today?   Yes _____   No _____
I prayed for somone today   Yes _____   No _____
I read my Bible today   Yes _____   No _____
I helped someone in need today   Yes _____   No _____
I got 6 1/2 to 8 hours of sleep last night   Yes _____   No _____
I know I ate right today   Yes _____   No _____
I ate breakfast today   Yes _____   No _____
I ate starches after 4:00 p.m. today   Yes _____   No _____
I ate at least 4 meals today   Yes _____   No _____
I drank at least a gallon of water today   Yes _____   No _____
I had Courage to Change today   Yes _____   No _____
Tonight I forgive… _____

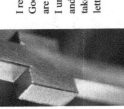

Captain's Log Statement of Faith

I realize that my actions don't earn my way into God's love or earn my way to heaven but that they are a reflection of my love affair with Jesus! I understand that by taking care of myself I honor and glorify God. I matter to God and the actions I take toward good health are daily written love letters telling God, "Thank you for my life"!

_____   **Signature**

"I press on toward the goal to win the prize for which God has called me heavenward in Christ Jesus."
Philippians 3:14

Captain's Log

Day: _____   Date: ____ / ____ / ____

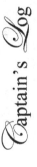
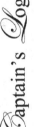

Nutrition Log

BREAKFAST   Time: _____

	Type	Amt:	Type	Amt:
Protein	1._____		2._____	
Complex Carbs	1._____		2._____	
Fruit	1._____		2._____	
Vegetables	1._____		2._____	
Fat	1._____		2._____	
Liquid/drink	1._____		2._____	
Meal Replace.	1._____		2._____	
Condiments	1._____		2._____	
Other	1._____		2._____	

LUNCH   Time: _____

	Type	Amt:	Type	Amt:
Protein	1._____		2._____	
Complex Carbs	1._____		2._____	
Fruit	1._____		2._____	
Vegetables	1._____		2._____	
Fat	1._____		2._____	
Liquid/drink	1._____		2._____	
Meal Replace.	1._____		2._____	
Condiments	1._____		2._____	
Other	1._____		2._____	

SNACK 3   Time: _____

	Type	Amt:	Type	Amt:
Protein	1._____		2._____	
Complex Carbs	1._____		2._____	
Fruit	1._____		2._____	
Vegetables	1._____		2._____	
Fat	1._____		2._____	
Liquid/drink	1._____		2._____	
Meal Replace.	1._____		2._____	
Condiments	1._____		2._____	
Other	1._____		2._____	

SNACK 1   Time: _____

	Type	Amt:	Type	Amt:
Protein	1._____		2._____	
Complex Carbs	1._____		2._____	
Fruit	1._____		2._____	
Vegetables	1._____		2._____	
Fat	1._____		2._____	
Liquid/drink	1._____		2._____	
Meal Replace.	1._____		2._____	
Condiments	1._____		2._____	
Other	1._____		2._____	

SNACK 2   Time: _____

	Type	Amt:	Type	Amt:
Protein	1._____		2._____	
Complex Carbs	1._____		2._____	
Fruit	1._____		2._____	
Vegetables	1._____		2._____	
Fat	1._____		2._____	
Liquid/drink	1._____		2._____	
Meal Replace.	1._____		2._____	
Condiments	1._____		2._____	
Other	1._____		2._____	

DINNER   Time: _____

	Type	Amt:	Type	Amt:
Protein	1._____		2._____	
Complex Carbs	1._____		2._____	
Fruit	1._____		2._____	
Vegetables	1._____		2._____	
Fat	1._____		2._____	
Liquid/drink	1._____		2._____	
Meal Replace.	1._____		2._____	
Condiments	1._____		2._____	
Other	1._____		2._____	

Resistance Training

Time of day: _____

Warmed up   Yes _____   No _____

	Weight:	Reps:
Name of exercise 1:	Set 1:	
	Set 2:	
Muscles worked:	Set 3:	
	Set 4:	
Stretched? Yes _____	No _____	

	Weight:	Reps:
Name of exercise 3:	Set 1:	
	Set 2:	
Muscles worked:	Set 3:	
	Set 4:	
Stretched? Yes _____	No _____	

	Weight:	Reps:
Name of exercise 5:	Set 1:	
	Set 2:	
Muscles worked:	Set 3:	
	Set 4:	
Stretched? Yes _____	No _____	

	Weight:	Reps:
Name of exercise 7:	Set 1:	
	Set 2:	
Muscles worked:	Set 3:	
	Set 4:	
Stretched? Yes _____	No _____	

	Weight:	Reps:
Name of exercise 9:	Set 1:	
	Set 2:	
Muscles worked:	Set 3:	
	Set 4:	
Stretched? Yes _____	No _____	

	Weight:	Reps:
Name of exercise 2:	Set 1:	
	Set 2:	
Muscles worked:	Set 3:	
	Set 4:	
Stretched? Yes _____	No _____	

	Weight:	Reps:
Name of exercise 4:	Set 1:	
	Set 2:	
Muscles worked:	Set 3:	
	Set 4:	
Stretched? Yes _____	No _____	

	Weight:	Reps:
Name of exercise 6:	Set 1:	
	Set 2:	
Muscles worked:	Set 3:	
	Set 4:	
Stretched? Yes _____	No _____	

	Weight:	Reps:
Name of exercise 8:	Set 1:	
	Set 2:	
Muscles worked:	Set 3:	
	Set 4:	
Stretched? Yes _____	No _____	

	Weight:	Reps:
Name of exercise 10:	Set 1:	
	Set 2:	
Muscles worked:	Set 3:	
	Set 4:	
Stretched? Yes _____	No _____	

Cardiovascular Training

Warmed up   Yes _____   No _____

	For how long?	Heart Rate
Time of day: _____		
Type 1:		
Type 2:		
Type 3:		
Type 4:		
Stretched? Yes _____	No _____	

Evening Reflection

Did I put my faith in Action today?	Yes _____	No _____
I prayed for somone today	Yes _____	No _____
I read my Bible today	Yes _____	No _____
I helped someone in need today	Yes _____	No _____
I got 6 1/2 to 8 hours of sleep last night	Yes _____	No _____
I know I ate right today	Yes _____	No _____
I ate breakfast today	Yes _____	No _____
I ate starches after 4:00 p.m. today	Yes _____	No _____
I ate at least 4 meals today	Yes _____	No _____
I drank at least a gallon of water today	Yes _____	No _____
I had Courage to Change today	Yes _____	No _____
Tonight I forgive... _____		

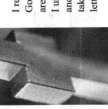

Captain's Log Statement of Faith

I realize that my actions don't earn my way into God's love or earn my way to heaven but that they are a reflection of my love affair with Jesus! I understand that by taking care of myself I honor and glorify God. I matter to God and the actions I take toward good health are daily written love letters telling God, "Thank you for my life"!

_____
Signature

"I press on toward the goal to win the prize for which God has called me heavenward in Christ Jesus."

Philippians 3:14

Captain's Log

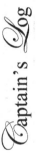

Day: _____   Date: _____ / _____ / _____

Nutrition Log

BREAKFAST Time: _____

	Type	Amt:	Type	Amt:
Protein	1.		2.	
Complex Carbs	1.		2.	
Fruit	1.		2.	
Vegetables	1.		2.	
Fat	1.		2.	
Liquid/drink	1.		2.	
Meal Replace.	1.		2.	
Condiments	1.		2.	
Other	1.		2.	

SNACK 1 Time: _____

	Type	Amt:	Type	Amt:
Protein	1.		2.	
Complex Carbs	1.		2.	
Fruit	1.		2.	
Vegetables	1.		2.	
Fat	1.		2.	
Liquid/drink	1.		2.	
Meal Replace.	1.		2.	
Condiments	1.		2.	
Other	1.		2.	

LUNCH Time: _____

	Type	Amt:	Type	Amt:
Protein	1.		2.	
Complex Carbs	1.		2.	
Fruit	1.		2.	
Vegetables	1.		2.	
Fat	1.		2.	
Liquid/drink	1.		2.	
Meal Replace.	1.		2.	
Condiments	1.		2.	
Other	1.		2.	

SNACK 2 Time: _____

	Type	Amt:	Type	Amt:
Protein	1.		2.	
Complex Carbs	1.		2.	
Fruit	1.		2.	
Vegetables	1.		2.	
Fat	1.		2.	
Liquid/drink	1.		2.	
Meal Replace.	1.		2.	
Condiments	1.		2.	
Other	1.		2.	

SNACK 3 Time: _____

	Type	Amt:	Type	Amt:
Protein	1.		2.	
Complex Carbs	1.		2.	
Fruit	1.		2.	
Vegetables	1.		2.	
Fat	1.		2.	
Liquid/drink	1.		2.	
Meal Replace.	1.		2.	
Condiments	1.		2.	
Other	1.		2.	

DINNER Time: _____

	Type	Amt:	Type	Amt:
Protein	1.		2.	
Complex Carbs	1.		2.	
Fruit	1.		2.	
Vegetables	1.		2.	
Fat	1.		2.	
Liquid/drink	1.		2.	
Meal Replace.	1.		2.	
Condiments	1.		2.	
Other	1.		2.	

Cardiovascular Training

Time of day: _____

Warmed up Yes _____ No _____

Type	For how long?	Heart Rate
Type 1:		
Type 2:		
Type 3:		
Type 4:		

Stretched? Yes _____ No _____

Evening Reflection

	Yes	No
Did I put my faith in Action today?	Yes _____	No _____
I prayed for somone today	Yes _____	No _____
I read my Bible today	Yes _____	No _____
I helped someone in need today	Yes _____	No _____
I got 6 1/2 to 8 hours of sleep last night	Yes _____	No _____
I know I ate right today	Yes _____	No _____
I ate breakfast today	Yes _____	No _____
I ate starches after 4:00 p.m. today	Yes _____	No _____
I ate at least 4 meals today	Yes _____	No _____
I drank at least a gallon of water today	Yes _____	No _____
I had Courage to Change today	Yes _____	No _____

Tonight I forgive...

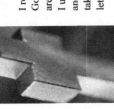

Captain's Log Statement of Faith

I realize that my actions don't earn my way into God's love or earn my way to heaven but that they are a reflection of my love affair with Jesus! I understand that by taking care of myself I honor and glorify God. I matter to God and the actions I take toward good health are daily written love letters telling God, "Thank you for my life"!

_____
Signature

Resistance Training

Time of day: _____

Warmed up Yes _____ No _____

Name of exercise 1: _____ Weight: _____ Reps: _____

Set 1: _____
Set 2: _____

Muscles worked: _____ Set 3: _____
Set 4: _____

Stretched? Yes _____ No _____

Name of exercise 2: _____ Weight: _____ Reps: _____

Set 1: _____
Set 2: _____

Muscles worked: _____ Set 3: _____
Set 4: _____

Stretched? Yes _____ No _____

Name of exercise 3: _____ Weight: _____ Reps: _____

Set 1: _____
Set 2: _____

Muscles worked: _____ Set 3: _____
Set 4: _____

Stretched? Yes _____ No _____

Name of exercise 4: _____ Weight: _____ Reps: _____

Set 1: _____
Set 2: _____

Muscles worked: _____ Set 3: _____
Set 4: _____

Stretched? Yes _____ No _____

Name of exercise 5: _____ Weight: _____ Reps: _____

Set 1: _____
Set 2: _____

Muscles worked: _____ Set 3: _____
Set 4: _____

Stretched? Yes _____ No _____

Name of exercise 6: _____ Weight: _____ Reps: _____

Set 1: _____
Set 2: _____

Muscles worked: _____ Set 3: _____
Set 4: _____

Stretched? Yes _____ No _____

Name of exercise 7: _____ Weight: _____ Reps: _____

Set 1: _____
Set 2: _____

Muscles worked: _____ Set 3: _____
Set 4: _____

Stretched? Yes _____ No _____

Name of exercise 8: _____ Weight: _____ Reps: _____

Set 1: _____
Set 2: _____

Muscles worked: _____ Set 3: _____
Set 4: _____

Stretched? Yes _____ No _____

Name of exercise 9: _____ Weight: _____ Reps: _____

Set 1: _____
Set 2: _____

Muscles worked: _____ Set 3: _____
Set 4: _____

Stretched? Yes _____ No _____

Name of exercise 10: _____ Weight: _____ Reps: _____

Set 1: _____
Set 2: _____

Muscles worked: _____ Set 3: _____
Set 4: _____

Stretched? Yes _____ No _____

"I press on toward the goal to win the prize for which God has called me heavenward in Christ Jesus."
Philippians 3:14

CONQUERING CONTROL and ADDICTION

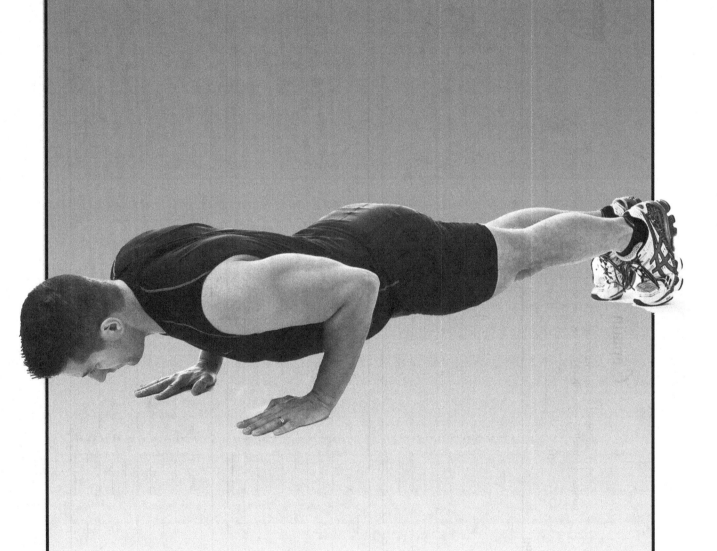

"This is love for God: to obey his commands. And his commands are not burdensome, for everyone born of God overcomes the world. This is the victory that has overcome the world, even our faith." (1 John 5:3-4)

WEEK NINE

Captain's Log

Day: _____ Date: _____ / _____ / _____

Nutrition Log

BREAKFAST Time: _____

	Type	Amt:
Protein	1. _____	_____
	2. _____	_____
Complex Carbs	1. _____	_____
	2. _____	_____
Fruit	1. _____	_____
	2. _____	_____
Vegetables	1. _____	_____
	2. _____	_____
Fat	1. _____	_____
	2. _____	_____
Liquid/drink	1. _____	_____
	2. _____	_____
Meal Replace.	1. _____	_____
	2. _____	_____
Condiments	1. _____	_____
	2. _____	_____
Other	1. _____	_____
	2. _____	_____

SNACK 1 Time: _____

	Type	Amt:
Protein	1. _____	_____
	2. _____	_____
Complex Carbs	1. _____	_____
	2. _____	_____
Fruit	1. _____	_____
	2. _____	_____
Vegetables	1. _____	_____
	2. _____	_____
Fat	1. _____	_____
	2. _____	_____
Liquid/drink	1. _____	_____
	2. _____	_____
Meal Replace.	1. _____	_____
	2. _____	_____
Condiments	1. _____	_____
	2. _____	_____
Other	1. _____	_____
	2. _____	_____

LUNCH Time: _____

	Type	Amt:
Protein	1. _____	_____
	2. _____	_____
Complex Carbs	1. _____	_____
	2. _____	_____
Fruit	1. _____	_____
	2. _____	_____
Vegetables	1. _____	_____
	2. _____	_____
Fat	1. _____	_____
	2. _____	_____
Liquid/drink	1. _____	_____
	2. _____	_____
Meal Replace.	1. _____	_____
	2. _____	_____
Condiments	1. _____	_____
	2. _____	_____
Other	1. _____	_____
	2. _____	_____

SNACK 2 Time: _____

	Type	Amt:
Protein	1. _____	_____
	2. _____	_____
Complex Carbs	1. _____	_____
	2. _____	_____
Fruit	1. _____	_____
	2. _____	_____
Vegetables	1. _____	_____
	2. _____	_____
Fat	1. _____	_____
	2. _____	_____
Liquid/drink	1. _____	_____
	2. _____	_____
Meal Replace.	1. _____	_____
	2. _____	_____
Condiments	1. _____	_____
	2. _____	_____
Other	1. _____	_____
	2. _____	_____

SNACK 3 Time: _____

	Type	Amt:
Protein	1. _____	_____
	2. _____	_____
Complex Carbs	1. _____	_____
	2. _____	_____
Fruit	1. _____	_____
	2. _____	_____
Vegetables	1. _____	_____
	2. _____	_____
Fat	1. _____	_____
	2. _____	_____
Liquid/drink	1. _____	_____
	2. _____	_____
Meal Replace.	1. _____	_____
	2. _____	_____
Condiments	1. _____	_____
	2. _____	_____
Other	1. _____	_____
	2. _____	_____

DINNER Time: _____

	Type	Amt:
Protein	1. _____	_____
	2. _____	_____
Complex Carbs	1. _____	_____
	2. _____	_____
Fruit	1. _____	_____
	2. _____	_____
Vegetables	1. _____	_____
	2. _____	_____
Fat	1. _____	_____
	2. _____	_____
Liquid/drink	1. _____	_____
	2. _____	_____
Meal Replace.	1. _____	_____
	2. _____	_____
Condiments	1. _____	_____
	2. _____	_____
Other	1. _____	_____
	2. _____	_____

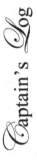
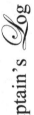

Resistance Training

Time of day: _____

Warmed up   Yes _____   No _____

Name of exercise 1: _____

	Weight:	Reps:
Set 1:		
Set 2:		
Muscles worked:	Set 3:	
	Set 4:	

Stretched?   Yes _____   No _____

Name of exercise 2: _____

	Weight:	Reps:
Set 1:		
Set 2:		
Muscles worked:	Set 3:	
	Set 4:	

Stretched?   Yes _____   No _____

Name of exercise 3: _____

	Weight:	Reps:
Set 1:		
Set 2:		
Muscles worked:	Set 3:	
	Set 4:	

Stretched?   Yes _____   No _____

Name of exercise 4: _____

	Weight:	Reps:
Set 1:		
Set 2:		
Muscles worked:	Set 3:	
	Set 4:	

Stretched?   Yes _____   No _____

Name of exercise 5: _____

	Weight:	Reps:
Set 1:		
Set 2:		
Muscles worked:	Set 3:	
	Set 4:	

Stretched?   Yes _____   No _____

Name of exercise 6: _____

	Weight:	Reps:
Set 1:		
Set 2:		
Muscles worked:	Set 3:	
	Set 4:	

Stretched?   Yes _____   No _____

Name of exercise 7: _____

	Weight:	Reps:
Set 1:		
Set 2:		
Muscles worked:	Set 3:	
	Set 4:	

Stretched?   Yes _____   No _____

Name of exercise 8: _____

	Weight:	Reps:
Set 1:		
Set 2:		
Muscles worked:	Set 3:	
	Set 4:	

Stretched?   Yes _____   No _____

Name of exercise 9: _____

	Weight:	Reps:
Set 1:		
Set 2:		
Muscles worked:	Set 3:	
	Set 4:	

Stretched?   Yes _____   No _____

Name of exercise 10: _____

	Weight:	Reps:
Set 1:		
Set 2:		
Muscles worked:	Set 3:	
	Set 4:	

Stretched?   Yes _____   No _____

Cardiovascular Training

Warmed up   Yes _____   No _____

Time of day:	For how long?	Heart Rate
Type 1:		
Type 2:		
Type 3:		
Type 4:		

Stretched?   Yes _____   No _____

Evening Reflection

Did I put my faith in Action today?	Yes _____	No _____
I prayed for somone today	Yes _____	No _____
I read my Bible today	Yes _____	No _____
I helped someone in need today	Yes _____	No _____
I got 6 1/2 to 8 hours of sleep last night	Yes _____	No _____
I know I ate right today	Yes _____	No _____
I ate breakfast today	Yes _____	No _____
I ate starches after 4:00 p.m. today	Yes _____	No _____
I ate at least 4 meals today	Yes _____	No _____
I drank at least a gallon of water today	Yes _____	No _____
I had Courage to Change today	Yes _____	No _____
Tonight I forgive…		

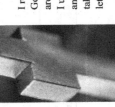

Captain's Log Statement of Faith

I realize that my actions don't earn my way into God's love or earn my way to heaven but that they are a reflection of my love affair with Jesus! I understand that by taking care of myself I honor and glorify God. I matter to God and the actions I take toward good health are daily written love letters telling God, "Thank you for my life"!

_____
Signature

"I press on toward the goal to win the prize for which God has called me heavenward in Christ Jesus."
Philippians 3:14

Captain's Log

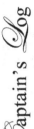

"Each one should test his own actions. Then he can take pride in himself without comparing himself to somebody else, for each one should carry his own load." (Galatians 6:40)

Day: _____ Date: _____ / _____ / _____

Nutrition Log

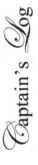

BREAKFAST	Time: _____					SNACK 1	Time: _____				
	Type	Amt:		Type	Amt:		Type	Amt:		Type	Amt:
Protein	1. ____	____		2. ____	____	Protein	1. ____	____		2. ____	____
Complex Carbs	1. ____	____		2. ____	____	Complex Carbs	1. ____	____		2. ____	____
Fruit	1. ____	____		2. ____	____	Fruit	1. ____	____		2. ____	____
Vegetables	1. ____	____		2. ____	____	Vegetables	1. ____	____		2. ____	____
Fat	1. ____	____		2. ____	____	Fat	1. ____	____		2. ____	____
Liquid/drink	1. ____	____		2. ____	____	Liquid/drink	1. ____	____		2. ____	____
Meal Replace.	1. ____	____		2. ____	____	Meal Replace.	1. ____	____		2. ____	____
Condiments	1. ____	____		2. ____	____	Condiments	1. ____	____		2. ____	____
Other	1. ____	____		2. ____	____	Other	1. ____	____		2. ____	____

LUNCH	Time: _____					SNACK 2	Time: _____				
	Type	Amt:		Type	Amt:		Type	Amt:		Type	Amt:
Protein	1. ____	____		2. ____	____	Protein	1. ____	____		2. ____	____
Complex Carbs	1. ____	____		2. ____	____	Complex Carbs	1. ____	____		2. ____	____
Fruit	1. ____	____		2. ____	____	Fruit	1. ____	____		2. ____	____
Vegetables	1. ____	____		2. ____	____	Vegetables	1. ____	____		2. ____	____
Fat	1. ____	____		2. ____	____	Fat	1. ____	____		2. ____	____
Liquid/drink	1. ____	____		2. ____	____	Liquid/drink	1. ____	____		2. ____	____
Meal Replace.	1. ____	____		2. ____	____	Meal Replace.	1. ____	____		2. ____	____
Condiments	1. ____	____		2. ____	____	Condiments	1. ____	____		2. ____	____
Other	1. ____	____		2. ____	____	Other	1. ____	____		2. ____	____

SNACK 3	Time: _____					DINNER	Time: _____				
	Type	Amt:		Type	Amt:		Type	Amt:		Type	Amt:
Protein	1. ____	____		2. ____	____	Protein	1. ____	____		2. ____	____
Complex Carbs	1. ____	____		2. ____	____	Complex Carbs	1. ____	____		2. ____	____
Fruit	1. ____	____		2. ____	____	Fruit	1. ____	____		2. ____	____
Vegetables	1. ____	____		2. ____	____	Vegetables	1. ____	____		2. ____	____
Fat	1. ____	____		2. ____	____	Fat	1. ____	____		2. ____	____
Liquid/drink	1. ____	____		2. ____	____	Liquid/drink	1. ____	____		2. ____	____
Meal Replace.	1. ____	____		2. ____	____	Meal Replace.	1. ____	____		2. ____	____
Condiments	1. ____	____		2. ____	____	Condiments	1. ____	____		2. ____	____
Other	1. ____	____		2. ____	____	Other	1. ____	____		2. ____	____

Cardiovascular Training

Warmed up   Yes _____   No _____

Time of day: _____	For how long?	Heart Rate
Type 1:	_____	_____
Type 2:	_____	_____
Type 3:	_____	_____
Type 4:	_____	_____

Stretched?   Yes _____   No _____

Evening Reflection

Did I put my faith in Action today?	Yes _____	No _____
I prayed for somone today	Yes _____	No _____
I read my Bible today	Yes _____	No _____
I helped someone in need today	Yes _____	No _____
I got 6 1/2 to 8 hours of sleep last night	Yes _____	No _____
I know I ate right today	Yes _____	No _____
I ate breakfast today	Yes _____	No _____
I ate starches after 4:00 p.m. today	Yes _____	No _____
I ate at least 4 meals today	Yes _____	No _____
I drank at least a gallon of water today	Yes _____	No _____
I had Courage to Change today	Yes _____	No _____
Tonight I forgive… _____		

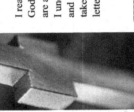

Captain's Log Statement of Faith

I realize that my actions don't earn my way into God's love or earn my way to heaven but that they are a reflection of my love affair with Jesus! I understand that by taking care of myself I honor and glorify God. I matter to God and the actions I take toward good health are daily written love letters telling God, "Thank you for my life"!

_____

Signature

Resistance Training

Time of day: _____

Warmed up   Yes _____   No _____

Name of exercise 1:

	Weight:	Reps:
Set 1:	_____	_____
Set 2:	_____	_____
Set 3:	_____	_____
Set 4:	_____	_____

Muscles worked:

Stretched?   Yes _____   No _____

Name of exercise 2:

	Weight:	Reps:
Set 1:	_____	_____
Set 2:	_____	_____
Set 3:	_____	_____
Set 4:	_____	_____

Muscles worked:

Stretched?   Yes _____   No _____

Name of exercise 3:

	Weight:	Reps:
Set 1:	_____	_____
Set 2:	_____	_____
Set 3:	_____	_____
Set 4:	_____	_____

Muscles worked:

Stretched?   Yes _____   No _____

Name of exercise 4:

	Weight:	Reps:
Set 1:	_____	_____
Set 2:	_____	_____
Set 3:	_____	_____
Set 4:	_____	_____

Muscles worked:

Stretched?   Yes _____   No _____

Name of exercise 5:

	Weight:	Reps:
Set 1:	_____	_____
Set 2:	_____	_____
Set 3:	_____	_____
Set 4:	_____	_____

Muscles worked:

Stretched?   Yes _____   No _____

Name of exercise 6:

	Weight:	Reps:
Set 1:	_____	_____
Set 2:	_____	_____
Set 3:	_____	_____
Set 4:	_____	_____

Muscles worked:

Stretched?   Yes _____   No _____

Name of exercise 7:

	Weight:	Reps:
Set 1:	_____	_____
Set 2:	_____	_____
Set 3:	_____	_____
Set 4:	_____	_____

Muscles worked:

Stretched?   Yes _____   No _____

Name of exercise 8:

	Weight:	Reps:
Set 1:	_____	_____
Set 2:	_____	_____
Set 3:	_____	_____
Set 4:	_____	_____

Muscles worked:

Stretched?   Yes _____   No _____

Name of exercise 9:

	Weight:	Reps:
Set 1:	_____	_____
Set 2:	_____	_____
Set 3:	_____	_____
Set 4:	_____	_____

Muscles worked:

Stretched?   Yes _____   No _____

Name of exercise 10:

	Weight:	Reps:
Set 1:	_____	_____
Set 2:	_____	_____
Set 3:	_____	_____
Set 4:	_____	_____

Muscles worked:

Stretched?   Yes _____   No _____

"I press on toward the goal to win the prize for which God has called me heavenward in Christ Jesus."
Philippians 3:14

Captain's Log

"Each one should test his own actions. Then he can take pride in himself without comparing himself to somebody else, for each one should carry his own load." (Galatians 6:40)

Day: _____ Date: _____ / _____ / _____

Nutrition Log

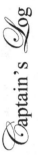

BREAKFAST Time: _____

	Type	Amt:		Type	Amt:
Protein	1.			2.	
Complex Carbs	1.			2.	
Fruit	1.			2.	
Vegetables	1.			2.	
Fat	1.			2.	
Liquid/drink	1.			2.	
Meal Replace.	1.			2.	
Condiments	1.			2.	
Other	1.			2.	

LUNCH Time: _____

	Type	Amt:		Type	Amt:
Protein	1.			2.	
Complex Carbs	1.			2.	
Fruit	1.			2.	
Vegetables	1.			2.	
Fat	1.			2.	
Liquid/drink	1.			2.	
Meal Replace.	1.			2.	
Condiments	1.			2.	
Other	1.			2.	

SNACK 3 Time: _____

	Type	Amt:		Type	Amt:
Protein	1.			2.	
Complex Carbs	1.			2.	
Fruit	1.			2.	
Vegetables	1.			2.	
Fat	1.			2.	
Liquid/drink	1.			2.	
Meal Replace.	1.			2.	
Condiments	1.			2.	
Other	1.			2.	

SNACK 1 Time: _____

	Type	Amt:		Type	Amt:
Protein	1.			2.	
Complex Carbs	1.			2.	
Fruit	1.			2.	
Vegetables	1.			2.	
Fat	1.			2.	
Liquid/drink	1.			2.	
Meal Replace.	1.			2.	
Condiments	1.			2.	
Other	1.			2.	

SNACK 2 Time: _____

	Type	Amt:		Type	Amt:
Protein	1.			2.	
Complex Carbs	1.			2.	
Fruit	1.			2.	
Vegetables	1.			2.	
Fat	1.			2.	
Liquid/drink	1.			2.	
Meal Replace.	1.			2.	
Condiments	1.			2.	
Other	1.			2.	

DINNER Time: _____

	Type	Amt:		Type	Amt:
Protein	1.			2.	
Complex Carbs	1.			2.	
Fruit	1.			2.	
Vegetables	1.			2.	
Fat	1.			2.	
Liquid/drink	1.			2.	
Meal Replace.	1.			2.	
Condiments	1.			2.	
Other	1.			2.	

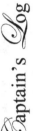

Cardiovascular Training

Warmed up   Yes _____   No _____

Time of day:	For how long?	Heart Rate
Type 1:		
Type 2:		
Type 3:		
Type 4:		

Stretched?   Yes _____   No _____

Evening Reflection

Did I put my faith in Action today?	Yes _____	No _____
I prayed for somone today	Yes _____	No _____
I read my Bible today	Yes _____	No _____
I helped someone in need today	Yes _____	No _____
I got 6 1/2 to 8 hours of sleep last night	Yes _____	No _____
I know I ate right today	Yes _____	No _____
I ate breakfast today	Yes _____	No _____
I ate starches after 4:00 p.m. today	Yes _____	No _____
I ate at least 4 meals today	Yes _____	No _____
I drank at least a gallon of water today	Yes _____	No _____
I had Courage to Change today	Yes _____	No _____
Tonight I forgive…		

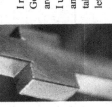

Captain's Log Statement of Faith

I realize that my actions don't earn my way into God's love or earn my way to heaven but that they are a reflection of my love affair with Jesus! I understand that by taking care of myself I honor and glorify God. I matter to God and the actions I take toward good health are daily written love letters telling God, "Thank you for my life"!

_____   **Signature**

Resistance Training

Time of day: _____

Warmed up   Yes _____   No _____

Name of exercise 1: Weight: _____ Reps: _____
Set 1: _____
Set 2: _____
Muscles worked: _____ Set 3: _____
Set 4: _____
Stretched?   Yes _____   No _____

Name of exercise 2: Weight: _____ Reps: _____
Set 1: _____
Set 2: _____
Muscles worked: _____ Set 3: _____
Set 4: _____
Stretched?   Yes _____   No _____

Name of exercise 3: Weight: _____ Reps: _____
Set 1: _____
Set 2: _____
Muscles worked: _____ Set 3: _____
Set 4: _____
Stretched?   Yes _____   No _____

Name of exercise 4: Weight: _____ Reps: _____
Set 1: _____
Set 2: _____
Muscles worked: _____ Set 3: _____
Set 4: _____
Stretched?   Yes _____   No _____

Name of exercise 5: Weight: _____ Reps: _____
Set 1: _____
Set 2: _____
Muscles worked: _____ Set 3: _____
Set 4: _____
Stretched?   Yes _____   No _____

Name of exercise 6: Weight: _____ Reps: _____
Set 1: _____
Set 2: _____
Muscles worked: _____ Set 3: _____
Set 4: _____
Stretched?   Yes _____   No _____

Name of exercise 7: Weight: _____ Reps: _____
Set 1: _____
Set 2: _____
Muscles worked: _____ Set 3: _____
Set 4: _____
Stretched?   Yes _____   No _____

Name of exercise 8: Weight: _____ Reps: _____
Set 1: _____
Set 2: _____
Muscles worked: _____ Set 3: _____
Set 4: _____
Stretched?   Yes _____   No _____

Name of exercise 9: Weight: _____ Reps: _____
Set 1: _____
Set 2: _____
Muscles worked: _____ Set 3: _____
Set 4: _____
Stretched?   Yes _____   No _____

Name of exercise 10: Weight: _____ Reps: _____
Set 1: _____
Set 2: _____
Muscles worked: _____ Set 3: _____
Set 4: _____
Stretched?   Yes _____   No _____

"I press on toward the goal to win the prize for which God has called me heavenward in Christ Jesus."
Philippians 3:14

Captain's Log

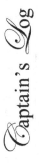
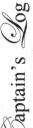

Day: _____   Date: ____ / ____ / ____

Nutrition Log

BREAKFAST	Time: _____				SNACK 1	Time: _____		
	Type	Amt:	Type	Amt:		Type	Amt:	Type	Amt:
Protein	1. _____	_____	2. _____	_____	Protein	1. _____	_____	2. _____	_____
Complex Carbs	1. _____	_____	2. _____	_____	Complex Carbs	1. _____	_____	2. _____	_____
Fruit	1. _____	_____	2. _____	_____	Fruit	1. _____	_____	2. _____	_____
Vegetables	1. _____	_____	2. _____	_____	Vegetables	1. _____	_____	2. _____	_____
Fat	1. _____	_____	2. _____	_____	Fat	1. _____	_____	2. _____	_____
Liquid/drink	1. _____	_____	2. _____	_____	Liquid/drink	1. _____	_____	2. _____	_____
Meal Replace.	1. _____	_____	2. _____	_____	Meal Replace.	1. _____	_____	2. _____	_____
Condiments	1. _____	_____	2. _____	_____	Condiments	1. _____	_____	2. _____	_____
Other	1. _____	_____	2. _____	_____	Other	1. _____	_____	2. _____	_____

LUNCH	Time: _____				SNACK 2	Time: _____		
	Type	Amt:	Type	Amt:		Type	Amt:	Type	Amt:
Protein	1. _____	_____	2. _____	_____	Protein	1. _____	_____	2. _____	_____
Complex Carbs	1. _____	_____	2. _____	_____	Complex Carbs	1. _____	_____	2. _____	_____
Fruit	1. _____	_____	2. _____	_____	Fruit	1. _____	_____	2. _____	_____
Vegetables	1. _____	_____	2. _____	_____	Vegetables	1. _____	_____	2. _____	_____
Fat	1. _____	_____	2. _____	_____	Fat	1. _____	_____	2. _____	_____
Liquid/drink	1. _____	_____	2. _____	_____	Liquid/drink	1. _____	_____	2. _____	_____
Meal Replace.	1. _____	_____	2. _____	_____	Meal Replace.	1. _____	_____	2. _____	_____
Condiments	1. _____	_____	2. _____	_____	Condiments	1. _____	_____	2. _____	_____
Other	1. _____	_____	2. _____	_____	Other	1. _____	_____	2. _____	_____

SNACK 3	Time: _____				DINNER	Time: _____		
	Type	Amt:	Type	Amt:		Type	Amt:	Type	Amt:
Protein	1. _____	_____	2. _____	_____	Protein	1. _____	_____	2. _____	_____
Complex Carbs	1. _____	_____	2. _____	_____	Complex Carbs	1. _____	_____	2. _____	_____
Fruit	1. _____	_____	2. _____	_____	Fruit	1. _____	_____	2. _____	_____
Vegetables	1. _____	_____	2. _____	_____	Vegetables	1. _____	_____	2. _____	_____
Fat	1. _____	_____	2. _____	_____	Fat	1. _____	_____	2. _____	_____
Liquid/drink	1. _____	_____	2. _____	_____	Liquid/drink	1. _____	_____	2. _____	_____
Meal Replace.	1. _____	_____	2. _____	_____	Meal Replace.	1. _____	_____	2. _____	_____
Condiments	1. _____	_____	2. _____	_____	Condiments	1. _____	_____	2. _____	_____
Other	1. _____	_____	2. _____	_____	Other	1. _____	_____	2. _____	_____

Cardiovascular Training

Time of day: _____

Warmed up   Yes _____   No _____

Type of day:	For how long?	Heart Rate
Type 1:		
Type 2:		
Type 3:		
Type 4:		

Stretched?   Yes _____   No _____

Evening Reflection

Did I put my faith in Action today?	Yes _____	No _____
I prayed for somone today	Yes _____	No _____
I read my Bible today	Yes _____	No _____
I helped someone in need today	Yes _____	No _____
I got 6 1/2 to 8 hours of sleep last night	Yes _____	No _____
I know I ate right today	Yes _____	No _____
I ate breakfast today	Yes _____	No _____
I ate starches after 4:00 p.m. today	Yes _____	No _____
I ate at least 4 meals today	Yes _____	No _____
I drank at least a gallon of water today	Yes _____	No _____
I had Courage to Change today	Yes _____	No _____
Tonight I forgive…		

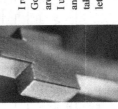

Captain's Log Statement of Faith

I realize that my actions don't earn my way into God's love or earn my way to heaven but that they are a reflection of my love affair with Jesus! I understand that by taking care of myself I honor and glorify God. I matter to God and the actions I take toward good health are daily written love letters telling God, "Thank you for my life"!

_____
Signature

Resistance Training

Time of day: _____

Warmed up   Yes _____   No _____

Name of exercise 1: _____
Weight: _____   Reps: _____

Set 1: _____
Set 2: _____
Set 3: _____
Set 4: _____

Muscles worked: _____

Stretched?   Yes _____   No _____

Name of exercise 2: _____
Weight: _____   Reps: _____

Set 1: _____
Set 2: _____
Set 3: _____
Set 4: _____

Muscles worked: _____

Stretched?   Yes _____   No _____

Name of exercise 3: _____
Weight: _____   Reps: _____

Set 1: _____
Set 2: _____
Set 3: _____
Set 4: _____

Muscles worked: _____

Stretched?   Yes _____   No _____

Name of exercise 4: _____
Weight: _____   Reps: _____

Set 1: _____
Set 2: _____
Set 3: _____
Set 4: _____

Muscles worked: _____

Stretched?   Yes _____   No _____

Name of exercise 5: _____
Weight: _____   Reps: _____

Set 1: _____
Set 2: _____
Set 3: _____
Set 4: _____

Muscles worked: _____

Stretched?   Yes _____   No _____

Name of exercise 6: _____
Weight: _____   Reps: _____

Set 1: _____
Set 2: _____
Set 3: _____
Set 4: _____

Muscles worked: _____

Stretched?   Yes _____   No _____

Name of exercise 7: _____
Weight: _____   Reps: _____

Set 1: _____
Set 2: _____
Set 3: _____
Set 4: _____

Muscles worked: _____

Stretched?   Yes _____   No _____

Name of exercise 8: _____
Weight: _____   Reps: _____

Set 1: _____
Set 2: _____
Set 3: _____
Set 4: _____

Muscles worked: _____

Stretched?   Yes _____   No _____

Name of exercise 9: _____
Weight: _____   Reps: _____

Set 1: _____
Set 2: _____
Set 3: _____
Set 4: _____

Muscles worked: _____

Stretched?   Yes _____   No _____

Name of exercise 10: _____
Weight: _____   Reps: _____

Set 1: _____
Set 2: _____
Set 3: _____
Set 4: _____

Muscles worked: _____

Stretched?   Yes _____   No _____

"I press on toward the goal to win the prize for which God has called me heavenward in Christ Jesus."
Philippians 3:14

Captain's Log

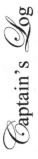
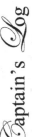

"Each one should test his own actions. Then he can take pride in himself without comparing himself to somebody else, for each one should carry his own load." (Galatians 6:40)

Day: _____ Date: _____ / _____ / _____

Nutrition Log

BREAKFAST   Time: _____

	Type	Amt:		Type	Amt:
Protein	1.			2.	
Complex Carbs	1.			2.	
Fruit	1.			2.	
Vegetables	1.			2.	
Fat	1.			2.	
Liquid/drink	1.			2.	
Meal Replace.	1.			2.	
Condiments	1.			2.	
Other	1.			2.	

SNACK 1   Time: _____

	Type	Amt:		Type	Amt:
Protein	1.			2.	
Complex Carbs	1.			2.	
Fruit	1.			2.	
Vegetables	1.			2.	
Fat	1.			2.	
Liquid/drink	1.			2.	
Meal Replace.	1.			2.	
Condiments	1.			2.	
Other	1.			2.	

LUNCH   Time: _____

	Type	Amt:		Type	Amt:
Protein	1.			2.	
Complex Carbs	1.			2.	
Fruit	1.			2.	
Vegetables	1.			2.	
Fat	1.			2.	
Liquid/drink	1.			2.	
Meal Replace.	1.			2.	
Condiments	1.			2.	
Other	1.			2.	

SNACK 2   Time: _____

	Type	Amt:		Type	Amt:
Protein	1.			2.	
Complex Carbs	1.			2.	
Fruit	1.			2.	
Vegetables	1.			2.	
Fat	1.			2.	
Liquid/drink	1.			2.	
Meal Replace.	1.			2.	
Condiments	1.			2.	
Other	1.			2.	

SNACK 3   Time: _____

	Type	Amt:		Type	Amt:
Protein	1.			2.	
Complex Carbs	1.			2.	
Fruit	1.			2.	
Vegetables	1.			2.	
Fat	1.			2.	
Liquid/drink	1.			2.	
Meal Replace.	1.			2.	
Condiments	1.			2.	
Other	1.			2.	

DINNER   Time: _____

	Type	Amt:		Type	Amt:
Protein	1.			2.	
Complex Carbs	1.			2.	
Fruit	1.			2.	
Vegetables	1.			2.	
Fat	1.			2.	
Liquid/drink	1.			2.	
Meal Replace.	1.			2.	
Condiments	1.			2.	
Other	1.			2.	

Resistance Training

Time of day: _____

Warmed up: Yes ___ No ___

Name of exercise 1: _____ Weight: ___ Reps: ___
- Set 1: ___
- Set 2: ___
- Set 3: ___
- Set 4: ___

Muscles worked: _____

Stretched? Yes ___ No ___

Name of exercise 3: _____ Weight: ___ Reps: ___
- Set 1: ___
- Set 2: ___
- Set 3: ___
- Set 4: ___

Muscles worked: _____

Stretched? Yes ___ No ___

Name of exercise 5: _____ Weight: ___ Reps: ___
- Set 1: ___
- Set 2: ___
- Set 3: ___
- Set 4: ___

Muscles worked: _____

Stretched? Yes ___ No ___

Name of exercise 7: _____ Weight: ___ Reps: ___
- Set 1: ___
- Set 2: ___
- Set 3: ___
- Set 4: ___

Muscles worked: _____

Stretched? Yes ___ No ___

Name of exercise 9: _____ Weight: ___ Reps: ___
- Set 1: ___
- Set 2: ___
- Set 3: ___
- Set 4: ___

Muscles worked: _____

Stretched? Yes ___ No ___

Name of exercise 2: _____ Weight: ___ Reps: ___
- Set 1: ___
- Set 2: ___
- Set 3: ___
- Set 4: ___

Muscles worked: _____

Stretched? Yes ___ No ___

Name of exercise 4: _____ Weight: ___ Reps: ___
- Set 1: ___
- Set 2: ___
- Set 3: ___
- Set 4: ___

Muscles worked: _____

Stretched? Yes ___ No ___

Name of exercise 6: _____ Weight: ___ Reps: ___
- Set 1: ___
- Set 2: ___
- Set 3: ___
- Set 4: ___

Muscles worked: _____

Stretched? Yes ___ No ___

Name of exercise 8: _____ Weight: ___ Reps: ___
- Set 1: ___
- Set 2: ___
- Set 3: ___
- Set 4: ___

Muscles worked: _____

Stretched? Yes ___ No ___

Name of exercise 10: _____ Weight: ___ Reps: ___
- Set 1: ___
- Set 2: ___
- Set 3: ___
- Set 4: ___

Muscles worked: _____

Stretched? Yes ___ No ___

Cardiovascular Training

Warmed up: Yes ___ No ___

Time of day: _____

	For how long?	Heart Rate
Type 1:		
Type 2:		
Type 3:		
Type 4:		

Stretched? Yes ___ No ___

Evening Reflection

Did I put my faith in Action today?	Yes ___	No ___
I prayed for somone today	Yes ___	No ___
I read my Bible today	Yes ___	No ___
I helped someone in need today	Yes ___	No ___
I got 6 1/2 to 8 hours of sleep last night	Yes ___	No ___
I know I ate right today	Yes ___	No ___
I ate breakfast today	Yes ___	No ___
I ate starches after 4:00 p.m. today	Yes ___	No ___
I ate at least 4 meals today	Yes ___	No ___
I drank at least a gallon of water today	Yes ___	No ___
I had Courage to Change today	Yes ___	No ___

Tonight I forgive… _____

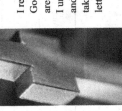

Captain's Log Statement of Faith

I realize that my actions don't earn my way into God's love or earn my way to heaven but that they are a reflection of my love affair with Jesus! I understand that by taking care of myself I honor and glorify God. I matter to God and the actions I take toward good health are daily written love letters telling God, "Thank you for my life"!

Signature _____

"I press on toward the goal to win the prize for which God has called me heavenward in Christ Jesus."
Philippians 3:14

Captain's Log

"Each one should test his own actions. Then he can take pride in himself without comparing himself to somebody else, for each one should carry his own load." (Galatians 6:40)

Day: _____   Date: ____ / ____ / ____

Nutrition Log

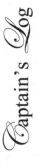

BREAKFAST	Time: _____				Time: _____			
	Type	Amt:	Type	Amt:	SNACK 1	Type	Amt:	Type	Amt:

BREAKFAST — Time: _____

	Type	Amt:	Type	Amt:
Protein	1. ___	___	2. ___	___
Complex Carbs	1. ___	___	2. ___	___
Fruit	1. ___	___	2. ___	___
Vegetables	1. ___	___	2. ___	___
Fat	1. ___	___	2. ___	___
Liquid/drink	1. ___	___	2. ___	___
Meal Replace.	1. ___	___	2. ___	___
Condiments	1. ___	___	2. ___	___
Other	1. ___	___	2. ___	___

SNACK 1 — Time: _____

	Type	Amt:	Type	Amt:
Protein	1. ___	___	2. ___	___
Complex Carbs	1. ___	___	2. ___	___
Fruit	1. ___	___	2. ___	___
Vegetables	1. ___	___	2. ___	___
Fat	1. ___	___	2. ___	___
Liquid/drink	1. ___	___	2. ___	___
Meal Replace.	1. ___	___	2. ___	___
Condiments	1. ___	___	2. ___	___
Other	1. ___	___	2. ___	___

LUNCH — Time: _____

	Type	Amt:	Type	Amt:
Protein	1. ___	___	2. ___	___
Complex Carbs	1. ___	___	2. ___	___
Fruit	1. ___	___	2. ___	___
Vegetables	1. ___	___	2. ___	___
Fat	1. ___	___	2. ___	___
Liquid/drink	1. ___	___	2. ___	___
Meal Replace.	1. ___	___	2. ___	___
Condiments	1. ___	___	2. ___	___
Other	1. ___	___	2. ___	___

SNACK 2 — Time: _____

	Type	Amt:	Type	Amt:
Protein	1. ___	___	2. ___	___
Complex Carbs	1. ___	___	2. ___	___
Fruit	1. ___	___	2. ___	___
Vegetables	1. ___	___	2. ___	___
Fat	1. ___	___	2. ___	___
Liquid/drink	1. ___	___	2. ___	___
Meal Replace.	1. ___	___	2. ___	___
Condiments	1. ___	___	2. ___	___
Other	1. ___	___	2. ___	___

SNACK 3 — Time: _____

	Type	Amt:	Type	Amt:
Protein	1. ___	___	2. ___	___
Complex Carbs	1. ___	___	2. ___	___
Fruit	1. ___	___	2. ___	___
Vegetables	1. ___	___	2. ___	___
Fat	1. ___	___	2. ___	___
Liquid/drink	1. ___	___	2. ___	___
Meal Replace.	1. ___	___	2. ___	___
Condiments	1. ___	___	2. ___	___
Other	1. ___	___	2. ___	___

DINNER — Time: _____

	Type	Amt:	Type	Amt:
Protein	1. ___	___	2. ___	___
Complex Carbs	1. ___	___	2. ___	___
Fruit	1. ___	___	2. ___	___
Vegetables	1. ___	___	2. ___	___
Fat	1. ___	___	2. ___	___
Liquid/drink	1. ___	___	2. ___	___
Meal Replace.	1. ___	___	2. ___	___
Condiments	1. ___	___	2. ___	___
Other	1. ___	___	2. ___	___

Cardiovascular Training

Time of day: _____
Warmed up   Yes _____   No _____

	For how long?	Heart Rate
Type 1:		
Type 2:		
Type 3:		
Type 4:		
Stretched?	Yes _____	No _____

Evening Reflection

Did I put my faith in Action today?	Yes _____	No _____
I prayed for somone today	Yes _____	No _____
I read my Bible today	Yes _____	No _____
I helped someone in need today	Yes _____	No _____
I got 6 1/2 to 8 hours of sleep last night	Yes _____	No _____
I know I ate right today	Yes _____	No _____
I ate breakfast today	Yes _____	No _____
I ate starches after 4:00 p.m. today	Yes _____	No _____
I ate at least 4 meals today	Yes _____	No _____
I drank at least a gallon of water today	Yes _____	No _____
I had Courage to Change today	Yes _____	No _____
Tonight I forgive…		

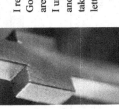

Captain's Log Statement of Faith

I realize that my actions don't earn my way into God's love or earn my way to heaven but that they are a reflection of my love affair with Jesus! I understand that by taking care of myself I honor and glorify God. I matter to God and the actions I take toward good health are daily written love letters telling God, "Thank you for my life"!

_____
Signature

Resistance Training

Time of day: _____
Warmed up   Yes _____   No _____

Name of exercise 1:

	Weight:	Reps:
Set 1:		
Set 2:		
Set 3:		
Set 4:		

Muscles worked: _____

Stretched?   Yes _____   No _____

Name of exercise 2:

	Weight:	Reps:
Set 1:		
Set 2:		
Set 3:		
Set 4:		

Muscles worked: _____

Stretched?   Yes _____   No _____

Name of exercise 3:

	Weight:	Reps:
Set 1:		
Set 2:		
Set 3:		
Set 4:		

Muscles worked: _____

Stretched?   Yes _____   No _____

Name of exercise 4:

	Weight:	Reps:
Set 1:		
Set 2:		
Set 3:		
Set 4:		

Muscles worked: _____

Stretched?   Yes _____   No _____

Name of exercise 5:

	Weight:	Reps:
Set 1:		
Set 2:		
Set 3:		
Set 4:		

Muscles worked: _____

Stretched?   Yes _____   No _____

Name of exercise 6:

	Weight:	Reps:
Set 1:		
Set 2:		
Set 3:		
Set 4:		

Muscles worked: _____

Stretched?   Yes _____   No _____

Name of exercise 7:

	Weight:	Reps:
Set 1:		
Set 2:		
Set 3:		
Set 4:		

Muscles worked: _____

Stretched?   Yes _____   No _____

Name of exercise 8:

	Weight:	Reps:
Set 1:		
Set 2:		
Set 3:		
Set 4:		

Muscles worked: _____

Stretched?   Yes _____   No _____

Name of exercise 9:

	Weight:	Reps:
Set 1:		
Set 2:		
Set 3:		
Set 4:		

Muscles worked: _____

Stretched?   Yes _____   No _____

Name of exercise 10:

	Weight:	Reps:
Set 1:		
Set 2:		
Set 3:		
Set 4:		

Muscles worked: _____

Stretched?   Yes _____   No _____

"I press on toward the goal to win the prize for which God has called me heavenward in Christ Jesus."
Philippians 3:14

Captain's Log

"Each one should test his own actions. Then he can take pride in himself without comparing himself to somebody else, for each one should carry his own load." (Galatians 6:40)

Day: _____   Date: _____ / _____ / _____

Nutrition Log

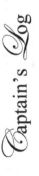

BREAKFAST   Time: _____

	Type	Amt:	Type	Amt:
Protein	1.		2.	
Complex Carbs	1.		2.	
Fruit	1.		2.	
Vegetables	1.		2.	
Fat	1.		2.	
Liquid/drink	1.		2.	
Meal Replace.	1.		2.	
Condiments	1.		2.	
Other	1.		2.	

LUNCH   Time: _____

	Type	Amt:	Type	Amt:
Protein	1.		2.	
Complex Carbs	1.		2.	
Fruit	1.		2.	
Vegetables	1.		2.	
Fat	1.		2.	
Liquid/drink	1.		2.	
Meal Replace.	1.		2.	
Condiments	1.		2.	
Other	1.		2.	

SNACK 3   Time: _____

	Type	Amt:	Type	Amt:
Protein	1.		2.	
Complex Carbs	1.		2.	
Fruit	1.		2.	
Vegetables	1.		2.	
Fat	1.		2.	
Liquid/drink	1.		2.	
Meal Replace.	1.		2.	
Condiments	1.		2.	
Other	1.		2.	

SNACK 1   Time: _____

	Type	Amt:	Type	Amt:
Protein	1.		2.	
Complex Carbs	1.		2.	
Fruit	1.		2.	
Vegetables	1.		2.	
Fat	1.		2.	
Liquid/drink	1.		2.	
Meal Replace.	1.		2.	
Condiments	1.		2.	
Other	1.		2.	

SNACK 2   Time: _____

	Type	Amt:	Type	Amt:
Protein	1.		2.	
Complex Carbs	1.		2.	
Fruit	1.		2.	
Vegetables	1.		2.	
Fat	1.		2.	
Liquid/drink	1.		2.	
Meal Replace.	1.		2.	
Condiments	1.		2.	
Other	1.		2.	

DINNER   Time: _____

	Type	Amt:	Type	Amt:
Protein	1.		2.	
Complex Carbs	1.		2.	
Fruit	1.		2.	
Vegetables	1.		2.	
Fat	1.		2.	
Liquid/drink	1.		2.	
Meal Replace.	1.		2.	
Condiments	1.		2.	
Other	1.		2.	

Resistance Training

Time of day: _____

Warmed up   Yes _____   No _____

Name of exercise 1: _____

	Weight:	Reps:
Set 1:		
Set 2:		
Set 3:		
Set 4:		

Muscles worked: _____

Stretched?   Yes _____   No _____

Name of exercise 3: _____

	Weight:	Reps:
Set 1:		
Set 2:		
Set 3:		
Set 4:		

Muscles worked: _____

Stretched?   Yes _____   No _____

Name of exercise 5: _____

	Weight:	Reps:
Set 1:		
Set 2:		
Set 3:		
Set 4:		

Muscles worked: _____

Stretched?   Yes _____   No _____

Name of exercise 7: _____

	Weight:	Reps:
Set 1:		
Set 2:		
Set 3:		
Set 4:		

Muscles worked: _____

Stretched?   Yes _____   No _____

Name of exercise 9: _____

	Weight:	Reps:
Set 1:		
Set 2:		
Set 3:		
Set 4:		

Muscles worked: _____

Stretched?   Yes _____   No _____

Name of exercise 2: _____

	Weight:	Reps:
Set 1:		
Set 2:		
Set 3:		
Set 4:		

Muscles worked: _____

Stretched?   Yes _____   No _____

Name of exercise 4: _____

	Weight:	Reps:
Set 1:		
Set 2:		
Set 3:		
Set 4:		

Muscles worked: _____

Stretched?   Yes _____   No _____

Name of exercise 6: _____

	Weight:	Reps:
Set 1:		
Set 2:		
Set 3:		
Set 4:		

Muscles worked: _____

Stretched?   Yes _____   No _____

Name of exercise 8: _____

	Weight:	Reps:
Set 1:		
Set 2:		
Set 3:		
Set 4:		

Muscles worked: _____

Stretched?   Yes _____   No _____

Name of exercise 10: _____

	Weight:	Reps:
Set 1:		
Set 2:		
Set 3:		
Set 4:		

Muscles worked: _____

Stretched?   Yes _____   No _____

Cardiovascular Training

Warmed up   Yes _____   No _____

Time of day: _____	For how long?	Heart Rate
Type 1:		
Type 2:		
Type 3:		
Type 4:		

Stretched?   Yes _____   No _____

Evening Reflection

Did I put my faith in Action today?	Yes _____	No _____
I prayed for somone today	Yes _____	No _____
I read my Bible today	Yes _____	No _____
I helped someone in need today	Yes _____	No _____
I got 6 1/2 to 8 hours of sleep last night	Yes _____	No _____
I know I ate right today	Yes _____	No _____
I ate breakfast today	Yes _____	No _____
I ate starches after 4:00 p.m. today	Yes _____	No _____
I ate at least 4 meals today	Yes _____	No _____
I drank at least a gallon of water today	Yes _____	No _____
I had Courage to Change today	Yes _____	No _____
Tonight I forgive…		

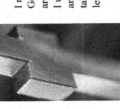

Captain's Log Statement of Faith

I realize that my actions don't earn my way into God's love or earn my way to heaven but that they are a reflection of my love affair with Jesus! I understand that by taking care of myself I honor and glorify God. I matter to God and the actions I take toward good health are daily written love letters telling God, "Thank you for my life"!

_____
Signature

"I press on toward the goal to win the prize for which God has called me heavenward in Christ Jesus."
Philippians 3:14

BUILDING RELATIONSHIPS

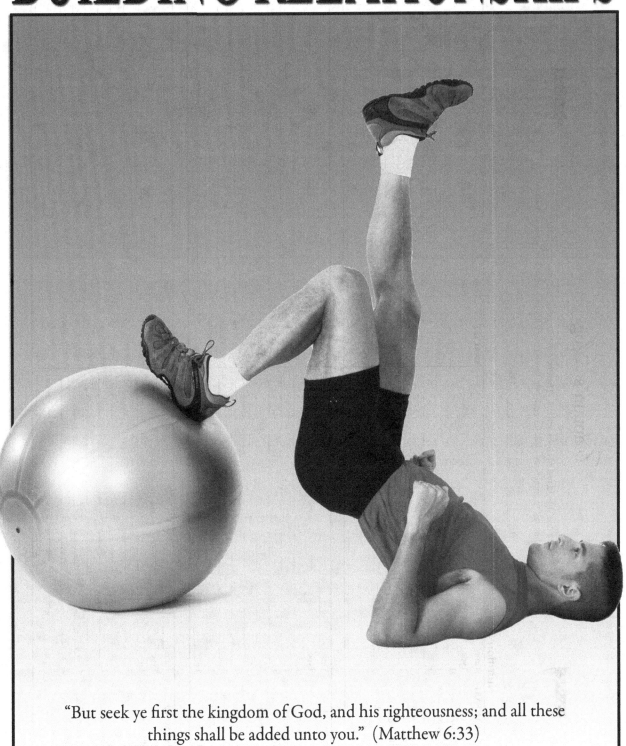

"But seek ye first the kingdom of God, and his righteousness; and all these things shall be added unto you." (Matthew 6:33)

WEEK TEN

Captain's Log

"Each one should test his own actions. Then he can take pride in himself without comparing himself to somebody else, for each one should carry his own load." (Galatians 6:40)

Day: _____ Date: _____ / _____ / _____

Nutrition Log

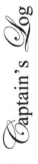

BREAKFAST	Time: _____				SNACK 1	Time: _____			
	Type	Amt:	Type	Amt:		Type	Amt:	Type	Amt:
Protein	1. _____	_____	2. _____	_____	Protein	1. _____	_____	2. _____	_____
Complex Carbs	1. _____	_____	2. _____	_____	Complex Carbs	1. _____	_____	2. _____	_____
Fruit	1. _____	_____	2. _____	_____	Fruit	1. _____	_____	2. _____	_____
Vegetables	1. _____	_____	2. _____	_____	Vegetables	1. _____	_____	2. _____	_____
Fat	1. _____	_____	2. _____	_____	Fat	1. _____	_____	2. _____	_____
Liquid/drink	1. _____	_____	2. _____	_____	Liquid/drink	1. _____	_____	2. _____	_____
Meal Replace.	1. _____	_____	2. _____	_____	Meal Replace.	1. _____	_____	2. _____	_____
Condiments	1. _____	_____	2. _____	_____	Condiments	1. _____	_____	2. _____	_____
Other	1. _____	_____	2. _____	_____	Other	1. _____	_____	2. _____	_____

LUNCH	Time: _____				SNACK 2	Time: _____			
	Type	Amt:	Type	Amt:		Type	Amt:	Type	Amt:
Protein	1. _____	_____	2. _____	_____	Protein	1. _____	_____	2. _____	_____
Complex Carbs	1. _____	_____	2. _____	_____	Complex Carbs	1. _____	_____	2. _____	_____
Fruit	1. _____	_____	2. _____	_____	Fruit	1. _____	_____	2. _____	_____
Vegetables	1. _____	_____	2. _____	_____	Vegetables	1. _____	_____	2. _____	_____
Fat	1. _____	_____	2. _____	_____	Fat	1. _____	_____	2. _____	_____
Liquid/drink	1. _____	_____	2. _____	_____	Liquid/drink	1. _____	_____	2. _____	_____
Meal Replace.	1. _____	_____	2. _____	_____	Meal Replace.	1. _____	_____	2. _____	_____
Condiments	1. _____	_____	2. _____	_____	Condiments	1. _____	_____	2. _____	_____
Other	1. _____	_____	2. _____	_____	Other	1. _____	_____	2. _____	_____

SNACK 3	Time: _____				DINNER	Time: _____			
	Type	Amt:	Type	Amt:		Type	Amt:	Type	Amt:
Protein	1. _____	_____	2. _____	_____	Protein	1. _____	_____	2. _____	_____
Complex Carbs	1. _____	_____	2. _____	_____	Complex Carbs	1. _____	_____	2. _____	_____
Fruit	1. _____	_____	2. _____	_____	Fruit	1. _____	_____	2. _____	_____
Vegetables	1. _____	_____	2. _____	_____	Vegetables	1. _____	_____	2. _____	_____
Fat	1. _____	_____	2. _____	_____	Fat	1. _____	_____	2. _____	_____
Liquid/drink	1. _____	_____	2. _____	_____	Liquid/drink	1. _____	_____	2. _____	_____
Meal Replace.	1. _____	_____	2. _____	_____	Meal Replace.	1. _____	_____	2. _____	_____
Condiments	1. _____	_____	2. _____	_____	Condiments	1. _____	_____	2. _____	_____
Other	1. _____	_____	2. _____	_____	Other	1. _____	_____	2. _____	_____

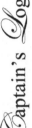

Cardiovascular Training

Warmed up   Yes _____   No _____

Time of day: _____	For how long?	Heart Rate
Type 1:	_____	_____
Type 2:	_____	_____
Type 3:	_____	_____
Type 4:	_____	_____
Stretched? Yes _____ No _____		

Evening Reflection

Did I put my faith in Action today?	Yes _____	No _____
I prayed for somone today	Yes _____	No _____
I read my Bible today	Yes _____	No _____
I helped someone in need today	Yes _____	No _____
I got 6 1/2 to 8 hours of sleep last night	Yes _____	No _____
I know I ate right today	Yes _____	No _____
I ate breakfast today	Yes _____	No _____
I ate starches after 4:00 p.m. today	Yes _____	No _____
I ate at least 4 meals today	Yes _____	No _____
I drank at least a gallon of water today	Yes _____	No _____
I had Courage to Change today	Yes _____	No _____
Tonight I forgive….		

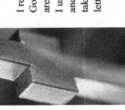

Captain's Log Statement of Faith

I realize that my actions don't earn my way into God's love or earn my way to heaven but that they are a reflection of my love affair with Jesus! I understand that by taking care of myself I honor and glorify God. I matter to God and the actions I take toward good health are daily written love letters telling God, "Thank you for my life"!

_____   **Signature**

Resistance Training

Time of day: _____

Warmed up   Yes _____   No _____

Name of exercise 1:	Weight:	Reps:
	Set 1: _____	
	Set 2: _____	
Muscles worked:	Set 3: _____	
	Set 4: _____	
Stretched? Yes _____	No _____	

Name of exercise 2:	Weight:	Reps:
	Set 1: _____	
	Set 2: _____	
Muscles worked:	Set 3: _____	
	Set 4: _____	
Stretched? Yes _____	No _____	

Name of exercise 3:	Weight:	Reps:
	Set 1: _____	
	Set 2: _____	
Muscles worked:	Set 3: _____	
	Set 4: _____	
Stretched? Yes _____	No _____	

Name of exercise 4:	Weight:	Reps:
	Set 1: _____	
	Set 2: _____	
Muscles worked:	Set 3: _____	
	Set 4: _____	
Stretched? Yes _____	No _____	

Name of exercise 5:	Weight:	Reps:
	Set 1: _____	
	Set 2: _____	
Muscles worked:	Set 3: _____	
	Set 4: _____	
Stretched? Yes _____	No _____	

Name of exercise 6:	Weight:	Reps:
	Set 1: _____	
	Set 2: _____	
Muscles worked:	Set 3: _____	
	Set 4: _____	
Stretched? Yes _____	No _____	

Name of exercise 7:	Weight:	Reps:
	Set 1: _____	
	Set 2: _____	
Muscles worked:	Set 3: _____	
	Set 4: _____	
Stretched? Yes _____	No _____	

Name of exercise 8:	Weight:	Reps:
	Set 1: _____	
	Set 2: _____	
Muscles worked:	Set 3: _____	
	Set 4: _____	
Stretched? Yes _____	No _____	

Name of exercise 9:	Weight:	Reps:
	Set 1: _____	
	Set 2: _____	
Muscles worked:	Set 3: _____	
	Set 4: _____	
Stretched? Yes _____	No _____	

Name of exercise 10:	Weight:	Reps:
	Set 1: _____	
	Set 2: _____	
Muscles worked:	Set 3: _____	
	Set 4: _____	
Stretched? Yes _____	No _____	

"I press on toward the goal to win the prize for which God has called me heavenward in Christ Jesus."
Philippians 3:14

Captain's Log

Day: _____ Date: _____ / _____ / _____

Nutrition Log

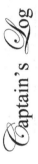

BREAKFAST Time: _____

	Type	Amt:	Type	Amt:
Protein	1.		2.	
Complex Carbs	1.		2.	
Fruit	1.		2.	
Vegetables	1.		2.	
Fat	1.		2.	
Liquid/drink	1.		2.	
Meal Replace.	1.		2.	
Condiments	1.		2.	
Other	1.		2.	

LUNCH Time: _____

	Type	Amt:	Type	Amt:
Protein	1.		2.	
Complex Carbs	1.		2.	
Fruit	1.		2.	
Vegetables	1.		2.	
Fat	1.		2.	
Liquid/drink	1.		2.	
Meal Replace.	1.		2.	
Condiments	1.		2.	
Other	1.		2.	

SNACK 3 Time: _____

	Type	Amt:	Type	Amt:
Protein	1.		2.	
Complex Carbs	1.		2.	
Fruit	1.		2.	
Vegetables	1.		2.	
Fat	1.		2.	
Liquid/drink	1.		2.	
Meal Replace.	1.		2.	
Condiments	1.		2.	
Other	1.		2.	

SNACK 1 Time: _____

	Type	Amt:	Type	Amt:
Protein	1.		2.	
Complex Carbs	1.		2.	
Fruit	1.		2.	
Vegetables	1.		2.	
Fat	1.		2.	
Liquid/drink	1.		2.	
Meal Replace.	1.		2.	
Condiments	1.		2.	
Other	1.		2.	

SNACK 2 Time: _____

	Type	Amt:	Type	Amt:
Protein	1.		2.	
Complex Carbs	1.		2.	
Fruit	1.		2.	
Vegetables	1.		2.	
Fat	1.		2.	
Liquid/drink	1.		2.	
Meal Replace.	1.		2.	
Condiments	1.		2.	
Other	1.		2.	

DINNER Time: _____

	Type	Amt:	Type	Amt:
Protein	1.		2.	
Complex Carbs	1.		2.	
Fruit	1.		2.	
Vegetables	1.		2.	
Fat	1.		2.	
Liquid/drink	1.		2.	
Meal Replace.	1.		2.	
Condiments	1.		2.	
Other	1.		2.	

Cardiovascular Training

Warmed up   Yes _____   No _____

Time of day: _____	For how long?	Heart Rate
Type 1:	_____	_____
Type 2:	_____	_____
Type 3:	_____	_____
Type 4:	_____	_____

Stretched?   Yes _____   No _____

Evening Reflection

Did I put my faith in Action today?	Yes _____	No _____
I prayed for somone today	Yes _____	No _____
I read my Bible today	Yes _____	No _____
I helped someone in need today	Yes _____	No _____
I got 6 1/2 to 8 hours of sleep last night	Yes _____	No _____
I know I ate right today	Yes _____	No _____
I ate breakfast today	Yes _____	No _____
I ate starches after 4:00 p.m. today	Yes _____	No _____
I ate at least 4 meals today	Yes _____	No _____
I drank at least a gallon of water today	Yes _____	No _____
I had Courage to Change today	Yes _____	No _____
Tonight I forgive... _____		

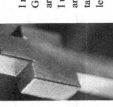

Captain's Log Statement of Faith

I realize that my actions don't earn my way into God's love or earn my way to heaven but that they are a reflection of my love affair with Jesus! I understand that by taking care of myself I honor and glorify God. I matter to God and the actions I take toward good health are daily written love letters telling God, "Thank you for my life"!

_____
Signature

Resistance Training

Time of day: _____

Warmed up   Yes _____   No _____

Name of exercise 1:
_____

	Weight:	Reps:
Set 1:	_____	_____
Set 2:	_____	_____
Set 3:	_____	_____
Set 4:	_____	_____

Muscles worked:
_____

Stretched?   Yes _____   No _____

Name of exercise 2:
_____

	Weight:	Reps:
Set 1:	_____	_____
Set 2:	_____	_____
Set 3:	_____	_____
Set 4:	_____	_____

Muscles worked:
_____

Stretched?   Yes _____   No _____

Name of exercise 3:
_____

	Weight:	Reps:
Set 1:	_____	_____
Set 2:	_____	_____
Set 3:	_____	_____
Set 4:	_____	_____

Muscles worked:
_____

Stretched?   Yes _____   No _____

Name of exercise 4:
_____

	Weight:	Reps:
Set 1:	_____	_____
Set 2:	_____	_____
Set 3:	_____	_____
Set 4:	_____	_____

Muscles worked:
_____

Stretched?   Yes _____   No _____

Name of exercise 5:
_____

	Weight:	Reps:
Set 1:	_____	_____
Set 2:	_____	_____
Set 3:	_____	_____
Set 4:	_____	_____

Muscles worked:
_____

Stretched?   Yes _____   No _____

Name of exercise 6:
_____

	Weight:	Reps:
Set 1:	_____	_____
Set 2:	_____	_____
Set 3:	_____	_____
Set 4:	_____	_____

Muscles worked:
_____

Stretched?   Yes _____   No _____

Name of exercise 7:
_____

	Weight:	Reps:
Set 1:	_____	_____
Set 2:	_____	_____
Set 3:	_____	_____
Set 4:	_____	_____

Muscles worked:
_____

Stretched?   Yes _____   No _____

Name of exercise 8:
_____

	Weight:	Reps:
Set 1:	_____	_____
Set 2:	_____	_____
Set 3:	_____	_____
Set 4:	_____	_____

Muscles worked:
_____

Stretched?   Yes _____   No _____

Name of exercise 9:
_____

	Weight:	Reps:
Set 1:	_____	_____
Set 2:	_____	_____
Set 3:	_____	_____
Set 4:	_____	_____

Muscles worked:
_____

Stretched?   Yes _____   No _____

Name of exercise 10:
_____

	Weight:	Reps:
Set 1:	_____	_____
Set 2:	_____	_____
Set 3:	_____	_____
Set 4:	_____	_____

Muscles worked:
_____

Stretched?   Yes _____   No _____

"I press on toward the goal to win the prize for which God has called me heavenward in Christ Jesus."
Philippians 3:14

Captain's Log

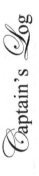

"Each one should test his own actions. Then he can take pride in himself without comparing himself to somebody else, for each one should carry his own load." (Galatians 6:40)

Day: _____   Date: _____ / _____ / _____

Nutrition Log

BREAKFAST   Time: _____

	Type	Amt:	Type	Amt:
Protein	1.		2.	
Complex Carbs	1.		2.	
Fruit	1.		2.	
Vegetables	1.		2.	
Fat	1.		2.	
Liquid/drink	1.		2.	
Meal Replace.	1.		2.	
Condiments	1.		2.	
Other	1.		2.	

SNACK 1   Time: _____

	Type	Amt:	Type	Amt:
Protein	1.		2.	
Complex Carbs	1.		2.	
Fruit	1.		2.	
Vegetables	1.		2.	
Fat	1.		2.	
Liquid/drink	1.		2.	
Meal Replace.	1.		2.	
Condiments	1.		2.	
Other	1.		2.	

LUNCH   Time: _____

	Type	Amt:	Type	Amt:
Protein	1.		2.	
Complex Carbs	1.		2.	
Fruit	1.		2.	
Vegetables	1.		2.	
Fat	1.		2.	
Liquid/drink	1.		2.	
Meal Replace.	1.		2.	
Condiments	1.		2.	
Other	1.		2.	

SNACK 2   Time: _____

	Type	Amt:	Type	Amt:
Protein	1.		2.	
Complex Carbs	1.		2.	
Fruit	1.		2.	
Vegetables	1.		2.	
Fat	1.		2.	
Liquid/drink	1.		2.	
Meal Replace.	1.		2.	
Condiments	1.		2.	
Other	1.		2.	

SNACK 3   Time: _____

	Type	Amt:	Type	Amt:
Protein	1.		2.	
Complex Carbs	1.		2.	
Fruit	1.		2.	
Vegetables	1.		2.	
Fat	1.		2.	
Liquid/drink	1.		2.	
Meal Replace.	1.		2.	
Condiments	1.		2.	
Other	1.		2.	

DINNER   Time: _____

	Type	Amt:	Type	Amt:
Protein	1.		2.	
Complex Carbs	1.		2.	
Fruit	1.		2.	
Vegetables	1.		2.	
Fat	1.		2.	
Liquid/drink	1.		2.	
Meal Replace.	1.		2.	
Condiments	1.		2.	
Other	1.		2.	

Cardiovascular Training

Warmed up   Yes _____   No _____

Time of day: _____	For how long?	Heart Rate
Type 1: _____	_____	_____
Type 2: _____	_____	_____
Type 3: _____	_____	_____
Type 4: _____	_____	_____
Stretched? Yes _____ No _____		

Evening Reflection

Did I put my faith in Action today?	Yes _____	No _____
I prayed for somone today	Yes _____	No _____
I read my Bible today	Yes _____	No _____
I helped someone in need today	Yes _____	No _____
I got 6 1/2 to 8 hours of sleep last night	Yes _____	No _____
I know I ate right today	Yes _____	No _____
I ate breakfast today	Yes _____	No _____
I ate starches after 4:00 p.m. today	Yes _____	No _____
I ate at least 4 meals today	Yes _____	No _____
I drank at least a gallon of water today	Yes _____	No _____
I had Courage to Change today	Yes _____	No _____
Tonight I forgive…		

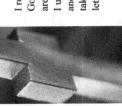

Captain's Log Statement of Faith

I realize that my actions don't earn my way into God's love or earn my way to heaven but that they are a reflection of my love affair with Jesus! I understand that by taking care of myself I honor and glorify God. I matter to God and the actions I take toward good health are daily written love letters telling God, "Thank you for my life"!

_____   **Signature**

Resistance Training

Time of day: _____

Warmed up   Yes _____   No _____

Name of exercise 1:
_____
	Weight:	Reps:
Set 1:	_____	_____
Set 2:	_____	_____
Set 3:	_____	_____
Set 4:	_____	_____

Muscles worked:
_____

Stretched?   Yes _____   No _____

Name of exercise 2:
_____
	Weight:	Reps:
Set 1:	_____	_____
Set 2:	_____	_____
Set 3:	_____	_____
Set 4:	_____	_____

Muscles worked:
_____

Stretched?   Yes _____   No _____

Name of exercise 3:
_____
	Weight:	Reps:
Set 1:	_____	_____
Set 2:	_____	_____
Set 3:	_____	_____
Set 4:	_____	_____

Muscles worked:
_____

Stretched?   Yes _____   No _____

Name of exercise 4:
_____
	Weight:	Reps:
Set 1:	_____	_____
Set 2:	_____	_____
Set 3:	_____	_____
Set 4:	_____	_____

Muscles worked:
_____

Stretched?   Yes _____   No _____

Name of exercise 5:
_____
	Weight:	Reps:
Set 1:	_____	_____
Set 2:	_____	_____
Set 3:	_____	_____
Set 4:	_____	_____

Muscles worked:
_____

Stretched?   Yes _____   No _____

Name of exercise 6:
_____
	Weight:	Reps:
Set 1:	_____	_____
Set 2:	_____	_____
Set 3:	_____	_____
Set 4:	_____	_____

Muscles worked:
_____

Stretched?   Yes _____   No _____

Name of exercise 7:
_____
	Weight:	Reps:
Set 1:	_____	_____
Set 2:	_____	_____
Set 3:	_____	_____
Set 4:	_____	_____

Muscles worked:
_____

Stretched?   Yes _____   No _____

Name of exercise 8:
_____
	Weight:	Reps:
Set 1:	_____	_____
Set 2:	_____	_____
Set 3:	_____	_____
Set 4:	_____	_____

Muscles worked:
_____

Stretched?   Yes _____   No _____

Name of exercise 9:
_____
	Weight:	Reps:
Set 1:	_____	_____
Set 2:	_____	_____
Set 3:	_____	_____
Set 4:	_____	_____

Muscles worked:
_____

Stretched?   Yes _____   No _____

Name of exercise 10:
_____
	Weight:	Reps:
Set 1:	_____	_____
Set 2:	_____	_____
Set 3:	_____	_____
Set 4:	_____	_____

Muscles worked:
_____

Stretched?   Yes _____   No _____

"I press on toward the goal to win the prize for which God has called me heavenward in Christ Jesus."
Philippians 3:14

Captain's Log

"Each one should test his own actions. Then he can take pride in himself without comparing himself to somebody else, for each one should carry his own load." (Galatians 6:40)

Day: _____ Date: _____ / _____ / _____

Nutrition Log

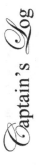
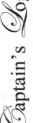

BREAKFAST   Time: _____

	Type	Amt:		Type	Amt:
Protein	1.			2.	
Complex Carbs	1.			2.	
Fruit	1.			2.	
Vegetables	1.			2.	
Fat	1.			2.	
Liquid/drink	1.			2.	
Meal Replace.	1.			2.	
Condiments	1.			2.	
Other	1.			2.	

SNACK 1   Time: _____

	Type	Amt:		Type	Amt:
Protein	1.			2.	
Complex Carbs	1.			2.	
Fruit	1.			2.	
Vegetables	1.			2.	
Fat	1.			2.	
Liquid/drink	1.			2.	
Meal Replace.	1.			2.	
Condiments	1.			2.	
Other	1.			2.	

LUNCH   Time: _____

	Type	Amt:		Type	Amt:
Protein	1.			2.	
Complex Carbs	1.			2.	
Fruit	1.			2.	
Vegetables	1.			2.	
Fat	1.			2.	
Liquid/drink	1.			2.	
Meal Replace.	1.			2.	
Condiments	1.			2.	
Other	1.			2.	

SNACK 2   Time: _____

	Type	Amt:		Type	Amt:
Protein	1.			2.	
Complex Carbs	1.			2.	
Fruit	1.			2.	
Vegetables	1.			2.	
Fat	1.			2.	
Liquid/drink	1.			2.	
Meal Replace.	1.			2.	
Condiments	1.			2.	
Other	1.			2.	

SNACK 3   Time: _____

	Type	Amt:		Type	Amt:
Protein	1.			2.	
Complex Carbs	1.			2.	
Fruit	1.			2.	
Vegetables	1.			2.	
Fat	1.			2.	
Liquid/drink	1.			2.	
Meal Replace.	1.			2.	
Condiments	1.			2.	
Other	1.			2.	

DINNER   Time: _____

	Type	Amt:		Type	Amt:
Protein	1.			2.	
Complex Carbs	1.			2.	
Fruit	1.			2.	
Vegetables	1.			2.	
Fat	1.			2.	
Liquid/drink	1.			2.	
Meal Replace.	1.			2.	
Condiments	1.			2.	
Other	1.			2.	

Resistance Training

Time of day: _____

Warmed up   Yes _____   No _____

Name of exercise 1: _____   Weight: _____   Reps: _____
Set 1: _____
Set 2: _____
Muscles worked: _____   Set 3: _____
Set 4: _____
Stretched?   Yes _____   No _____

Name of exercise 3: _____   Weight: _____   Reps: _____
Set 1: _____
Set 2: _____
Muscles worked: _____   Set 3: _____
Set 4: _____
Stretched?   Yes _____   No _____

Name of exercise 5: _____   Weight: _____   Reps: _____
Set 1: _____
Set 2: _____
Muscles worked: _____   Set 3: _____
Set 4: _____
Stretched?   Yes _____   No _____

Name of exercise 7: _____   Weight: _____   Reps: _____
Set 1: _____
Set 2: _____
Muscles worked: _____   Set 3: _____
Set 4: _____
Stretched?   Yes _____   No _____

Name of exercise 9: _____   Weight: _____   Reps: _____
Set 1: _____
Set 2: _____
Muscles worked: _____   Set 3: _____
Set 4: _____
Stretched?   Yes _____   No _____

Cardiovascular Training

Warmed up   Yes _____   No _____

Time of day: _____   For how long?   Heart Rate
Type 1: _____
Type 2: _____
Type 3: _____
Type 4: _____
Stretched?   Yes _____   No _____

Name of exercise 2: _____   Weight: _____   Reps: _____
Set 1: _____
Set 2: _____
Muscles worked: _____   Set 3: _____
Set 4: _____
Stretched?   Yes _____   No _____

Name of exercise 4: _____   Weight: _____   Reps: _____
Set 1: _____
Set 2: _____
Muscles worked: _____   Set 3: _____
Set 4: _____
Stretched?   Yes _____   No _____

Name of exercise 6: _____   Weight: _____   Reps: _____
Set 1: _____
Set 2: _____
Muscles worked: _____   Set 3: _____
Set 4: _____
Stretched?   Yes _____   No _____

Name of exercise 8: _____   Weight: _____   Reps: _____
Set 1: _____
Set 2: _____
Muscles worked: _____   Set 3: _____
Set 4: _____
Stretched?   Yes _____   No _____

Name of exercise 10: _____   Weight: _____   Reps: _____
Set 1: _____
Set 2: _____
Muscles worked: _____   Set 3: _____
Set 4: _____
Stretched?   Yes _____   No _____

Evening Reflection

Did I put my faith in Action today?   Yes _____   No _____
I prayed for somone today   Yes _____   No _____
I read my Bible today   Yes _____   No _____
I helped someone in need today   Yes _____   No _____
I got 6 1/2 to 8 hours of sleep last night   Yes _____   No _____
I know I ate right today   Yes _____   No _____
I ate breakfast today   Yes _____   No _____
I ate starches after 4:00 p.m. today   Yes _____   No _____
I ate at least 4 meals today   Yes _____   No _____
I drank at least a gallon of water today   Yes _____   No _____
I had Courage to Change today   Yes _____   No _____
Tonight I forgive...

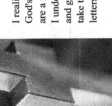

Captain's Log Statement of Faith

I realize that my actions don't earn my way into God's love or earn my way to heaven but that they are a reflection of my love affair with Jesus! I understand that by taking care of myself I honor and glorify God. I matter to God and the actions I take toward good health are daily written love letters telling God, "Thank you for my life"!

_____   **Signature**

"I press on toward the goal to win the prize for which God has called me heavenward in Christ Jesus."
Philippians 3:14

Captain's Log

"Each one should test his own actions. Then he can take pride in himself without comparing himself to somebody else, for each one should carry his own load." (Galatians 6:40)

Day: _____   Date: _____ / _____ / _____

Nutrition Log

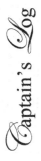
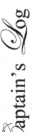

BREAKFAST	Time: _____				Type	Amt:
	Type	Amt:				
Protein	1.		2.			
Complex Carbs	1.		2.			
Fruit	1.		2.			
Vegetables	1.		2.			
Fat	1.		2.			
Liquid/drink	1.		2.			
Meal Replace.	1.		2.			
Condiments	1.		2.			
Other	1.		2.			

SNACK 1	Time: _____					
	Type	Amt:		Type	Amt:	
Protein	1.			2.		
Complex Carbs	1.			2.		
Fruit	1.			2.		
Vegetables	1.			2.		
Fat	1.			2.		
Liquid/drink	1.			2.		
Meal Replace.	1.			2.		
Condiments	1.			2.		
Other	1.			2.		

LUNCH	Time: _____					
	Type	Amt:		Type	Amt:	
Protein	1.			2.		
Complex Carbs	1.			2.		
Fruit	1.			2.		
Vegetables	1.			2.		
Fat	1.			2.		
Liquid/drink	1.			2.		
Meal Replace.	1.			2.		
Condiments	1.			2.		
Other	1.			2.		

SNACK 2	Time: _____					
	Type	Amt:		Type	Amt:	
Protein	1.			2.		
Complex Carbs	1.			2.		
Fruit	1.			2.		
Vegetables	1.			2.		
Fat	1.			2.		
Liquid/drink	1.			2.		
Meal Replace.	1.			2.		
Condiments	1.			2.		
Other	1.			2.		

SNACK 3	Time: _____					
	Type	Amt:		Type	Amt:	
Protein	1.			2.		
Complex Carbs	1.			2.		
Fruit	1.			2.		
Vegetables	1.			2.		
Fat	1.			2.		
Liquid/drink	1.			2.		
Meal Replace.	1.			2.		
Condiments	1.			2.		
Other	1.			2.		

DINNER	Time: _____					
	Type	Amt:		Type	Amt:	
Protein	1.			2.		
Complex Carbs	1.			2.		
Fruit	1.			2.		
Vegetables	1.			2.		
Fat	1.			2.		
Liquid/drink	1.			2.		
Meal Replace.	1.			2.		
Condiments	1.			2.		
Other	1.			2.		

Cardiovascular Training

Warmed up   Yes _____   No _____

Time of day: _____		For how long?	Heart Rate
Type 1:		_____	_____
Type 2:		_____	_____
Type 3:		_____	_____
Type 4:		_____	_____
Stretched? Yes _____ No _____			

Evening Reflection

Did I put my faith in Action today?	Yes _____	No _____
I prayed for somone today	Yes _____	No _____
I read my Bible today	Yes _____	No _____
I helped someone in need today	Yes _____	No _____
I got 6 1/2 to 8 hours of sleep last night	Yes _____	No _____
I know I ate right today	Yes _____	No _____
I ate breakfast today	Yes _____	No _____
I ate starches after 4:00 p.m. today	Yes _____	No _____
I ate at least 4 meals today	Yes _____	No _____
I drank at least a gallon of water today	Yes _____	No _____
I had Courage to Change today	Yes _____	No _____
Tonight I forgive…		

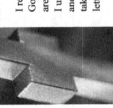

Captain's Log Statement of Faith

I realize that my actions don't earn my way into God's love or earn my way to heaven but that they are a reflection of my love affair with Jesus! I understand that by taking care of myself I honor and glorify God. I matter to God and the actions I take toward good health are daily written love letters telling God, "Thank you for my life"!

_____   Signature

Resistance Training

Time of day: _____

Warmed up   Yes _____   No _____

Name of exercise 1:

	Weight:	Reps:
Set 1:	_____	_____
Set 2:	_____	_____
Set 3:	_____	_____
Set 4:	_____	_____

Muscles worked: _____

Stretched?   Yes _____   No _____

Name of exercise 2:

	Weight:	Reps:
Set 1:	_____	_____
Set 2:	_____	_____
Set 3:	_____	_____
Set 4:	_____	_____

Muscles worked: _____

Stretched?   Yes _____   No _____

Name of exercise 3:

	Weight:	Reps:
Set 1:	_____	_____
Set 2:	_____	_____
Set 3:	_____	_____
Set 4:	_____	_____

Muscles worked: _____

Stretched?   Yes _____   No _____

Name of exercise 4:

	Weight:	Reps:
Set 1:	_____	_____
Set 2:	_____	_____
Set 3:	_____	_____
Set 4:	_____	_____

Muscles worked: _____

Stretched?   Yes _____   No _____

Name of exercise 5:

	Weight:	Reps:
Set 1:	_____	_____
Set 2:	_____	_____
Set 3:	_____	_____
Set 4:	_____	_____

Muscles worked: _____

Stretched?   Yes _____   No _____

Name of exercise 6:

	Weight:	Reps:
Set 1:	_____	_____
Set 2:	_____	_____
Set 3:	_____	_____
Set 4:	_____	_____

Muscles worked: _____

Stretched?   Yes _____   No _____

Name of exercise 7:

	Weight:	Reps:
Set 1:	_____	_____
Set 2:	_____	_____
Set 3:	_____	_____
Set 4:	_____	_____

Muscles worked: _____

Stretched?   Yes _____   No _____

Name of exercise 8:

	Weight:	Reps:
Set 1:	_____	_____
Set 2:	_____	_____
Set 3:	_____	_____
Set 4:	_____	_____

Muscles worked: _____

Stretched?   Yes _____   No _____

Name of exercise 9:

	Weight:	Reps:
Set 1:	_____	_____
Set 2:	_____	_____
Set 3:	_____	_____
Set 4:	_____	_____

Muscles worked: _____

Stretched?   Yes _____   No _____

Name of exercise 10:

	Weight:	Reps:
Set 1:	_____	_____
Set 2:	_____	_____
Set 3:	_____	_____
Set 4:	_____	_____

Muscles worked: _____

Stretched?   Yes _____   No _____

"I press on toward the goal to win the prize for which God has called me heavenward in Christ Jesus."
Philippians 3:14

Captain's Log

Day: _____ Date: _____ / _____ / _____

Nutrition Log

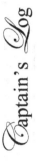
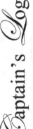

BREAKFAST   Time: _____

	Type	Amt:	Type	Amt:
Protein	1.		2.	
Complex Carbs	1.		2.	
Fruit	1.		2.	
Vegetables	1.		2.	
Fat	1.		2.	
Liquid/drink	1.		2.	
Meal Replace.	1.		2.	
Condiments	1.		2.	
Other	1.		2.	

SNACK 1   Time: _____

	Type	Amt:	Type	Amt:
Protein	1.		2.	
Complex Carbs	1.		2.	
Fruit	1.		2.	
Vegetables	1.		2.	
Fat	1.		2.	
Liquid/drink	1.		2.	
Meal Replace.	1.		2.	
Condiments	1.		2.	
Other	1.		2.	

LUNCH   Time: _____

	Type	Amt:	Type	Amt:
Protein	1.		2.	
Complex Carbs	1.		2.	
Fruit	1.		2.	
Vegetables	1.		2.	
Fat	1.		2.	
Liquid/drink	1.		2.	
Meal Replace.	1.		2.	
Condiments	1.		2.	
Other	1.		2.	

SNACK 2   Time: _____

	Type	Amt:	Type	Amt:
Protein	1.		2.	
Complex Carbs	1.		2.	
Fruit	1.		2.	
Vegetables	1.		2.	
Fat	1.		2.	
Liquid/drink	1.		2.	
Meal Replace.	1.		2.	
Condiments	1.		2.	
Other	1.		2.	

SNACK 3   Time: _____

	Type	Amt:	Type	Amt:
Protein	1.		2.	
Complex Carbs	1.		2.	
Fruit	1.		2.	
Vegetables	1.		2.	
Fat	1.		2.	
Liquid/drink	1.		2.	
Meal Replace.	1.		2.	
Condiments	1.		2.	
Other	1.		2.	

DINNER   Time: _____

	Type	Amt:	Type	Amt:
Protein	1.		2.	
Complex Carbs	1.		2.	
Fruit	1.		2.	
Vegetables	1.		2.	
Fat	1.		2.	
Liquid/drink	1.		2.	
Meal Replace.	1.		2.	
Condiments	1.		2.	
Other	1.		2.	

Resistance Training

Time of day: _____

Warmed up   Yes _____   No _____

Name of exercise 1:
_____
Muscles worked: _____
Stretched?   Yes _____   No _____

	Weight:	Reps:
Set 1:	_____	_____
Set 2:	_____	_____
Set 3:	_____	_____
Set 4:	_____	_____

Name of exercise 2:
_____
Muscles worked: _____
Stretched?   Yes _____   No _____

	Weight:	Reps:
Set 1:	_____	_____
Set 2:	_____	_____
Set 3:	_____	_____
Set 4:	_____	_____

Name of exercise 3:
_____
Muscles worked: _____
Stretched?   Yes _____   No _____

	Weight:	Reps:
Set 1:	_____	_____
Set 2:	_____	_____
Set 3:	_____	_____
Set 4:	_____	_____

Name of exercise 4:
_____
Muscles worked: _____
Stretched?   Yes _____   No _____

	Weight:	Reps:
Set 1:	_____	_____
Set 2:	_____	_____
Set 3:	_____	_____
Set 4:	_____	_____

Name of exercise 5:
_____
Muscles worked: _____
Stretched?   Yes _____   No _____

	Weight:	Reps:
Set 1:	_____	_____
Set 2:	_____	_____
Set 3:	_____	_____
Set 4:	_____	_____

Name of exercise 6:
_____
Muscles worked: _____
Stretched?   Yes _____   No _____

	Weight:	Reps:
Set 1:	_____	_____
Set 2:	_____	_____
Set 3:	_____	_____
Set 4:	_____	_____

Name of exercise 7:
_____
Muscles worked: _____
Stretched?   Yes _____   No _____

	Weight:	Reps:
Set 1:	_____	_____
Set 2:	_____	_____
Set 3:	_____	_____
Set 4:	_____	_____

Name of exercise 8:
_____
Muscles worked: _____
Stretched?   Yes _____   No _____

	Weight:	Reps:
Set 1:	_____	_____
Set 2:	_____	_____
Set 3:	_____	_____
Set 4:	_____	_____

Name of exercise 9:
_____
Muscles worked: _____
Stretched?   Yes _____   No _____

	Weight:	Reps:
Set 1:	_____	_____
Set 2:	_____	_____
Set 3:	_____	_____
Set 4:	_____	_____

Name of exercise 10:
_____
Muscles worked: _____
Stretched?   Yes _____   No _____

	Weight:	Reps:
Set 1:	_____	_____
Set 2:	_____	_____
Set 3:	_____	_____
Set 4:	_____	_____

Cardiovascular Training

Warmed up   Yes _____   No _____

Time of day:	For how long?	Heart Rate
Type 1:	_____	_____
Type 2:	_____	_____
Type 3:	_____	_____
Type 4:	_____	_____

Stretched?   Yes _____   No _____

Evening Reflection

Did I put my faith in Action today?	Yes _____	No _____
I prayed for somone today	Yes _____	No _____
I read my Bible today	Yes _____	No _____
I helped someone in need today	Yes _____	No _____
I got 6 1/2 to 8 hours of sleep last night	Yes _____	No _____
I know I ate right today	Yes _____	No _____
I ate breakfast today	Yes _____	No _____
I ate starches after 4:00 p.m. today	Yes _____	No _____
I ate at least 4 meals today	Yes _____	No _____
I drank at least a gallon of water today	Yes _____	No _____
I had Courage to Change today	Yes _____	No _____

Tonight I forgive…

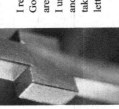

Captain's Log Statement of Faith

I realize that my actions don't earn my way into God's love or earn my way to heaven but that they are a reflection of my love affair with Jesus! I understand that by taking care of myself I honor and glorify God. I matter to God and the actions I take toward good health are daily written love letters telling God, "Thank you for my life"!

_____
Signature

"I press on toward the goal to win the prize for which God has called me heavenward in Christ Jesus."
Philippians 3:14

Captain's Log

"Each one should test his own actions. Then he can take pride in himself without comparing himself to somebody else, for each one should carry his own load." (Galatians 6:40)

Day: _____ Date: _____ / _____ / _____

Nutrition Log

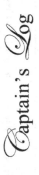

BREAKFAST	Time:				Type	Amt:
	Type	Amt:				
Protein	1.				2.	
Complex Carbs	1.				2.	
Fruit	1.				2.	
Vegetables	1.				2.	
Fat	1.				2.	
Liquid/drink	1.				2.	
Meal Replace.	1.				2.	
Condiments	1.				2.	
Other	1.				2.	

LUNCH	Time:				Type	Amt:
	Type	Amt:				
Protein	1.				2.	
Complex Carbs	1.				2.	
Fruit	1.				2.	
Vegetables	1.				2.	
Fat	1.				2.	
Liquid/drink	1.				2.	
Meal Replace.	1.				2.	
Condiments	1.				2.	
Other	1.				2.	

SNACK 3	Time:				Type	Amt:
	Type	Amt:				
Protein	1.				2.	
Complex Carbs	1.				2.	
Fruit	1.				2.	
Vegetables	1.				2.	
Fat	1.				2.	
Liquid/drink	1.				2.	
Meal Replace.	1.				2.	
Condiments	1.				2.	
Other	1.				2.	

SNACK 1	Time:				Type	Amt:
	Type	Amt:				
Protein	1.				2.	
Complex Carbs	1.				2.	
Fruit	1.				2.	
Vegetables	1.				2.	
Fat	1.				2.	
Liquid/drink	1.				2.	
Meal Replace.	1.				2.	
Condiments	1.				2.	
Other	1.				2.	

SNACK 2	Time:				Type	Amt:
	Type	Amt:				
Protein	1.				2.	
Complex Carbs	1.				2.	
Fruit	1.				2.	
Vegetables	1.				2.	
Fat	1.				2.	
Liquid/drink	1.				2.	
Meal Replace.	1.				2.	
Condiments	1.				2.	
Other	1.				2.	

DINNER	Time:				Type	Amt:
	Type	Amt:				
Protein	1.				2.	
Complex Carbs	1.				2.	
Fruit	1.				2.	
Vegetables	1.				2.	
Fat	1.				2.	
Liquid/drink	1.				2.	
Meal Replace.	1.				2.	
Condiments	1.				2.	
Other	1.				2.	

Cardiovascular Training

Warmed up   Yes _____   No _____

Time of day: _____	For how long?	Heart Rate
Type 1:	_____	_____
Type 2:	_____	_____
Type 3:	_____	_____
Type 4:	_____	_____
Stretched? Yes _____ No _____		

Resistance Training

Time of day: _____

Warmed up   Yes _____   No _____

Name of exercise 1: _____
	Weight:	Reps:
Set 1:	_____	_____
Set 2:	_____	_____
Set 3:	_____	_____
Set 4:	_____	_____

Muscles worked: _____

Stretched?   Yes _____   No _____

Name of exercise 2: _____
	Weight:	Reps:
Set 1:	_____	_____
Set 2:	_____	_____
Set 3:	_____	_____
Set 4:	_____	_____

Muscles worked: _____

Stretched?   Yes _____   No _____

Name of exercise 3: _____
	Weight:	Reps:
Set 1:	_____	_____
Set 2:	_____	_____
Set 3:	_____	_____
Set 4:	_____	_____

Muscles worked: _____

Stretched?   Yes _____   No _____

Name of exercise 4: _____
	Weight:	Reps:
Set 1:	_____	_____
Set 2:	_____	_____
Set 3:	_____	_____
Set 4:	_____	_____

Muscles worked: _____

Stretched?   Yes _____   No _____

Name of exercise 5: _____
	Weight:	Reps:
Set 1:	_____	_____
Set 2:	_____	_____
Set 3:	_____	_____
Set 4:	_____	_____

Muscles worked: _____

Stretched?   Yes _____   No _____

Name of exercise 6: _____
	Weight:	Reps:
Set 1:	_____	_____
Set 2:	_____	_____
Set 3:	_____	_____
Set 4:	_____	_____

Muscles worked: _____

Stretched?   Yes _____   No _____

Name of exercise 7: _____
	Weight:	Reps:
Set 1:	_____	_____
Set 2:	_____	_____
Set 3:	_____	_____
Set 4:	_____	_____

Muscles worked: _____

Stretched?   Yes _____   No _____

Name of exercise 8: _____
	Weight:	Reps:
Set 1:	_____	_____
Set 2:	_____	_____
Set 3:	_____	_____
Set 4:	_____	_____

Muscles worked: _____

Stretched?   Yes _____   No _____

Name of exercise 9: _____
	Weight:	Reps:
Set 1:	_____	_____
Set 2:	_____	_____
Set 3:	_____	_____
Set 4:	_____	_____

Muscles worked: _____

Stretched?   Yes _____   No _____

Name of exercise 10: _____
	Weight:	Reps:
Set 1:	_____	_____
Set 2:	_____	_____
Set 3:	_____	_____
Set 4:	_____	_____

Muscles worked: _____

Stretched?   Yes _____   No _____

Evening Reflection

Did I put my faith in Action today?	Yes _____	No _____
I prayed for somone today	Yes _____	No _____
I read my Bible today	Yes _____	No _____
I helped someone in need today	Yes _____	No _____
I got 6 1/2 to 8 hours of sleep last night	Yes _____	No _____
I know I ate right today	Yes _____	No _____
I ate breakfast today	Yes _____	No _____
I ate starches after 4:00 p.m. today	Yes _____	No _____
I ate at least 4 meals today	Yes _____	No _____
I drank at least a gallon of water today	Yes _____	No _____
I had Courage to Change today	Yes _____	No _____
Tonight I forgive... _____		

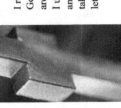

Captain's Log Statement of Faith

I realize that my actions don't earn my way into God's love or earn my way to heaven but that they are a reflection of my love affair with Jesus! I understand that by taking care of myself I honor and glorify God. I matter to God and the actions I take toward good health are daily written love letters telling God, "Thank you for my life"!

_____
Signature

"I press on toward the goal to win the prize for which God has called me heavenward in Christ Jesus."
Philippians 3:14

A CALL TO ACTION

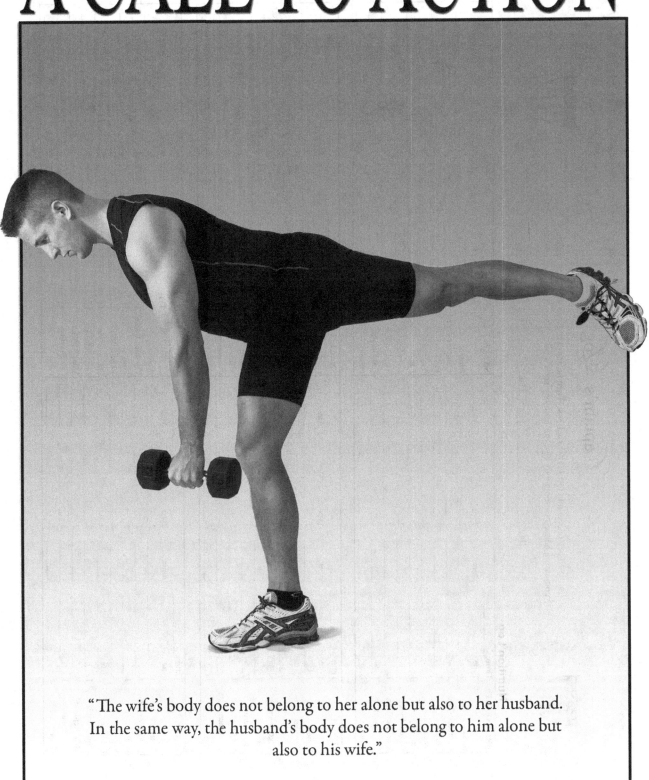

"The wife's body does not belong to her alone but also to her husband. In the same way, the husband's body does not belong to him alone but also to his wife."

WEEK ELEVEN

Captain's Log

Day: _____ Date: _____ / _____ / _____

Nutrition Log

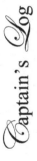

BREAKFAST — Time: _____

	Type	Amt:	Type	Amt:
Protein	1.		2.	
Complex Carbs	1.		2.	
Fruit	1.		2.	
Vegetables	1.		2.	
Fat	1.		2.	
Liquid/drink	1.		2.	
Meal Replace.	1.		2.	
Condiments	1.		2.	
Other	1.		2.	

LUNCH — Time: _____

	Type	Amt:	Type	Amt:
Protein	1.		2.	
Complex Carbs	1.		2.	
Fruit	1.		2.	
Vegetables	1.		2.	
Fat	1.		2.	
Liquid/drink	1.		2.	
Meal Replace.	1.		2.	
Condiments	1.		2.	
Other	1.		2.	

SNACK 3 — Time: _____

	Type	Amt:	Type	Amt:
Protein	1.		2.	
Complex Carbs	1.		2.	
Fruit	1.		2.	
Vegetables	1.		2.	
Fat	1.		2.	
Liquid/drink	1.		2.	
Meal Replace.	1.		2.	
Condiments	1.		2.	
Other	1.		2.	

SNACK 1 — Time: _____

	Type	Amt:	Type	Amt:
Protein	1.		2.	
Complex Carbs	1.		2.	
Fruit	1.		2.	
Vegetables	1.		2.	
Fat	1.		2.	
Liquid/drink	1.		2.	
Meal Replace.	1.		2.	
Condiments	1.		2.	
Other	1.		2.	

SNACK 2 — Time: _____

	Type	Amt:	Type	Amt:
Protein	1.		2.	
Complex Carbs	1.		2.	
Fruit	1.		2.	
Vegetables	1.		2.	
Fat	1.		2.	
Liquid/drink	1.		2.	
Meal Replace.	1.		2.	
Condiments	1.		2.	
Other	1.		2.	

DINNER — Time: _____

	Type	Amt:	Type	Amt:
Protein	1.		2.	
Complex Carbs	1.		2.	
Fruit	1.		2.	
Vegetables	1.		2.	
Fat	1.		2.	
Liquid/drink	1.		2.	
Meal Replace.	1.		2.	
Condiments	1.		2.	
Other	1.		2.	

Cardiovascular Training

Warmed up   Yes _____   No _____

	For how long?	Heart Rate
Time of day: _____		
Type 1: _____	_____	_____
Type 2: _____	_____	_____
Type 3: _____	_____	_____
Type 4: _____	_____	_____
Stretched? Yes _____ No _____		

Evening Reflection

Did I put my faith in Action today?	Yes _____	No _____
I prayed for somone today	Yes _____	No _____
I read my Bible today	Yes _____	No _____
I helped someone in need today	Yes _____	No _____
I got 6 1/2 to 8 hours of sleep last night	Yes _____	No _____
I know I ate right today	Yes _____	No _____
I ate breakfast today	Yes _____	No _____
I ate starches after 4:00 p.m. today	Yes _____	No _____
I ate at least 4 meals today	Yes _____	No _____
I drank at least a gallon of water today	Yes _____	No _____
I had Courage to Change today	Yes _____	No _____
Tonight I forgive… _____		

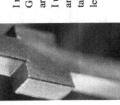

Captain's Log Statement of Faith

I realize that my actions don't earn my way into
God's love or earn my way to heaven but that they
are a reflection of my love affair with Jesus!
I understand that by taking care of myself I honor
and glorify God. I matter to God and the actions I
take toward good health are daily written love
letters telling God, "Thank you for my life"!

_____

Signature

Resistance Training

Time of day: _____

Warmed up   Yes _____   No _____

Name of exercise 1: _____

	Weight:	Reps:
Set 1:	_____	_____
Set 2:	_____	_____
Muscles worked:	Set 3:	_____	_____
	Set 4:	_____	_____
Stretched? Yes _____	No _____	

Name of exercise 2: _____

	Weight:	Reps:
Set 1:	_____	_____
Set 2:	_____	_____
Muscles worked:	Set 3:	_____	_____
	Set 4:	_____	_____
Stretched? Yes _____	No _____	

Name of exercise 3: _____

	Weight:	Reps:
Set 1:	_____	_____
Set 2:	_____	_____
Muscles worked:	Set 3:	_____	_____
	Set 4:	_____	_____
Stretched? Yes _____	No _____	

Name of exercise 4: _____

	Weight:	Reps:
Set 1:	_____	_____
Set 2:	_____	_____
Muscles worked:	Set 3:	_____	_____
	Set 4:	_____	_____
Stretched? Yes _____	No _____	

Name of exercise 5: _____

	Weight:	Reps:
Set 1:	_____	_____
Set 2:	_____	_____
Muscles worked:	Set 3:	_____	_____
	Set 4:	_____	_____
Stretched? Yes _____	No _____	

Name of exercise 6: _____

	Weight:	Reps:
Set 1:	_____	_____
Set 2:	_____	_____
Muscles worked:	Set 3:	_____	_____
	Set 4:	_____	_____
Stretched? Yes _____	No _____	

Name of exercise 7: _____

	Weight:	Reps:
Set 1:	_____	_____
Set 2:	_____	_____
Muscles worked:	Set 3:	_____	_____
	Set 4:	_____	_____
Stretched? Yes _____	No _____	

Name of exercise 8: _____

	Weight:	Reps:
Set 1:	_____	_____
Set 2:	_____	_____
Muscles worked:	Set 3:	_____	_____
	Set 4:	_____	_____
Stretched? Yes _____	No _____	

Name of exercise 9: _____

	Weight:	Reps:
Set 1:	_____	_____
Set 2:	_____	_____
Muscles worked:	Set 3:	_____	_____
	Set 4:	_____	_____
Stretched? Yes _____	No _____	

Name of exercise 10: _____

	Weight:	Reps:
Set 1:	_____	_____
Set 2:	_____	_____
Muscles worked:	Set 3:	_____	_____
	Set 4:	_____	_____
Stretched? Yes _____	No _____	

"I press on toward the goal to win the prize for which God has called me heavenward in Christ Jesus."
Philippians 3:14

Captain's Log

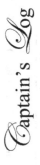 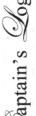

Day: _____   Date: _____ / _____ / _____

Nutrition Log

BREAKFAST   Time: _____

	Type	Amt:	Type	Amt:
Protein	1. _____	_____	2. _____	_____
Complex Carbs	1. _____	_____	2. _____	_____
Fruit	1. _____	_____	2. _____	_____
Vegetables	1. _____	_____	2. _____	_____
Fat	1. _____	_____	2. _____	_____
Liquid/drink	1. _____	_____	2. _____	_____
Meal Replace.	1. _____	_____	2. _____	_____
Condiments	1. _____	_____	2. _____	_____
Other	1. _____	_____	2. _____	_____

SNACK 1   Time: _____

	Type	Amt:	Type	Amt:
Protein	1. _____	_____	2. _____	_____
Complex Carbs	1. _____	_____	2. _____	_____
Fruit	1. _____	_____	2. _____	_____
Vegetables	1. _____	_____	2. _____	_____
Fat	1. _____	_____	2. _____	_____
Liquid/drink	1. _____	_____	2. _____	_____
Meal Replace.	1. _____	_____	2. _____	_____
Condiments	1. _____	_____	2. _____	_____
Other	1. _____	_____	2. _____	_____

LUNCH   Time: _____

	Type	Amt:	Type	Amt:
Protein	1. _____	_____	2. _____	_____
Complex Carbs	1. _____	_____	2. _____	_____
Fruit	1. _____	_____	2. _____	_____
Vegetables	1. _____	_____	2. _____	_____
Fat	1. _____	_____	2. _____	_____
Liquid/drink	1. _____	_____	2. _____	_____
Meal Replace.	1. _____	_____	2. _____	_____
Condiments	1. _____	_____	2. _____	_____
Other	1. _____	_____	2. _____	_____

SNACK 2   Time: _____

	Type	Amt:	Type	Amt:
Protein	1. _____	_____	2. _____	_____
Complex Carbs	1. _____	_____	2. _____	_____
Fruit	1. _____	_____	2. _____	_____
Vegetables	1. _____	_____	2. _____	_____
Fat	1. _____	_____	2. _____	_____
Liquid/drink	1. _____	_____	2. _____	_____
Meal Replace.	1. _____	_____	2. _____	_____
Condiments	1. _____	_____	2. _____	_____
Other	1. _____	_____	2. _____	_____

SNACK 3   Time: _____

	Type	Amt:	Type	Amt:
Protein	1. _____	_____	2. _____	_____
Complex Carbs	1. _____	_____	2. _____	_____
Fruit	1. _____	_____	2. _____	_____
Vegetables	1. _____	_____	2. _____	_____
Fat	1. _____	_____	2. _____	_____
Liquid/drink	1. _____	_____	2. _____	_____
Meal Replace.	1. _____	_____	2. _____	_____
Condiments	1. _____	_____	2. _____	_____
Other	1. _____	_____	2. _____	_____

DINNER   Time: _____

	Type	Amt:	Type	Amt:
Protein	1. _____	_____	2. _____	_____
Complex Carbs	1. _____	_____	2. _____	_____
Fruit	1. _____	_____	2. _____	_____
Vegetables	1. _____	_____	2. _____	_____
Fat	1. _____	_____	2. _____	_____
Liquid/drink	1. _____	_____	2. _____	_____
Meal Replace.	1. _____	_____	2. _____	_____
Condiments	1. _____	_____	2. _____	_____
Other	1. _____	_____	2. _____	_____

Cardiovascular Training

Warmed up   Yes _____   No _____

Time of day:		For how long?	Heart Rate
Type 1:			
Type 2:			
Type 3:			
Type 4:			

Stretched?   Yes _____   No _____

Resistance Training

Time of day: _____
Warmed up   Yes _____   No _____

Name of exercise 1:

_____   Weight: Reps:
Set 1: _____
Set 2: _____
Set 3: _____
Set 4: _____
Muscles worked: _____
Stretched?   Yes _____   No _____

Name of exercise 2:

_____   Weight: Reps:
Set 1: _____
Set 2: _____
Set 3: _____
Set 4: _____
Muscles worked: _____
Stretched?   Yes _____   No _____

Name of exercise 3:

_____   Weight: Reps:
Set 1: _____
Set 2: _____
Set 3: _____
Set 4: _____
Muscles worked: _____
Stretched?   Yes _____   No _____

Name of exercise 4:

_____   Weight: Reps:
Set 1: _____
Set 2: _____
Set 3: _____
Set 4: _____
Muscles worked: _____
Stretched?   Yes _____   No _____

Name of exercise 5:

_____   Weight: Reps:
Set 1: _____
Set 2: _____
Set 3: _____
Set 4: _____
Muscles worked: _____
Stretched?   Yes _____   No _____

Name of exercise 6:

_____   Weight: Reps:
Set 1: _____
Set 2: _____
Set 3: _____
Set 4: _____
Muscles worked: _____
Stretched?   Yes _____   No _____

Name of exercise 7:

_____   Weight: Reps:
Set 1: _____
Set 2: _____
Set 3: _____
Set 4: _____
Muscles worked: _____
Stretched?   Yes _____   No _____

Name of exercise 8:

_____   Weight: Reps:
Set 1: _____
Set 2: _____
Set 3: _____
Set 4: _____
Muscles worked: _____
Stretched?   Yes _____   No _____

Name of exercise 9:

_____   Weight: Reps:
Set 1: _____
Set 2: _____
Set 3: _____
Set 4: _____
Muscles worked: _____
Stretched?   Yes _____   No _____

Name of exercise 10:

_____   Weight: Reps:
Set 1: _____
Set 2: _____
Set 3: _____
Set 4: _____
Muscles worked: _____
Stretched?   Yes _____   No _____

Evening Reflection

Did I put my faith in Action today?	Yes _____	No _____
I prayed for somone today	Yes _____	No _____
I read my Bible today	Yes _____	No _____
I helped someone in need today	Yes _____	No _____
I got 6 1/2 to 8 hours of sleep last night	Yes _____	No _____
I know I ate right today	Yes _____	No _____
I ate breakfast today	Yes _____	No _____
I ate starches after 4:00 p.m. today	Yes _____	No _____
I ate at least 4 meals today	Yes _____	No _____
I drank at least a gallon of water today	Yes _____	No _____
I had Courage to Change today	Yes _____	No _____
Tonight I forgive…		

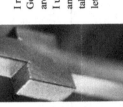

Captain's Log Statement of Faith

I realize that my actions don't earn my way into God's love or earn my way to heaven but that they are a reflection of my love affair with Jesus! I understand that by taking care of myself I honor and glorify God. I matter to God and the actions I take toward good health are daily written love letters telling God, "Thank you for my life"!

_____
Signature

"I press on toward the goal to win the prize for which God has called me heavenward in Christ Jesus."
Philippians 3:14

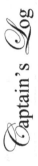

Captain's Log

"Each one should test his own actions. Then he can take pride in himself without comparing himself to somebody else, for each one should carry his own load." (Galatians 6:40)

Day: _____   Date: _____ / _____ / _____

Nutrition Log

BREAKFAST Time: _____

Type		Amt:	Type		Amt:
Protein	1. _____	_____		2. _____	_____
Complex Carbs	1. _____	_____		2. _____	_____
Fruit	1. _____	_____		2. _____	_____
Vegetables	1. _____	_____		2. _____	_____
Fat	1. _____	_____		2. _____	_____
Liquid/drink	1. _____	_____		2. _____	_____
Meal Replace.	1. _____	_____		2. _____	_____
Condiments	1. _____	_____		2. _____	_____
Other	1. _____	_____		2. _____	_____

LUNCH Time: _____

Type		Amt:	Type		Amt:
Protein	1. _____	_____		2. _____	_____
Complex Carbs	1. _____	_____		2. _____	_____
Fruit	1. _____	_____		2. _____	_____
Vegetables	1. _____	_____		2. _____	_____
Fat	1. _____	_____		2. _____	_____
Liquid/drink	1. _____	_____		2. _____	_____
Meal Replace.	1. _____	_____		2. _____	_____
Condiments	1. _____	_____		2. _____	_____
Other	1. _____	_____		2. _____	_____

SNACK 3 Time: _____

Type		Amt:	Type		Amt:
Protein	1. _____	_____		2. _____	_____
Complex Carbs	1. _____	_____		2. _____	_____
Fruit	1. _____	_____		2. _____	_____
Vegetables	1. _____	_____		2. _____	_____
Fat	1. _____	_____		2. _____	_____
Liquid/drink	1. _____	_____		2. _____	_____
Meal Replace.	1. _____	_____		2. _____	_____
Condiments	1. _____	_____		2. _____	_____
Other	1. _____	_____		2. _____	_____

SNACK 1 Time: _____

Type		Amt:	Type		Amt:
Protein	1. _____	_____		2. _____	_____
Complex Carbs	1. _____	_____		2. _____	_____
Fruit	1. _____	_____		2. _____	_____
Vegetables	1. _____	_____		2. _____	_____
Fat	1. _____	_____		2. _____	_____
Liquid/drink	1. _____	_____		2. _____	_____
Meal Replace.	1. _____	_____		2. _____	_____
Condiments	1. _____	_____		2. _____	_____
Other	1. _____	_____		2. _____	_____

SNACK 2 Time: _____

Type		Amt:	Type		Amt:
Protein	1. _____	_____		2. _____	_____
Complex Carbs	1. _____	_____		2. _____	_____
Fruit	1. _____	_____		2. _____	_____
Vegetables	1. _____	_____		2. _____	_____
Fat	1. _____	_____		2. _____	_____
Liquid/drink	1. _____	_____		2. _____	_____
Meal Replace.	1. _____	_____		2. _____	_____
Condiments	1. _____	_____		2. _____	_____
Other	1. _____	_____		2. _____	_____

DINNER Time: _____

Type		Amt:	Type		Amt:
Protein	1. _____	_____		2. _____	_____
Complex Carbs	1. _____	_____		2. _____	_____
Fruit	1. _____	_____		2. _____	_____
Vegetables	1. _____	_____		2. _____	_____
Fat	1. _____	_____		2. _____	_____
Liquid/drink	1. _____	_____		2. _____	_____
Meal Replace.	1. _____	_____		2. _____	_____
Condiments	1. _____	_____		2. _____	_____
Other	1. _____	_____		2. _____	_____

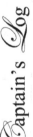

Resistance Training

Time of day: _____ **No** _____

Warmed up Yes _____ No _____

Name of exercise 1:
_____

Weight: _____ Reps: _____
Set 1: _____
Set 2: _____

Muscles worked: _____
Set 3: _____
Set 4: _____

Stretched? Yes _____ No _____

Name of exercise 3:
_____

Weight: _____ Reps: _____
Set 1: _____
Set 2: _____

Muscles worked: _____
Set 3: _____
Set 4: _____

Stretched? Yes _____ No _____

Name of exercise 5:
_____

Weight: _____ Reps: _____
Set 1: _____
Set 2: _____

Muscles worked: _____
Set 3: _____
Set 4: _____

Stretched? Yes _____ No _____

Name of exercise 7:
_____

Weight: _____ Reps: _____
Set 1: _____
Set 2: _____

Muscles worked: _____
Set 3: _____
Set 4: _____

Stretched? Yes _____ No _____

Name of exercise 9:
_____

Weight: _____ Reps: _____
Set 1: _____
Set 2: _____

Muscles worked: _____
Set 3: _____
Set 4: _____

Stretched? Yes _____ No _____

Name of exercise 2:
_____

Weight: _____ Reps: _____
Set 1: _____
Set 2: _____

Muscles worked: _____
Set 3: _____
Set 4: _____

Stretched? Yes _____ No _____

Name of exercise 4:
_____

Weight: _____ Reps: _____
Set 1: _____
Set 2: _____

Muscles worked: _____
Set 3: _____
Set 4: _____

Stretched? Yes _____ No _____

Name of exercise 6:
_____

Weight: _____ Reps: _____
Set 1: _____
Set 2: _____

Muscles worked: _____
Set 3: _____
Set 4: _____

Stretched? Yes _____ No _____

Name of exercise 8:
_____

Weight: _____ Reps: _____
Set 1: _____
Set 2: _____

Muscles worked: _____
Set 3: _____
Set 4: _____

Stretched? Yes _____ No _____

Name of exercise 10:
_____

Weight: _____ Reps: _____
Set 1: _____
Set 2: _____

Muscles worked: _____
Set 3: _____
Set 4: _____

Stretched? Yes _____ No _____

Cardiovascular Training

Warmed up Yes _____ No _____

Time of day: _____ **For how long?** **Heart Rate**
Type 1: _____
Type 2: _____
Type 3: _____
Type 4: _____

Stretched? Yes _____ No _____

Evening Reflection

Did I put my faith in Action today?	Yes _____	No _____
I prayed for somone today	Yes _____	No _____
I read my Bible today	Yes _____	No _____
I helped someone in need today	Yes _____	No _____
I got 6 1/2 to 8 hours of sleep last night	Yes _____	No _____
I know I ate right today	Yes _____	No _____
I ate breakfast today	Yes _____	No _____
I ate starches after 4:00 p.m. today	Yes _____	No _____
I ate at least 4 meals today	Yes _____	No _____
I drank at least a gallon of water today	Yes _____	No _____
I had Courage to Change today	Yes _____	No _____
Tonight I forgive… _____		

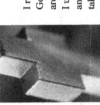

Captain's Log Statement of Faith

I realize that my actions don't earn my way into God's love or earn my way to heaven but that they are a reflection of my love affair with Jesus! I understand that by taking care of myself I honor and glorify God. I matter to God and the actions I take toward good health are daily written love letters telling God, "Thank you for my life"!

_____
Signature

"I press on toward the goal to win the prize for which God has called me heavenward in Christ Jesus."
Philippians 3:14

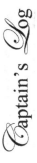

Captain's Log

"Each one should test his own actions. Then he can take pride in himself without comparing himself to somebody else, for each one should carry his own load." (Galatians 6:40)

Day: _____   Date: ____ / ____ / ____

Nutrition Log

BREAKFAST	Time: _____		
	Type	Amt:	
Protein	1.		
Complex Carbs	1.		2.
Fruit	1.		2.
Vegetables	1.		2.
Fat	1.		2.
Liquid/drink	1.		2.
Meal Replace.	1.		2.
Condiments	1.		2.
Other	1.		2.

SNACK 1	Time: _____		
	Type	Amt:	
Protein	1.		2.
Complex Carbs	1.		2.
Fruit	1.		2.
Vegetables	1.		2.
Fat	1.		2.
Liquid/drink	1.		2.
Meal Replace.	1.		2.
Condiments	1.		2.
Other	1.		2.

LUNCH	Time: _____		
	Type	Amt:	
Protein	1.		2.
Complex Carbs	1.		2.
Fruit	1.		2.
Vegetables	1.		2.
Fat	1.		2.
Liquid/drink	1.		2.
Meal Replace.	1.		2.
Condiments	1.		2.
Other	1.		2.

SNACK 2	Time: _____		
	Type	Amt:	
Protein	1.		2.
Complex Carbs	1.		2.
Fruit	1.		2.
Vegetables	1.		2.
Fat	1.		2.
Liquid/drink	1.		2.
Meal Replace.	1.		2.
Condiments	1.		2.
Other	1.		2.

SNACK 3	Time: _____		
	Type	Amt:	
Protein	1.		2.
Complex Carbs	1.		2.
Fruit	1.		2.
Vegetables	1.		2.
Fat	1.		2.
Liquid/drink	1.		2.
Meal Replace.	1.		2.
Condiments	1.		2.
Other	1.		2.

DINNER	Time: _____		
	Type	Amt:	
Protein	1.		2.
Complex Carbs	1.		2.
Fruit	1.		2.
Vegetables	1.		2.
Fat	1.		2.
Liquid/drink	1.		2.
Meal Replace.	1.		2.
Condiments	1.		2.
Other	1.		2.

Cardiovascular Training

Warmed up Yes _____ No _____

Time of day: _____	For how long?	Heart Rate
Type 1:	_____	_____
Type 2:	_____	_____
Type 3:	_____	_____
Type 4:	_____	_____

Stretched? Yes _____ No _____

Evening Reflection

Did I put my faith in Action today?	Yes _____	No _____
I prayed for somone today	Yes _____	No _____
I read my Bible today	Yes _____	No _____
I helped someone in need today	Yes _____	No _____
I got 6 1/2 to 8 hours of sleep last night	Yes _____	No _____
I know I ate right today	Yes _____	No _____
I ate breakfast today	Yes _____	No _____
I ate starches after 4:00 p.m. today	Yes _____	No _____
I ate at least 4 meals today	Yes _____	No _____
I drank at least a gallon of water today	Yes _____	No _____
I had Courage to Change today	Yes _____	No _____
Tonight I forgive…		

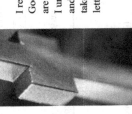

Captain's Log Statement of Faith

I realize that my actions don't earn my way into God's love or earn my way to heaven but that they are a reflection of my love affair with Jesus! I understand that by taking care of myself I honor and glorify God. I matter to God and the actions I take toward good health are daily written love letters telling God, "Thank you for my life"!

_____ **Signature**

Resistance Training

Time of day: _____

Warmed up Yes _____ No _____

Name of exercise 1: _____
Muscles worked: _____

	Weight:	Reps:
Set 1:	_____	_____
Set 2:	_____	_____
Set 3:	_____	_____
Set 4:	_____	_____

Stretched? Yes _____ No _____

Name of exercise 2: _____
Muscles worked: _____

	Weight:	Reps:
Set 1:	_____	_____
Set 2:	_____	_____
Set 3:	_____	_____
Set 4:	_____	_____

Stretched? Yes _____ No _____

Name of exercise 3: _____
Muscles worked: _____

	Weight:	Reps:
Set 1:	_____	_____
Set 2:	_____	_____
Set 3:	_____	_____
Set 4:	_____	_____

Stretched? Yes _____ No _____

Name of exercise 4: _____
Muscles worked: _____

	Weight:	Reps:
Set 1:	_____	_____
Set 2:	_____	_____
Set 3:	_____	_____
Set 4:	_____	_____

Stretched? Yes _____ No _____

Name of exercise 5: _____
Muscles worked: _____

	Weight:	Reps:
Set 1:	_____	_____
Set 2:	_____	_____
Set 3:	_____	_____
Set 4:	_____	_____

Stretched? Yes _____ No _____

Name of exercise 6: _____
Muscles worked: _____

	Weight:	Reps:
Set 1:	_____	_____
Set 2:	_____	_____
Set 3:	_____	_____
Set 4:	_____	_____

Stretched? Yes _____ No _____

Name of exercise 7: _____
Muscles worked: _____

	Weight:	Reps:
Set 1:	_____	_____
Set 2:	_____	_____
Set 3:	_____	_____
Set 4:	_____	_____

Stretched? Yes _____ No _____

Name of exercise 8: _____
Muscles worked: _____

	Weight:	Reps:
Set 1:	_____	_____
Set 2:	_____	_____
Set 3:	_____	_____
Set 4:	_____	_____

Stretched? Yes _____ No _____

Name of exercise 9: _____
Muscles worked: _____

	Weight:	Reps:
Set 1:	_____	_____
Set 2:	_____	_____
Set 3:	_____	_____
Set 4:	_____	_____

Stretched? Yes _____ No _____

Name of exercise 10: _____
Muscles worked: _____

	Weight:	Reps:
Set 1:	_____	_____
Set 2:	_____	_____
Set 3:	_____	_____
Set 4:	_____	_____

Stretched? Yes _____ No _____

"I press on toward the goal to win the prize for which God has called me heavenward in Christ Jesus."
Philippians 3:14

Captain's Log

"Each one should test his own actions. Then he can take pride in himself without comparing himself to somebody else, for each one should carry his own load." (Galatians 6:40)

Day: _____ Date: _____ / _____ / _____

Nutrition Log

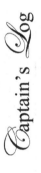

BREAKFAST	Time: _____			
	Type	Amt:	Type	Amt:
Protein	1.		2.	
Complex Carbs	1.		2.	
Fruit	1.		2.	
Vegetables	1.		2.	
Fat	1.		2.	
Liquid/drink	1.		2.	
Meal Replace.	1.		2.	
Condiments	1.		2.	
Other	1.		2.	

SNACK 1	Time: _____			
	Type	Amt:	Type	Amt:
Protein	1.		2.	
Complex Carbs	1.		2.	
Fruit	1.		2.	
Vegetables	1.		2.	
Fat	1.		2.	
Liquid/drink	1.		2.	
Meal Replace.	1.		2.	
Condiments	1.		2.	
Other	1.		2.	

LUNCH	Time: _____			
	Type	Amt:	Type	Amt:
Protein	1.		2.	
Complex Carbs	1.		2.	
Fruit	1.		2.	
Vegetables	1.		2.	
Fat	1.		2.	
Liquid/drink	1.		2.	
Meal Replace.	1.		2.	
Condiments	1.		2.	
Other	1.		2.	

SNACK 2	Time: _____			
	Type	Amt:	Type	Amt:
Protein	1.		2.	
Complex Carbs	1.		2.	
Fruit	1.		2.	
Vegetables	1.		2.	
Fat	1.		2.	
Liquid/drink	1.		2.	
Meal Replace.	1.		2.	
Condiments	1.		2.	
Other	1.		2.	

SNACK 3	Time: _____			
	Type	Amt:	Type	Amt:
Protein	1.		2.	
Complex Carbs	1.		2.	
Fruit	1.		2.	
Vegetables	1.		2.	
Fat	1.		2.	
Liquid/drink	1.		2.	
Meal Replace.	1.		2.	
Condiments	1.		2.	
Other	1.		2.	

DINNER	Time: _____			
	Type	Amt:	Type	Amt:
Protein	1.		2.	
Complex Carbs	1.		2.	
Fruit	1.		2.	
Vegetables	1.		2.	
Fat	1.		2.	
Liquid/drink	1.		2.	
Meal Replace.	1.		2.	
Condiments	1.		2.	
Other	1.		2.	

Cardiovascular Training

Warmed up   Yes _____   No _____

Time of day: _____	For how long?	Heart Rate
Type 1: _____	_____	_____
Type 2: _____	_____	_____
Type 3: _____	_____	_____
Type 4: _____	_____	_____
Stretched? Yes _____ No _____		

Evening Reflection

Did I put my faith in Action today?	Yes _____	No _____
I prayed for somone today	Yes _____	No _____
I read my Bible today	Yes _____	No _____
I helped someone in need today	Yes _____	No _____
I got 6 1/2 to 8 hours of sleep last night	Yes _____	No _____
I know I ate right today	Yes _____	No _____
I ate breakfast today	Yes _____	No _____
I ate starches after 4:00 p.m. today	Yes _____	No _____
I ate at least 4 meals today	Yes _____	No _____
I drank at least a gallon of water today	Yes _____	No _____
I had Courage to Change today	Yes _____	No _____
Tonight I forgive…		

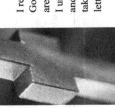

Captain's Log Statement of Faith

I realize that my actions don't earn my way into God's love or earn my way to heaven but that they are a reflection of my love affair with Jesus! I understand that by taking care of myself I honor and glorify God. I matter to God and the actions I take toward good health are daily written love letters telling God, "Thank you for my life"!

_____

Signature

Resistance Training

Time of day: _____

Warmed up   Yes _____   No _____

Name of exercise 1: _____

	Weight:	Reps:
Set 1:	_____	_____
Set 2:	_____	_____
Set 3:	_____	_____
Set 4:	_____	_____

Muscles worked: _____

Stretched?   Yes _____   No _____

Name of exercise 2: _____

	Weight:	Reps:
Set 1:	_____	_____
Set 2:	_____	_____
Set 3:	_____	_____
Set 4:	_____	_____

Muscles worked: _____

Stretched?   Yes _____   No _____

Name of exercise 3: _____

	Weight:	Reps:
Set 1:	_____	_____
Set 2:	_____	_____
Set 3:	_____	_____
Set 4:	_____	_____

Muscles worked: _____

Stretched?   Yes _____   No _____

Name of exercise 4: _____

	Weight:	Reps:
Set 1:	_____	_____
Set 2:	_____	_____
Set 3:	_____	_____
Set 4:	_____	_____

Muscles worked: _____

Stretched?   Yes _____   No _____

Name of exercise 5: _____

	Weight:	Reps:
Set 1:	_____	_____
Set 2:	_____	_____
Set 3:	_____	_____
Set 4:	_____	_____

Muscles worked: _____

Stretched?   Yes _____   No _____

Name of exercise 6: _____

	Weight:	Reps:
Set 1:	_____	_____
Set 2:	_____	_____
Set 3:	_____	_____
Set 4:	_____	_____

Muscles worked: _____

Stretched?   Yes _____   No _____

Name of exercise 7: _____

	Weight:	Reps:
Set 1:	_____	_____
Set 2:	_____	_____
Set 3:	_____	_____
Set 4:	_____	_____

Muscles worked: _____

Stretched?   Yes _____   No _____

Name of exercise 8: _____

	Weight:	Reps:
Set 1:	_____	_____
Set 2:	_____	_____
Set 3:	_____	_____
Set 4:	_____	_____

Muscles worked: _____

Stretched?   Yes _____   No _____

Name of exercise 9: _____

	Weight:	Reps:
Set 1:	_____	_____
Set 2:	_____	_____
Set 3:	_____	_____
Set 4:	_____	_____

Muscles worked: _____

Stretched?   Yes _____   No _____

Name of exercise 10: _____

	Weight:	Reps:
Set 1:	_____	_____
Set 2:	_____	_____
Set 3:	_____	_____
Set 4:	_____	_____

Muscles worked: _____

Stretched?   Yes _____   No _____

"I press on toward the goal to win the prize for which God has called me heavenward in Christ Jesus."

Philippians 3:14

Captain's Log

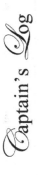

"Each one should test his own actions. Then he can take pride in himself without comparing himself to somebody else, for each one should carry his own load." (Galatians 6:40)

Day: _____ Date: _____ / _____ / _____

Nutrition Log

BREAKFAST   Time: _____

	Type	Amt:	Type	Amt:
Protein	1.		2.	
Complex Carbs	1.		2.	
Fruit	1.		2.	
Vegetables	1.		2.	
Fat	1.		2.	
Liquid/drink	1.		2.	
Meal Replace.	1.		2.	
Condiments	1.		2.	
Other	1.		2.	

SNACK 1   Time: _____

	Type	Amt:	Type	Amt:
Protein	1.		2.	
Complex Carbs	1.		2.	
Fruit	1.		2.	
Vegetables	1.		2.	
Fat	1.		2.	
Liquid/drink	1.		2.	
Meal Replace.	1.		2.	
Condiments	1.		2.	
Other	1.		2.	

LUNCH   Time: _____

	Type	Amt:	Type	Amt:
Protein	1.		2.	
Complex Carbs	1.		2.	
Fruit	1.		2.	
Vegetables	1.		2.	
Fat	1.		2.	
Liquid/drink	1.		2.	
Meal Replace.	1.		2.	
Condiments	1.		2.	
Other	1.		2.	

SNACK 2   Time: _____

	Type	Amt:	Type	Amt:
Protein	1.		2.	
Complex Carbs	1.		2.	
Fruit	1.		2.	
Vegetables	1.		2.	
Fat	1.		2.	
Liquid/drink	1.		2.	
Meal Replace.	1.		2.	
Condiments	1.		2.	
Other	1.		2.	

SNACK 3   Time: _____

	Type	Amt:	Type	Amt:
Protein	1.		2.	
Complex Carbs	1.		2.	
Fruit	1.		2.	
Vegetables	1.		2.	
Fat	1.		2.	
Liquid/drink	1.		2.	
Meal Replace.	1.		2.	
Condiments	1.		2.	
Other	1.		2.	

DINNER   Time: _____

	Type	Amt:	Type	Amt:
Protein	1.		2.	
Complex Carbs	1.		2.	
Fruit	1.		2.	
Vegetables	1.		2.	
Fat	1.		2.	
Liquid/drink	1.		2.	
Meal Replace.	1.		2.	
Condiments	1.		2.	
Other	1.		2.	

Cardiovascular Training

Warmed up   Yes _____   No _____

Time of day: _____			
		For how long?	Heart Rate
Type 1:	_____	_____	_____
Type 2:	_____	_____	_____
Type 3:	_____	_____	_____
Type 4:	_____	_____	_____
Stretched?	Yes _____	No _____	

Evening Reflection

Did I put my faith in Action today?	Yes _____	No _____
I prayed for somone today	Yes _____	No _____
I read my Bible today	Yes _____	No _____
I helped someone in need today	Yes _____	No _____
I got 6 1/2 to 8 hours of sleep last night	Yes _____	No _____
I know I ate right today	Yes _____	No _____
I ate breakfast today	Yes _____	No _____
I ate starches after 4:00 p.m. today	Yes _____	No _____
I ate at least 4 meals today	Yes _____	No _____
I drank at least a gallon of water today	Yes _____	No _____
I had Courage to Change today	Yes _____	No _____
Tonight I forgive... _____		

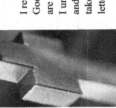

Captain's Log Statement of Faith

I realize that my actions don't earn my way into God's love or earn my way to heaven but that they are a reflection of my love affair with Jesus! I understand that by taking care of myself I honor and glorify God. I matter to God and the actions I take toward good health are daily written love letters telling God, "Thank you for my life"!

_____   **Signature**

Resistance Training

Time of day: _____

Warmed up   Yes _____   No _____

Name of exercise 1:
_____
_____

	Weight:	Reps:
Set 1:	_____	_____
Set 2:	_____	_____
Set 3:	_____	_____
Set 4:	_____	_____

Muscles worked:
_____
_____

Stretched?   Yes _____   No _____

Name of exercise 2:
_____
_____

	Weight:	Reps:
Set 1:	_____	_____
Set 2:	_____	_____
Set 3:	_____	_____
Set 4:	_____	_____

Muscles worked:
_____
_____

Stretched?   Yes _____   No _____

Name of exercise 3:
_____
_____

	Weight:	Reps:
Set 1:	_____	_____
Set 2:	_____	_____
Set 3:	_____	_____
Set 4:	_____	_____

Muscles worked:
_____
_____

Stretched?   Yes _____   No _____

Name of exercise 4:
_____
_____

	Weight:	Reps:
Set 1:	_____	_____
Set 2:	_____	_____
Set 3:	_____	_____
Set 4:	_____	_____

Muscles worked:
_____
_____

Stretched?   Yes _____   No _____

Name of exercise 5:
_____
_____

	Weight:	Reps:
Set 1:	_____	_____
Set 2:	_____	_____
Set 3:	_____	_____
Set 4:	_____	_____

Muscles worked:
_____
_____

Stretched?   Yes _____   No _____

Name of exercise 6:
_____
_____

	Weight:	Reps:
Set 1:	_____	_____
Set 2:	_____	_____
Set 3:	_____	_____
Set 4:	_____	_____

Muscles worked:
_____
_____

Stretched?   Yes _____   No _____

Name of exercise 7:
_____
_____

	Weight:	Reps:
Set 1:	_____	_____
Set 2:	_____	_____
Set 3:	_____	_____
Set 4:	_____	_____

Muscles worked:
_____
_____

Stretched?   Yes _____   No _____

Name of exercise 8:
_____
_____

	Weight:	Reps:
Set 1:	_____	_____
Set 2:	_____	_____
Set 3:	_____	_____
Set 4:	_____	_____

Muscles worked:
_____
_____

Stretched?   Yes _____   No _____

Name of exercise 9:
_____
_____

	Weight:	Reps:
Set 1:	_____	_____
Set 2:	_____	_____
Set 3:	_____	_____
Set 4:	_____	_____

Muscles worked:
_____
_____

Stretched?   Yes _____   No _____

Name of exercise 10:
_____
_____

	Weight:	Reps:
Set 1:	_____	_____
Set 2:	_____	_____
Set 3:	_____	_____
Set 4:	_____	_____

Muscles worked:
_____
_____

Stretched?   Yes _____   No _____

"I press on toward the goal to win the prize for which God has called me heavenward in Christ Jesus."

Philippians 3:14

Captain's Log

"Each one should test his own actions. Then he can take pride in himself without comparing himself to somebody else, for each one should carry his own load." (Galatians 6:40)

Day: _____   Date: ____ / ____ / ____

Nutrition Log

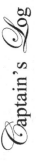

BREAKFAST	Time: _____		
	Type	Amt:	
Protein	1.		
Complex Carbs	1.		
Fruit	1.		
Vegetables	1.		
Fat	1.		
Liquid/drink	1.		
Meal Replace.	1.		
Condiments	1.		
Other	1.		
	Type	Amt:	
	2.		
	2.		
	2.		
	2.		
	2.		
	2.		
	2.		
	2.		
	2.		

SNACK 1	Time: _____		
	Type	Amt:	
Protein	1.		
Complex Carbs	1.		
Fruit	1.		
Vegetables	1.		
Fat	1.		
Liquid/drink	1.		
Meal Replace.	1.		
Condiments	1.		
Other	1.		
	Type	Amt:	
	2.		
	2.		
	2.		
	2.		
	2.		
	2.		
	2.		
	2.		
	2.		

LUNCH	Time: _____		
	Type	Amt:	
Protein	1.		
Complex Carbs	1.		
Fruit	1.		
Vegetables	1.		
Fat	1.		
Liquid/drink	1.		
Meal Replace.	1.		
Condiments	1.		
Other	1.		
	Type	Amt:	
	2.		
	2.		
	2.		
	2.		
	2.		
	2.		
	2.		
	2.		
	2.		

SNACK 2	Time: _____		
	Type	Amt:	
Protein	1.		
Complex Carbs	1.		
Fruit	1.		
Vegetables	1.		
Fat	1.		
Liquid/drink	1.		
Meal Replace.	1.		
Condiments	1.		
Other	1.		
	Type	Amt:	
	2.		
	2.		
	2.		
	2.		
	2.		
	2.		
	2.		
	2.		
	2.		

SNACK 3	Time: _____		
	Type	Amt:	
Protein	1.		
Complex Carbs	1.		
Fruit	1.		
Vegetables	1.		
Fat	1.		
Liquid/drink	1.		
Meal Replace.	1.		
Condiments	1.		
Other	1.		
	Type	Amt:	
	2.		
	2.		
	2.		
	2.		
	2.		
	2.		
	2.		
	2.		
	2.		

DINNER	Time: _____		
	Type	Amt:	
Protein	1.		
Complex Carbs	1.		
Fruit	1.		
Vegetables	1.		
Fat	1.		
Liquid/drink	1.		
Meal Replace.	1.		
Condiments	1.		
Other	1.		
	Type	Amt:	
	2.		
	2.		
	2.		
	2.		
	2.		
	2.		
	2.		
	2.		
	2.		

Cardiovascular Training

Time of day: _____
Warmed up Yes _____ No _____

Time of day:		For how long?	Heart Rate
Type 1:			
Type 2:			
Type 3:			
Type 4:			
Stretched?	Yes _____	No _____	

Evening Reflection

Did I put my faith in Action today?	Yes _____	No _____
I prayed for somone today	Yes _____	No _____
I read my Bible today	Yes _____	No _____
I helped someone in need today	Yes _____	No _____
I got 6 1/2 to 8 hours of sleep last night	Yes _____	No _____
I know I ate right today	Yes _____	No _____
I ate breakfast today	Yes _____	No _____
I ate starches after 4:00 p.m. today	Yes _____	No _____
I ate at least 4 meals today	Yes _____	No _____
I drank at least a gallon of water today	Yes _____	No _____
I had Courage to Change today	Yes _____	No _____
Tonight I forgive…		

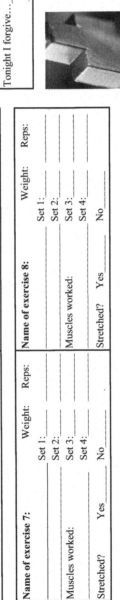

Captain's Log Statement of Faith

I realize that my actions don't earn my way into God's love or earn my way to heaven but that they are a reflection of my love affair with Jesus! I understand that by taking care of myself I honor and glorify God. I matter to God and the actions I take toward good health are daily written love letters telling God, "Thank you for my life"!

_____
Signature

Resistance Training

Time of day: _____
Warmed up Yes _____ No _____

Name of exercise 1: _____
Weight: Reps:
Set 1: _____
Set 2: _____
Muscles worked: _____ Set 3: _____
Set 4: _____
Stretched? Yes _____ No _____

Name of exercise 2: _____
Weight: Reps:
Set 1: _____
Set 2: _____
Muscles worked: _____ Set 3: _____
Set 4: _____
Stretched? Yes _____ No _____

Name of exercise 3: _____
Weight: Reps:
Set 1: _____
Set 2: _____
Muscles worked: _____ Set 3: _____
Set 4: _____
Stretched? Yes _____ No _____

Name of exercise 4: _____
Weight: Reps:
Set 1: _____
Set 2: _____
Muscles worked: _____ Set 3: _____
Set 4: _____
Stretched? Yes _____ No _____

Name of exercise 5: _____
Weight: Reps:
Set 1: _____
Set 2: _____
Muscles worked: _____ Set 3: _____
Set 4: _____
Stretched? Yes _____ No _____

Name of exercise 6: _____
Weight: Reps:
Set 1: _____
Set 2: _____
Muscles worked: _____ Set 3: _____
Set 4: _____
Stretched? Yes _____ No _____

Name of exercise 7: _____
Weight: Reps:
Set 1: _____
Set 2: _____
Muscles worked: _____ Set 3: _____
Set 4: _____
Stretched? Yes _____ No _____

Name of exercise 8: _____
Weight: Reps:
Set 1: _____
Set 2: _____
Muscles worked: _____ Set 3: _____
Set 4: _____
Stretched? Yes _____ No _____

Name of exercise 9: _____
Weight: Reps:
Set 1: _____
Set 2: _____
Muscles worked: _____ Set 3: _____
Set 4: _____
Stretched? Yes _____ No _____

Name of exercise 10: _____
Weight: Reps:
Set 1: _____
Set 2: _____
Muscles worked: _____ Set 3: _____
Set 4: _____
Stretched? Yes _____ No _____

"I press on toward the goal to win the prize for which God has called me heavenward in Christ Jesus."
Philippians 3:14

IMAGE OF GOD

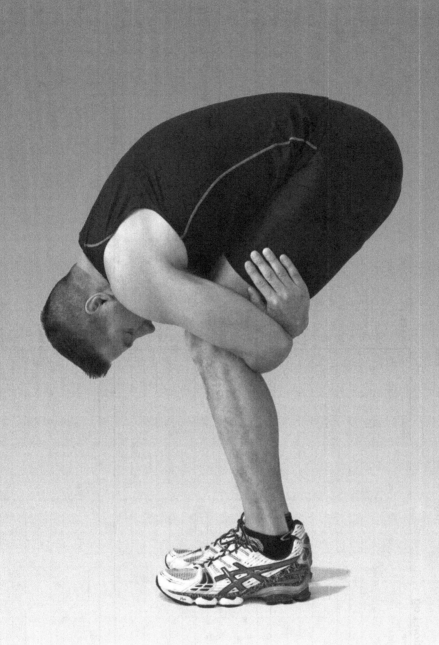

"Then God said, Let us make man in our image, in our likeness, and let them rule over the fish of the sea and the birds of the air, over the livestock, over all the earth, and over all the creatures that move along the ground." So God created him; male and female he created them.

WEEK TWELVE

Captain's Log

"Each one should test his own actions. Then he can take pride in himself without comparing himself to somebody else, for each one should carry his own load." (Galatians 6:40)

Day: _____   Date: _____ / _____ / _____

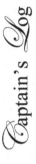
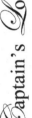

Nutrition Log

BREAKFAST   Time: _____

	Type	Amt:		Type	Amt:
Protein	1. ____ ____			2. ____ ____	
Complex Carbs	1. ____ ____			2. ____ ____	
Fruit	1. ____ ____			2. ____ ____	
Vegetables	1. ____ ____			2. ____ ____	
Fat	1. ____ ____			2. ____ ____	
Liquid/drink	1. ____ ____			2. ____ ____	
Meal Replace.	1. ____ ____			2. ____ ____	
Condiments	1. ____ ____			2. ____ ____	
Other	1. ____ ____			2. ____ ____	

LUNCH   Time: _____

	Type	Amt:		Type	Amt:
Protein	1. ____ ____			2. ____ ____	
Complex Carbs	1. ____ ____			2. ____ ____	
Fruit	1. ____ ____			2. ____ ____	
Vegetables	1. ____ ____			2. ____ ____	
Fat	1. ____ ____			2. ____ ____	
Liquid/drink	1. ____ ____			2. ____ ____	
Meal Replace.	1. ____ ____			2. ____ ____	
Condiments	1. ____ ____			2. ____ ____	
Other	1. ____ ____			2. ____ ____	

SNACK 3   Time: _____

	Type	Amt:		Type	Amt:
Protein	1. ____ ____			2. ____ ____	
Complex Carbs	1. ____ ____			2. ____ ____	
Fruit	1. ____ ____			2. ____ ____	
Vegetables	1. ____ ____			2. ____ ____	
Fat	1. ____ ____			2. ____ ____	
Liquid/drink	1. ____ ____			2. ____ ____	
Meal Replace.	1. ____ ____			2. ____ ____	
Condiments	1. ____ ____			2. ____ ____	
Other	1. ____ ____			2. ____ ____	

SNACK 1   Time: _____

	Type	Amt:		Type	Amt:
Protein	1. ____ ____			2. ____ ____	
Complex Carbs	1. ____ ____			2. ____ ____	
Fruit	1. ____ ____			2. ____ ____	
Vegetables	1. ____ ____			2. ____ ____	
Fat	1. ____ ____			2. ____ ____	
Liquid/drink	1. ____ ____			2. ____ ____	
Meal Replace.	1. ____ ____			2. ____ ____	
Condiments	1. ____ ____			2. ____ ____	
Other	1. ____ ____			2. ____ ____	

SNACK 2   Time: _____

	Type	Amt:		Type	Amt:
Protein	1. ____ ____			2. ____ ____	
Complex Carbs	1. ____ ____			2. ____ ____	
Fruit	1. ____ ____			2. ____ ____	
Vegetables	1. ____ ____			2. ____ ____	
Fat	1. ____ ____			2. ____ ____	
Liquid/drink	1. ____ ____			2. ____ ____	
Meal Replace.	1. ____ ____			2. ____ ____	
Condiments	1. ____ ____			2. ____ ____	
Other	1. ____ ____			2. ____ ____	

DINNER   Time: _____

	Type	Amt:		Type	Amt:
Protein	1. ____ ____			2. ____ ____	
Complex Carbs	1. ____ ____			2. ____ ____	
Fruit	1. ____ ____			2. ____ ____	
Vegetables	1. ____ ____			2. ____ ____	
Fat	1. ____ ____			2. ____ ____	
Liquid/drink	1. ____ ____			2. ____ ____	
Meal Replace.	1. ____ ____			2. ____ ____	
Condiments	1. ____ ____			2. ____ ____	
Other	1. ____ ____			2. ____ ____	

Cardiovascular Training

Warmed up   Yes _____   No _____

Time of day:	For how long?	Heart Rate
Type 1:	_____	_____
Type 2:	_____	_____
Type 3:	_____	_____
Type 4:	_____	_____
Stretched? Yes_____ No_____		

Evening Reflection

Did I put my faith in Action today?	Yes _____	No _____
I prayed for somone today	Yes _____	No _____
I read my Bible today	Yes _____	No _____
I helped someone in need today	Yes _____	No _____
I got 6 1/2 to 8 hours of sleep last night	Yes _____	No _____
I know I ate right today	Yes _____	No _____
I ate breakfast today	Yes _____	No _____
I ate starches after 4:00 p.m. today	Yes _____	No _____
I ate at least 4 meals today	Yes _____	No _____
I drank at least a gallon of water today	Yes _____	No _____
I had Courage to Change today	Yes _____	No _____
Tonight I forgive…		

Captain's Log Statement of Faith

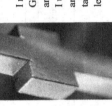

I realize that my actions don't earn my way into God's love or earn my way to heaven but that they are a reflection of my love affair with Jesus! I understand that by taking care of myself I honor and glorify God. I matter to God and the actions I take toward good health are daily written love letters telling God, "Thank you for my life"!

_____
Signature

"I press on toward the goal to win the prize for which God has called me heavenward in Christ Jesus."
Philippians 3:14

Resistance Training

Time of day: _____

Warmed up   Yes _____   No _____

Name of exercise 1:

	Weight:	Reps:
Set 1:	_____	_____
Set 2:	_____	_____
Set 3:	_____	_____
Set 4:	_____	_____

Muscles worked: _____

Stretched?   Yes_____   No _____

Name of exercise 2:

	Weight:	Reps:
Set 1:	_____	_____
Set 2:	_____	_____
Set 3:	_____	_____
Set 4:	_____	_____

Muscles worked: _____

Stretched?   Yes_____   No _____

Name of exercise 3:

	Weight:	Reps:
Set 1:	_____	_____
Set 2:	_____	_____
Set 3:	_____	_____
Set 4:	_____	_____

Muscles worked: _____

Stretched?   Yes_____   No _____

Name of exercise 4:

	Weight:	Reps:
Set 1:	_____	_____
Set 2:	_____	_____
Set 3:	_____	_____
Set 4:	_____	_____

Muscles worked: _____

Stretched?   Yes_____   No _____

Name of exercise 5:

	Weight:	Reps:
Set 1:	_____	_____
Set 2:	_____	_____
Set 3:	_____	_____
Set 4:	_____	_____

Muscles worked: _____

Stretched?   Yes_____   No _____

Name of exercise 6:

	Weight:	Reps:
Set 1:	_____	_____
Set 2:	_____	_____
Set 3:	_____	_____
Set 4:	_____	_____

Muscles worked: _____

Stretched?   Yes_____   No _____

Name of exercise 7:

	Weight:	Reps:
Set 1:	_____	_____
Set 2:	_____	_____
Set 3:	_____	_____
Set 4:	_____	_____

Muscles worked: _____

Stretched?   Yes_____   No _____

Name of exercise 8:

	Weight:	Reps:
Set 1:	_____	_____
Set 2:	_____	_____
Set 3:	_____	_____
Set 4:	_____	_____

Muscles worked: _____

Stretched?   Yes_____   No _____

Name of exercise 9:

	Weight:	Reps:
Set 1:	_____	_____
Set 2:	_____	_____
Set 3:	_____	_____
Set 4:	_____	_____

Muscles worked: _____

Stretched?   Yes_____   No _____

Name of exercise 10:

	Weight:	Reps:
Set 1:	_____	_____
Set 2:	_____	_____
Set 3:	_____	_____
Set 4:	_____	_____

Muscles worked: _____

Stretched?   Yes_____   No _____

Captain's Log

"Each one should test his own actions. Then he can take pride in himself without comparing himself to somebody else, for each one should carry his own load." (Galatians 6:40)

Day: _____ Date: _____ / _____ / _____

Nutrition Log

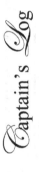

BREAKFAST	Time: _____				Time: _____			
	Type	Amt:	Type	Amt:	SNACK 1	Type	Amt:	Type	Amt:
Protein	1. _____	_____	2. _____	_____	Protein	1. _____	_____	2. _____	_____
Complex Carbs	1. _____	_____	2. _____	_____	Complex Carbs	1. _____	_____	2. _____	_____
Fruit	1. _____	_____	2. _____	_____	Fruit	1. _____	_____	2. _____	_____
Vegetables	1. _____	_____	2. _____	_____	Vegetables	1. _____	_____	2. _____	_____
Fat	1. _____	_____	2. _____	_____	Fat	1. _____	_____	2. _____	_____
Liquid/drink	1. _____	_____	2. _____	_____	Liquid/drink	1. _____	_____	2. _____	_____
Meal Replace.	1. _____	_____	2. _____	_____	Meal Replace.	1. _____	_____	2. _____	_____
Condiments	1. _____	_____	2. _____	_____	Condiments	1. _____	_____	2. _____	_____
Other	1. _____	_____	2. _____	_____	Other	1. _____	_____	2. _____	_____

LUNCH	Time: _____				SNACK 2	Time: _____			
	Type	Amt:	Type	Amt:		Type	Amt:	Type	Amt:
Protein	1. _____	_____	2. _____	_____	Protein	1. _____	_____	2. _____	_____
Complex Carbs	1. _____	_____	2. _____	_____	Complex Carbs	1. _____	_____	2. _____	_____
Fruit	1. _____	_____	2. _____	_____	Fruit	1. _____	_____	2. _____	_____
Vegetables	1. _____	_____	2. _____	_____	Vegetables	1. _____	_____	2. _____	_____
Fat	1. _____	_____	2. _____	_____	Fat	1. _____	_____	2. _____	_____
Liquid/drink	1. _____	_____	2. _____	_____	Liquid/drink	1. _____	_____	2. _____	_____
Meal Replace.	1. _____	_____	2. _____	_____	Meal Replace.	1. _____	_____	2. _____	_____
Condiments	1. _____	_____	2. _____	_____	Condiments	1. _____	_____	2. _____	_____
Other	1. _____	_____	2. _____	_____	Other	1. _____	_____	2. _____	_____

SNACK 3	Time: _____				DINNER	Time: _____			
	Type	Amt:	Type	Amt:		Type	Amt:	Type	Amt:
Protein	1. _____	_____	2. _____	_____	Protein	1. _____	_____	2. _____	_____
Complex Carbs	1. _____	_____	2. _____	_____	Complex Carbs	1. _____	_____	2. _____	_____
Fruit	1. _____	_____	2. _____	_____	Fruit	1. _____	_____	2. _____	_____
Vegetables	1. _____	_____	2. _____	_____	Vegetables	1. _____	_____	2. _____	_____
Fat	1. _____	_____	2. _____	_____	Fat	1. _____	_____	2. _____	_____
Liquid/drink	1. _____	_____	2. _____	_____	Liquid/drink	1. _____	_____	2. _____	_____
Meal Replace.	1. _____	_____	2. _____	_____	Meal Replace.	1. _____	_____	2. _____	_____
Condiments	1. _____	_____	2. _____	_____	Condiments	1. _____	_____	2. _____	_____
Other	1. _____	_____	2. _____	_____	Other	1. _____	_____	2. _____	_____

Cardiovascular Training

Warmed up   Yes _____   No _____

Time of day: _____	For how long?	Heart Rate
Type 1: _____	_____	_____
Type 2: _____	_____	_____
Type 3: _____	_____	_____
Type 4: _____	_____	_____

Stretched?   Yes _____   No _____

Resistance Training

Time of day: _____

Warmed up   Yes _____   No _____

Name of exercise 1: _____

	Weight:	Reps:
Set 1:	_____	_____
Set 2:	_____	_____
Set 3:	_____	_____
Set 4:	_____	_____

Muscles worked: _____

Stretched?   Yes _____   No _____

Name of exercise 2: _____

	Weight:	Reps:
Set 1:	_____	_____
Set 2:	_____	_____
Set 3:	_____	_____
Set 4:	_____	_____

Muscles worked: _____

Stretched?   Yes _____   No _____

Name of exercise 3: _____

	Weight:	Reps:
Set 1:	_____	_____
Set 2:	_____	_____
Set 3:	_____	_____
Set 4:	_____	_____

Muscles worked: _____

Stretched?   Yes _____   No _____

Name of exercise 4: _____

	Weight:	Reps:
Set 1:	_____	_____
Set 2:	_____	_____
Set 3:	_____	_____
Set 4:	_____	_____

Muscles worked: _____

Stretched?   Yes _____   No _____

Name of exercise 5: _____

	Weight:	Reps:
Set 1:	_____	_____
Set 2:	_____	_____
Set 3:	_____	_____
Set 4:	_____	_____

Muscles worked: _____

Stretched?   Yes _____   No _____

Name of exercise 6: _____

	Weight:	Reps:
Set 1:	_____	_____
Set 2:	_____	_____
Set 3:	_____	_____
Set 4:	_____	_____

Muscles worked: _____

Stretched?   Yes _____   No _____

Name of exercise 7: _____

	Weight:	Reps:
Set 1:	_____	_____
Set 2:	_____	_____
Set 3:	_____	_____
Set 4:	_____	_____

Muscles worked: _____

Stretched?   Yes _____   No _____

Name of exercise 8: _____

	Weight:	Reps:
Set 1:	_____	_____
Set 2:	_____	_____
Set 3:	_____	_____
Set 4:	_____	_____

Muscles worked: _____

Stretched?   Yes _____   No _____

Name of exercise 9: _____

	Weight:	Reps:
Set 1:	_____	_____
Set 2:	_____	_____
Set 3:	_____	_____
Set 4:	_____	_____

Muscles worked: _____

Stretched?   Yes _____   No _____

Name of exercise 10: _____

	Weight:	Reps:
Set 1:	_____	_____
Set 2:	_____	_____
Set 3:	_____	_____
Set 4:	_____	_____

Muscles worked: _____

Stretched?   Yes _____   No _____

Evening Reflection

Did I put my faith in Action today?	Yes _____	No _____
I prayed for somone today	Yes _____	No _____
I read my Bible today	Yes _____	No _____
I helped someone in need today	Yes _____	No _____
I got 6 1/2 to 8 hours of sleep last night	Yes _____	No _____
I know I ate right today	Yes _____	No _____
I ate breakfast today	Yes _____	No _____
I ate starches after 4:00 p.m. today	Yes _____	No _____
I ate at least 4 meals today	Yes _____	No _____
I drank at least a gallon of water today	Yes _____	No _____
I had Courage to Change today	Yes _____	No _____
Tonight I forgive…		

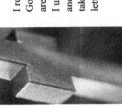

Captain's Log Statement of Faith

I realize that my actions don't earn my way into God's love or earn my way to heaven but that they are a reflection of my love affair with Jesus! I understand that by taking care of myself I honor and glorify God. I matter to God and the actions I take toward good health are daily written love letters telling God, "Thank you for my life"!

_____ Signature

"I press on toward the goal to win the prize for which God has called me heavenward in Christ Jesus."
Philippians 3:14

Captain's Log

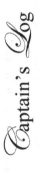

"Each one should test his own actions. Then he can take pride in himself without comparing himself to somebody else, for each one should carry his own load." (Galatians 6:40)

Day: _____ Date: _____ / _____ / _____

Nutrition Log

BREAKFAST Time: _____

	Type	Amt:		Type	Amt:
Protein	1. _____	_____		2. _____	_____
Complex Carbs	1. _____	_____		2. _____	_____
Fruit	1. _____	_____		2. _____	_____
Vegetables	1. _____	_____		2. _____	_____
Fat	1. _____	_____		2. _____	_____
Liquid/drink	1. _____	_____		2. _____	_____
Meal Replace.	1. _____	_____		2. _____	_____
Condiments	1. _____	_____		2. _____	_____
Other	1. _____	_____		2. _____	_____

SNACK 1 Time: _____

	Type	Amt:		Type	Amt:
Protein	1. _____	_____		2. _____	_____
Complex Carbs	1. _____	_____		2. _____	_____
Fruit	1. _____	_____		2. _____	_____
Vegetables	1. _____	_____		2. _____	_____
Fat	1. _____	_____		2. _____	_____
Liquid/drink	1. _____	_____		2. _____	_____
Meal Replace.	1. _____	_____		2. _____	_____
Condiments	1. _____	_____		2. _____	_____
Other	1. _____	_____		2. _____	_____

LUNCH Time: _____

	Type	Amt:		Type	Amt:
Protein	1. _____	_____		2. _____	_____
Complex Carbs	1. _____	_____		2. _____	_____
Fruit	1. _____	_____		2. _____	_____
Vegetables	1. _____	_____		2. _____	_____
Fat	1. _____	_____		2. _____	_____
Liquid/drink	1. _____	_____		2. _____	_____
Meal Replace.	1. _____	_____		2. _____	_____
Condiments	1. _____	_____		2. _____	_____
Other	1. _____	_____		2. _____	_____

SNACK 2 Time: _____

	Type	Amt:		Type	Amt:
Protein	1. _____	_____		2. _____	_____
Complex Carbs	1. _____	_____		2. _____	_____
Fruit	1. _____	_____		2. _____	_____
Vegetables	1. _____	_____		2. _____	_____
Fat	1. _____	_____		2. _____	_____
Liquid/drink	1. _____	_____		2. _____	_____
Meal Replace.	1. _____	_____		2. _____	_____
Condiments	1. _____	_____		2. _____	_____
Other	1. _____	_____		2. _____	_____

SNACK 3 Time: _____

	Type	Amt:		Type	Amt:
Protein	1. _____	_____		2. _____	_____
Complex Carbs	1. _____	_____		2. _____	_____
Fruit	1. _____	_____		2. _____	_____
Vegetables	1. _____	_____		2. _____	_____
Fat	1. _____	_____		2. _____	_____
Liquid/drink	1. _____	_____		2. _____	_____
Meal Replace.	1. _____	_____		2. _____	_____
Condiments	1. _____	_____		2. _____	_____
Other	1. _____	_____		2. _____	_____

DINNER Time: _____

	Type	Amt:		Type	Amt:
Protein	1. _____	_____		2. _____	_____
Complex Carbs	1. _____	_____		2. _____	_____
Fruit	1. _____	_____		2. _____	_____
Vegetables	1. _____	_____		2. _____	_____
Fat	1. _____	_____		2. _____	_____
Liquid/drink	1. _____	_____		2. _____	_____
Meal Replace.	1. _____	_____		2. _____	_____
Condiments	1. _____	_____		2. _____	_____
Other	1. _____	_____		2. _____	_____

Resistance Training

Time of day: _____
Warmed up   Yes _____   No _____

Name of exercise 1:
	Weight:	Reps:
Set 1:		
Set 2:		
Set 3:		
Set 4:		

Muscles worked: _____

Stretched?   Yes _____   No _____

Name of exercise 2:
	Weight:	Reps:
Set 1:		
Set 2:		
Set 3:		
Set 4:		

Muscles worked: _____

Stretched?   Yes _____   No _____

Name of exercise 3:
	Weight:	Reps:
Set 1:		
Set 2:		
Set 3:		
Set 4:		

Muscles worked: _____

Stretched?   Yes _____   No _____

Name of exercise 4:
	Weight:	Reps:
Set 1:		
Set 2:		
Set 3:		
Set 4:		

Muscles worked: _____

Stretched?   Yes _____   No _____

Name of exercise 5:
	Weight:	Reps:
Set 1:		
Set 2:		
Set 3:		
Set 4:		

Muscles worked: _____

Stretched?   Yes _____   No _____

Name of exercise 6:
	Weight:	Reps:
Set 1:		
Set 2:		
Set 3:		
Set 4:		

Muscles worked: _____

Stretched?   Yes _____   No _____

Name of exercise 7:
	Weight:	Reps:
Set 1:		
Set 2:		
Set 3:		
Set 4:		

Muscles worked: _____

Stretched?   Yes _____   No _____

Name of exercise 8:
	Weight:	Reps:
Set 1:		
Set 2:		
Set 3:		
Set 4:		

Muscles worked: _____

Stretched?   Yes _____   No _____

Name of exercise 9:
	Weight:	Reps:
Set 1:		
Set 2:		
Set 3:		
Set 4:		

Muscles worked: _____

Stretched?   Yes _____   No _____

Name of exercise 10:
	Weight:	Reps:
Set 1:		
Set 2:		
Set 3:		
Set 4:		

Muscles worked: _____

Stretched?   Yes _____   No _____

Cardiovascular Training

Warmed up   Yes _____   No _____

Time of day: _____

Type	For how long?	Heart Rate
Type 1:		
Type 2:		
Type 3:		
Type 4:		

Stretched?   Yes _____   No _____

Evening Reflection

Did I put my faith in Action today?	Yes _____	No _____
I prayed for somone today	Yes _____	No _____
I read my Bible today	Yes _____	No _____
I helped someone in need today	Yes _____	No _____
I got 6 1/2 to 8 hours of sleep last night	Yes _____	No _____
I know I ate right today	Yes _____	No _____
I ate breakfast today	Yes _____	No _____
I ate starches after 4:00 p.m. today	Yes _____	No _____
I ate at least 4 meals today	Yes _____	No _____
I drank at least a gallon of water today	Yes _____	No _____
I had Courage to Change today	Yes _____	No _____
Tonight I forgive...		

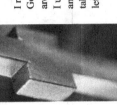

Captain's Log Statement of Faith

I realize that my actions don't earn my way into God's love or earn my way to heaven but that they are a reflection of my love affair with Jesus! I understand that by taking care of myself I honor and glorify God. I matter to God and the actions I take toward good health are daily written love letters telling God, "Thank you for my life"!

_____
Signature

"I press on toward the goal to win the prize for which God has called me heavenward in Christ Jesus."
Philippians 3:14

Captain's Log

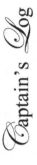 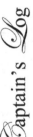

"Each one should test his own actions. Then he can take pride in himself without comparing himself to somebody else, for each one should carry his own load." (Galatians 6:40)

Day: _____   Date: ____ / ____ / ____

Nutrition Log

BREAKFAST	Time:				SNACK 1	Time:			
	Type 1.	Amt:	Type 2.	Amt:		Type 1.	Amt:	Type 2.	Amt:
Protein	1.		2.		Protein	1.		2.	
Complex Carbs	1.		2.		Complex Carbs	1.		2.	
Fruit	1.		2.		Fruit	1.		2.	
Vegetables	1.		2.		Vegetables	1.		2.	
Fat	1.		2.		Fat	1.		2.	
Liquid/drink	1.		2.		Liquid/drink	1.		2.	
Meal Replace.	1.		2.		Meal Replace.	1.		2.	
Condiments	1.		2.		Condiments	1.		2.	
Other	1.		2.		Other	1.		2.	

LUNCH	Time:				SNACK 2	Time:			
	Type 1.	Amt:	Type 2.	Amt:		Type 1.	Amt:	Type 2.	Amt:
Protein	1.		2.		Protein	1.		2.	
Complex Carbs	1.		2.		Complex Carbs	1.		2.	
Fruit	1.		2.		Fruit	1.		2.	
Vegetables	1.		2.		Vegetables	1.		2.	
Fat	1.		2.		Fat	1.		2.	
Liquid/drink	1.		2.		Liquid/drink	1.		2.	
Meal Replace.	1.		2.		Meal Replace.	1.		2.	
Condiments	1.		2.		Condiments	1.		2.	
Other	1.		2.		Other	1.		2.	

SNACK 3	Time:				DINNER	Time:			
	Type 1.	Amt:	Type 2.	Amt:		Type 1.	Amt:	Type 2.	Amt:
Protein	1.		2.		Protein	1.		2.	
Complex Carbs	1.		2.		Complex Carbs	1.		2.	
Fruit	1.		2.		Fruit	1.		2.	
Vegetables	1.		2.		Vegetables	1.		2.	
Fat	1.		2.		Fat	1.		2.	
Liquid/drink	1.		2.		Liquid/drink	1.		2.	
Meal Replace.	1.		2.		Meal Replace.	1.		2.	
Condiments	1.		2.		Condiments	1.		2.	
Other	1.		2.		Other	1.		2.	

Cardiovascular Training

Warmed up   Yes _____   No _____

Time of day: _____	For how long?	Heart Rate
Type 1:	_____	_____
Type 2:	_____	_____
Type 3:	_____	_____
Type 4:	_____	_____
Stretched? Yes _____ No _____		

Evening Reflection

Did I put my faith in Action today?	Yes _____	No _____
I prayed for somone today	Yes _____	No _____
I read my Bible today	Yes _____	No _____
I helped someone in need today	Yes _____	No _____
I got 6 1/2 to 8 hours of sleep last night	Yes _____	No _____
I know I ate right today	Yes _____	No _____
I ate breakfast today	Yes _____	No _____
I ate starches after 4:00 p.m. today	Yes _____	No _____
I ate at least 4 meals today	Yes _____	No _____
I drank at least a gallon of water today	Yes _____	No _____
I had Courage to Change today	Yes _____	No _____
Tonight I forgive… _____		

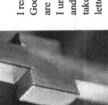

Captain's Log Statement of Faith

I realize that my actions don't earn my way into God's love or earn my way to heaven but that they are a reflection of my love affair with Jesus! I understand that by taking care of myself I honor and glorify God. I matter to God and the actions I take toward good health are daily written love letters telling God, "Thank you for my life"!

_____
Signature

Resistance Training

Time of day: _____
Warmed up   Yes _____   No _____

Name of exercise 1:	Weight:	Reps:
	Set 1: _____	
	Set 2: _____	
Muscles worked:	Set 3: _____	
	Set 4: _____	
Stretched? Yes _____ No _____		

Name of exercise 2:	Weight:	Reps:
	Set 1: _____	
	Set 2: _____	
Muscles worked:	Set 3: _____	
	Set 4: _____	
Stretched? Yes _____ No _____		

Name of exercise 3:	Weight:	Reps:
	Set 1: _____	
	Set 2: _____	
Muscles worked:	Set 3: _____	
	Set 4: _____	
Stretched? Yes _____ No _____		

Name of exercise 4:	Weight:	Reps:
	Set 1: _____	
	Set 2: _____	
Muscles worked:	Set 3: _____	
	Set 4: _____	
Stretched? Yes _____ No _____		

Name of exercise 5:	Weight:	Reps:
	Set 1: _____	
	Set 2: _____	
Muscles worked:	Set 3: _____	
	Set 4: _____	
Stretched? Yes _____ No _____		

Name of exercise 6:	Weight:	Reps:
	Set 1: _____	
	Set 2: _____	
Muscles worked:	Set 3: _____	
	Set 4: _____	
Stretched? Yes _____ No _____		

Name of exercise 7:	Weight:	Reps:
	Set 1: _____	
	Set 2: _____	
Muscles worked:	Set 3: _____	
	Set 4: _____	
Stretched? Yes _____ No _____		

Name of exercise 8:	Weight: ,	Reps:
	Set 1: _____	
	Set 2: _____	
Muscles worked:	Set 3: _____	
	Set 4: _____	
Stretched? Yes _____ No _____		

Name of exercise 9:	Weight:	Reps:
	Set 1: _____	
	Set 2: _____	
Muscles worked:	Set 3: _____	
	Set 4: _____	
Stretched? Yes _____ No _____		

Name of exercise 10:	Weight:	Reps:
	Set 1: _____	
	Set 2: _____	
Muscles worked:	Set 3: _____	
	Set 4: _____	
Stretched? Yes _____ No _____		

"I press on toward the goal to win the prize for which God has called me heavenward in Christ Jesus."
Philippians 3:14

Captain's Log

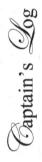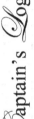

"Each one should test his own actions. Then he can take pride in himself without comparing himself to somebody else, for each one should carry his own load." (Galatians 6:40)

Day: _____   Date: ____ / ____ / ____

Nutrition Log

BREAKFAST   Time: _____

	Type	Amt:
Protein	1. _____ / 2. _____	_____
Complex Carbs	1. _____ / 2. _____	_____
Fruit	1. _____ / 2. _____	_____
Vegetables	1. _____ / 2. _____	_____
Fat	1. _____ / 2. _____	_____
Liquid/drink	1. _____ / 2. _____	_____
Meal Replace.	1. _____ / 2. _____	_____
Condiments	1. _____ / 2. _____	_____
Other	1. _____ / 2. _____	_____

SNACK 1   Time: _____

	Type	Amt:
Protein	1. _____ / 2. _____	_____
Complex Carbs	1. _____ / 2. _____	_____
Fruit	1. _____ / 2. _____	_____
Vegetables	1. _____ / 2. _____	_____
Fat	1. _____ / 2. _____	_____
Liquid/drink	1. _____ / 2. _____	_____
Meal Replace.	1. _____ / 2. _____	_____
Condiments	1. _____ / 2. _____	_____
Other	1. _____ / 2. _____	_____

LUNCH   Time: _____

	Type	Amt:
Protein	1. _____ / 2. _____	_____
Complex Carbs	1. _____ / 2. _____	_____
Fruit	1. _____ / 2. _____	_____
Vegetables	1. _____ / 2. _____	_____
Fat	1. _____ / 2. _____	_____
Liquid/drink	1. _____ / 2. _____	_____
Meal Replace.	1. _____ / 2. _____	_____
Condiments	1. _____ / 2. _____	_____
Other	1. _____ / 2. _____	_____

SNACK 2   Time: _____

	Type	Amt:
Protein	1. _____ / 2. _____	_____
Complex Carbs	1. _____ / 2. _____	_____
Fruit	1. _____ / 2. _____	_____
Vegetables	1. _____ / 2. _____	_____
Fat	1. _____ / 2. _____	_____
Liquid/drink	1. _____ / 2. _____	_____
Meal Replace.	1. _____ / 2. _____	_____
Condiments	1. _____ / 2. _____	_____
Other	1. _____ / 2. _____	_____

SNACK 3   Time: _____

	Type	Amt:
Protein	1. _____ / 2. _____	_____
Complex Carbs	1. _____ / 2. _____	_____
Fruit	1. _____ / 2. _____	_____
Vegetables	1. _____ / 2. _____	_____
Fat	1. _____ / 2. _____	_____
Liquid/drink	1. _____ / 2. _____	_____
Meal Replace.	1. _____ / 2. _____	_____
Condiments	1. _____ / 2. _____	_____
Other	1. _____ / 2. _____	_____

DINNER   Time: _____

	Type	Amt:
Protein	1. _____ / 2. _____	_____
Complex Carbs	1. _____ / 2. _____	_____
Fruit	1. _____ / 2. _____	_____
Vegetables	1. _____ / 2. _____	_____
Fat	1. _____ / 2. _____	_____
Liquid/drink	1. _____ / 2. _____	_____
Meal Replace.	1. _____ / 2. _____	_____
Condiments	1. _____ / 2. _____	_____
Other	1. _____ / 2. _____	_____

Cardiovascular Training

Warmed up   Yes _____   No _____

	For how long?	Heart Rate
Type 1:	_____	_____
Type 2:	_____	_____
Type 3:	_____	_____
Type 4:	_____	_____

Time of day: _____

Stretched?   Yes _____   No _____

Evening Reflection

Did I put my faith in Action today?	Yes _____	No _____
I prayed for somone today	Yes _____	No _____
I read my Bible today	Yes _____	No _____
I helped someone in need today	Yes _____	No _____
I got 6 1/2 to 8 hours of sleep last night	Yes _____	No _____
I know I ate right today	Yes _____	No _____
I ate breakfast today	Yes _____	No _____
I ate starches after 4:00 p.m. today	Yes _____	No _____
I ate at least 4 meals today	Yes _____	No _____
I drank at least a gallon of water today	Yes _____	No _____
I had Courage to Change today	Yes _____	No _____
Tonight I forgive…		

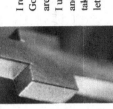

Captain's Log Statement of Faith

I realize that my actions don't earn my way into God's love or earn my way to heaven but that they are a reflection of my love affair with Jesus! I understand that by taking care of myself I honor and glorify God. I matter to God and the actions I take toward good health are daily written love letters telling God, "Thank you for my life"!

_____
Signature

Resistance Training

Time of day: _____

Warmed up   Yes _____   No _____

Name of exercise 1: _____

	Weight:	Reps:
Set 1:	_____	_____
Set 2:	_____	_____
Set 3:	_____	_____
Set 4:	_____	_____

Muscles worked: _____

Stretched?   Yes _____   No _____

Name of exercise 2: _____

	Weight:	Reps:
Set 1:	_____	_____
Set 2:	_____	_____
Set 3:	_____	_____
Set 4:	_____	_____

Muscles worked: _____

Stretched?   Yes _____   No _____

Name of exercise 3: _____

	Weight:	Reps:
Set 1:	_____	_____
Set 2:	_____	_____
Set 3:	_____	_____
Set 4:	_____	_____

Muscles worked: _____

Stretched?   Yes _____   No _____

Name of exercise 4: _____

	Weight:	Reps:
Set 1:	_____	_____
Set 2:	_____	_____
Set 3:	_____	_____
Set 4:	_____	_____

Muscles worked: _____

Stretched?   Yes _____   No _____

Name of exercise 5: _____

	Weight:	Reps:
Set 1:	_____	_____
Set 2:	_____	_____
Set 3:	_____	_____
Set 4:	_____	_____

Muscles worked: _____

Stretched?   Yes _____   No _____

Name of exercise 6: _____

	Weight:	Reps:
Set 1:	_____	_____
Set 2:	_____	_____
Set 3:	_____	_____
Set 4:	_____	_____

Muscles worked: _____

Stretched?   Yes _____   No _____

Name of exercise 7: _____

	Weight:	Reps:
Set 1:	_____	_____
Set 2:	_____	_____
Set 3:	_____	_____
Set 4:	_____	_____

Muscles worked: _____

Stretched?   Yes _____   No _____

Name of exercise 8: _____

	Weight:	Reps:
Set 1:	_____	_____
Set 2:	_____	_____
Set 3:	_____	_____
Set 4:	_____	_____

Muscles worked: _____

Stretched?   Yes _____   No _____

Name of exercise 9: _____

	Weight:	Reps:
Set 1:	_____	_____
Set 2:	_____	_____
Set 3:	_____	_____
Set 4:	_____	_____

Muscles worked: _____

Stretched?   Yes _____   No _____

Name of exercise 10: _____

	Weight:	Reps:
Set 1:	_____	_____
Set 2:	_____	_____
Set 3:	_____	_____
Set 4:	_____	_____

Muscles worked: _____

Stretched?   Yes _____   No _____

"I press on toward the goal to win the prize for which God has called me heavenward in Christ Jesus."
Philippians 3:14

Captain's Log

"Each one should test his own actions. Then he can take pride in himself without comparing himself to somebody else, for each one should carry his own load." (Galatians 6:40)

Day: _____   Date: _____ / _____ / _____

Nutrition Log

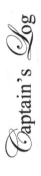

BREAKFAST	Time: _____		
	Type	Amt:	
Protein	1.		
Complex Carbs	1.		
Fruit	1.		
Vegetables	1.		
Fat	1.		
Liquid/drink	1.		
Meal Replace.	1.		
Condiments	1.		
Other	1.		

	Type	Amt:
	2.	
	2.	
	2.	
	2.	
	2.	
	2.	
	2.	
	2.	
	2.	

SNACK 1	Time: _____		
	Type	Amt:	
Protein	1.		
Complex Carbs	1.		
Fruit	1.		
Vegetables	1.		
Fat	1.		
Liquid/drink	1.		
Meal Replace.	1.		
Condiments	1.		
Other	1.		

	Type	Amt:
	2.	
	2.	
	2.	
	2.	
	2.	
	2.	
	2.	
	2.	
	2.	

LUNCH	Time: _____		
	Type	Amt:	
Protein	1.		
Complex Carbs	1.		
Fruit	1.		
Vegetables	1.		
Fat	1.		
Liquid/drink	1.		
Meal Replace.	1.		
Condiments	1.		
Other	1.		

	Type	Amt:
	2.	
	2.	
	2.	
	2.	
	2.	
	2.	
	2.	
	2.	
	2.	

SNACK 2	Time: _____		
	Type	Amt:	
Protein	1.		
Complex Carbs	1.		
Fruit	1.		
Vegetables	1.		
Fat	1.		
Liquid/drink	1.		
Meal Replace.	1.		
Condiments	1.		
Other	1.		

	Type	Amt:
	2.	
	2.	
	2.	
	2.	
	2.	
	2.	
	2.	
	2.	
	2.	

SNACK 3	Time: _____		
	Type	Amt:	
Protein	1.		
Complex Carbs	1.		
Fruit	1.		
Vegetables	1.		
Fat	1.		
Liquid/drink	1.		
Meal Replace.	1.		
Condiments	1.		
Other	1.		

	Type	Amt:
	2.	
	2.	
	2.	
	2.	
	2.	
	2.	
	2.	
	2.	
	2.	

DINNER	Time: _____		
	Type	Amt:	
Protein	1.		
Complex Carbs	1.		
Fruit	1.		
Vegetables	1.		
Fat	1.		
Liquid/drink	1.		
Meal Replace.	1.		
Condiments	1.		
Other	1.		

	Type	Amt:
	2.	
	2.	
	2.	
	2.	
	2.	
	2.	
	2.	
	2.	
	2.	

Cardiovascular Training

Warmed up Yes _____ No _____

Time of day: _____	For how long?	Heart Rate
Type 1:	_____	_____
Type 2:	_____	_____
Type 3:	_____	_____
Type 4:	_____	_____
Stretched? Yes _____ No _____		

Evening Reflection

Did I put my faith in Action today?	Yes _____	No _____
I prayed for somone today	Yes _____	No _____
I read my Bible today	Yes _____	No _____
I helped someone in need today	Yes _____	No _____
I got 6 1/2 to 8 hours of sleep last night	Yes _____	No _____
I know I ate right today	Yes _____	No _____
I ate breakfast today	Yes _____	No _____
I ate starches after 4:00 p.m. today	Yes _____	No _____
I ate at least 4 meals today	Yes _____	No _____
I drank at least a gallon of water today	Yes _____	No _____
I had Courage to Change today	Yes _____	No _____
Tonight I forgive……		

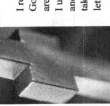

Captain's Log Statement of Faith

I realize that my actions don't earn my way into God's love or earn my way to heaven but that they are a reflection of my love affair with Jesus! I understand that by taking care of myself I honor and glorify God. I matter to God and the actions I take toward good health are daily written love letters telling God, "Thank you for my life"!

_____
Signature

Resistance Training

Time of day: _____

Warmed up Yes _____ No _____

Name of exercise 1:	Weight:	Reps:
_____	Set 1: _____	_____
_____	Set 2: _____	_____
Muscles worked:	Set 3: _____	_____
_____	Set 4: _____	_____
Stretched? Yes _____ No _____		

Name of exercise 2:	Weight:	Reps:
_____	Set 1: _____	_____
_____	Set 2: _____	_____
Muscles worked:	Set 3: _____	_____
_____	Set 4: _____	_____
Stretched? Yes _____ No _____		

Name of exercise 3:	Weight:	Reps:
_____	Set 1: _____	_____
_____	Set 2: _____	_____
Muscles worked:	Set 3: _____	_____
_____	Set 4: _____	_____
Stretched? Yes _____ No _____		

Name of exercise 4:	Weight:	Reps:
_____	Set 1: _____	_____
_____	Set 2: _____	_____
Muscles worked:	Set 3: _____	_____
_____	Set 4: _____	_____
Stretched? Yes _____ No _____		

Name of exercise 5:	Weight:	Reps:
_____	Set 1: _____	_____
_____	Set 2: _____	_____
Muscles worked:	Set 3: _____	_____
_____	Set 4: _____	_____
Stretched? Yes _____ No _____		

Name of exercise 6:	Weight:	Reps:
_____	Set 1: _____	_____
_____	Set 2: _____	_____
Muscles worked:	Set 3: _____	_____
_____	Set 4: _____	_____
Stretched? Yes _____ No _____		

Name of exercise 7:	Weight:	Reps:
_____	Set 1: _____	_____
_____	Set 2: _____	_____
Muscles worked:	Set 3: _____	_____
_____	Set 4: _____	_____
Stretched? Yes _____ No _____		

Name of exercise 8:	Weight:	Reps:
_____	Set 1: _____	_____
_____	Set 2: _____	_____
Muscles worked:	Set 3: _____	_____
_____	Set 4: _____	_____
Stretched? Yes _____ No _____		

Name of exercise 9:	Weight:	Reps:
_____	Set 1: _____	_____
_____	Set 2: _____	_____
Muscles worked:	Set 3: _____	_____
_____	Set 4: _____	_____
Stretched? Yes _____ No _____		

Name of exercise 10:	Weight:	Reps:
_____	Set 1: _____	_____
_____	Set 2: _____	_____
Muscles worked:	Set 3: _____	_____
_____	Set 4: _____	_____
Stretched? Yes _____ No _____		

"I press on toward the goal to win the prize for which God has called me heavenward in Christ Jesus."
Philippians 3:14

Captain's Log

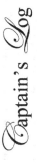

"Each one should test his own actions. Then he can take pride in himself without comparing himself to somebody else, for each one should carry his own load." (Galatians 6:40)

Day: _____ Date: _____ / _____ / _____

Nutrition Log

BREAKFAST	Time: _____				SNACK 1	Time: _____			
	Type	Amt:	Type	Amt:		Type	Amt:	Type	Amt:
Protein	1. _____	_____	2. _____	_____	Protein	1. _____	_____	2. _____	_____
Complex Carbs	1. _____	_____	2. _____	_____	Complex Carbs	1. _____	_____	2. _____	_____
Fruit	1. _____	_____	2. _____	_____	Fruit	1. _____	_____	2. _____	_____
Vegetables	1. _____	_____	2. _____	_____	Vegetables	1. _____	_____	2. _____	_____
Fat	1. _____	_____	2. _____	_____	Fat	1. _____	_____	2. _____	_____
Liquid/drink	1. _____	_____	2. _____	_____	Liquid/drink	1. _____	_____	2. _____	_____
Meal Replace.	1. _____	_____	2. _____	_____	Meal Replace.	1. _____	_____	2. _____	_____
Condiments	1. _____	_____	2. _____	_____	Condiments	1. _____	_____	2. _____	_____
Other	1. _____	_____	2. _____	_____	Other	1. _____	_____	2. _____	_____

LUNCH	Time: _____				SNACK 2	Time: _____			
	Type	Amt:	Type	Amt:		Type	Amt:	Type	Amt:
Protein	1. _____	_____	2. _____	_____	Protein	1. _____	_____	2. _____	_____
Complex Carbs	1. _____	_____	2. _____	_____	Complex Carbs	1. _____	_____	2. _____	_____
Fruit	1. _____	_____	2. _____	_____	Fruit	1. _____	_____	2. _____	_____
Vegetables	1. _____	_____	2. _____	_____	Vegetables	1. _____	_____	2. _____	_____
Fat	1. _____	_____	2. _____	_____	Fat	1. _____	_____	2. _____	_____
Liquid/drink	1. _____	_____	2. _____	_____	Liquid/drink	1. _____	_____	2. _____	_____
Meal Replace.	1. _____	_____	2. _____	_____	Meal Replace.	1. _____	_____	2. _____	_____
Condiments	1. _____	_____	2. _____	_____	Condiments	1. _____	_____	2. _____	_____
Other	1. _____	_____	2. _____	_____	Other	1. _____	_____	2. _____	_____

SNACK 3	Time: _____				DINNER	Time: _____			
	Type	Amt:	Type	Amt:		Type	Amt:	Type	Amt:
Protein	1. _____	_____	2. _____	_____	Protein	1. _____	_____	2. _____	_____
Complex Carbs	1. _____	_____	2. _____	_____	Complex Carbs	1. _____	_____	2. _____	_____
Fruit	1. _____	_____	2. _____	_____	Fruit	1. _____	_____	2. _____	_____
Vegetables	1. _____	_____	2. _____	_____	Vegetables	1. _____	_____	2. _____	_____
Fat	1. _____	_____	2. _____	_____	Fat	1. _____	_____	2. _____	_____
Liquid/drink	1. _____	_____	2. _____	_____	Liquid/drink	1. _____	_____	2. _____	_____
Meal Replace.	1. _____	_____	2. _____	_____	Meal Replace.	1. _____	_____	2. _____	_____
Condiments	1. _____	_____	2. _____	_____	Condiments	1. _____	_____	2. _____	_____
Other	1. _____	_____	2. _____	_____	Other	1. _____	_____	2. _____	_____

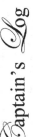

Cardiovascular Training

Warmed up   Yes _____   No _____

Time of day: _____	For how long?	Heart Rate
Type 1:	_____	_____
Type 2:	_____	_____
Type 3:	_____	_____
Type 4:	_____	_____

Stretched?   Yes _____   No _____

Evening Reflection

Did I put my faith in Action today?	Yes _____	No _____
I prayed for somone today	Yes _____	No _____
I read my Bible today	Yes _____	No _____
I helped someone in need today	Yes _____	No _____
I got 6 1/2 to 8 hours of sleep last night	Yes _____	No _____
I know I ate right today	Yes _____	No _____
I ate breakfast today	Yes _____	No _____
I ate starches after 4:00 p.m. today	Yes _____	No _____
I ate at least 4 meals today	Yes _____	No _____
I drank at least a gallon of water today	Yes _____	No _____
I had Courage to Change today	Yes _____	No _____

Tonight I forgive.…

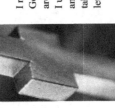

Captain's Log Statement of Faith

I realize that my actions don't earn my way into God's love or earn my way to heaven but that they are a reflection of my love affair with Jesus! I understand that by taking care of myself I honor and glorify God. I matter to God and the actions I take toward good health are daily written love letters telling God, "Thank you for my life"!

_____
Signature

Resistance Training

Time of day: _____

Warmed up   Yes _____   No _____

Name of exercise 1: _____

	Weight:	Reps:
Set 1:	_____	_____
Set 2:	_____	_____
Set 3:	_____	_____
Set 4:	_____	_____

Muscles worked: _____

Stretched?   Yes _____   No _____

Name of exercise 2: _____

	Weight:	Reps:
Set 1:	_____	_____
Set 2:	_____	_____
Set 3:	_____	_____
Set 4:	_____	_____

Muscles worked: _____

Stretched?   Yes _____   No _____

Name of exercise 3: _____

	Weight:	Reps:
Set 1:	_____	_____
Set 2:	_____	_____
Set 3:	_____	_____
Set 4:	_____	_____

Muscles worked: _____

Stretched?   Yes _____   No _____

Name of exercise 4: _____

	Weight:	Reps:
Set 1:	_____	_____
Set 2:	_____	_____
Set 3:	_____	_____
Set 4:	_____	_____

Muscles worked: _____

Stretched?   Yes _____   No _____

Name of exercise 5: _____

	Weight:	Reps:
Set 1:	_____	_____
Set 2:	_____	_____
Set 3:	_____	_____
Set 4:	_____	_____

Muscles worked: _____

Stretched?   Yes _____   No _____

Name of exercise 6: _____

	Weight:	Reps:
Set 1:	_____	_____
Set 2:	_____	_____
Set 3:	_____	_____
Set 4:	_____	_____

Muscles worked: _____

Stretched?   Yes _____   No _____

Name of exercise 7: _____

	Weight:	Reps:
Set 1:	_____	_____
Set 2:	_____	_____
Set 3:	_____	_____
Set 4:	_____	_____

Muscles worked: _____

Stretched?   Yes _____   No _____

Name of exercise 8: _____

	Weight:	Reps:
Set 1:	_____	_____
Set 2:	_____	_____
Set 3:	_____	_____
Set 4:	_____	_____

Muscles worked: _____

Stretched?   Yes _____   No _____

Name of exercise 9: _____

	Weight:	Reps:
Set 1:	_____	_____
Set 2:	_____	_____
Set 3:	_____	_____
Set 4:	_____	_____

Muscles worked: _____

Stretched?   Yes _____   No _____

Name of exercise 10: _____

	Weight:	Reps:
Set 1:	_____	_____
Set 2:	_____	_____
Set 3:	_____	_____
Set 4:	_____	_____

Muscles worked: _____

Stretched?   Yes _____   No _____

"I press on toward the goal to win the prize for which God has called me heavenward in Christ Jesus."
Philippians 3:14